COSMOPOLITAN
SHORT CUTS TO
LOOKING GOOD
& FEELING GREAT

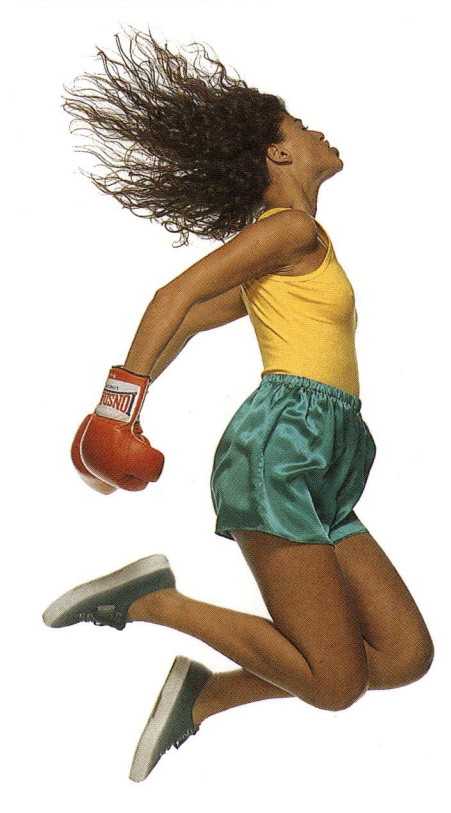

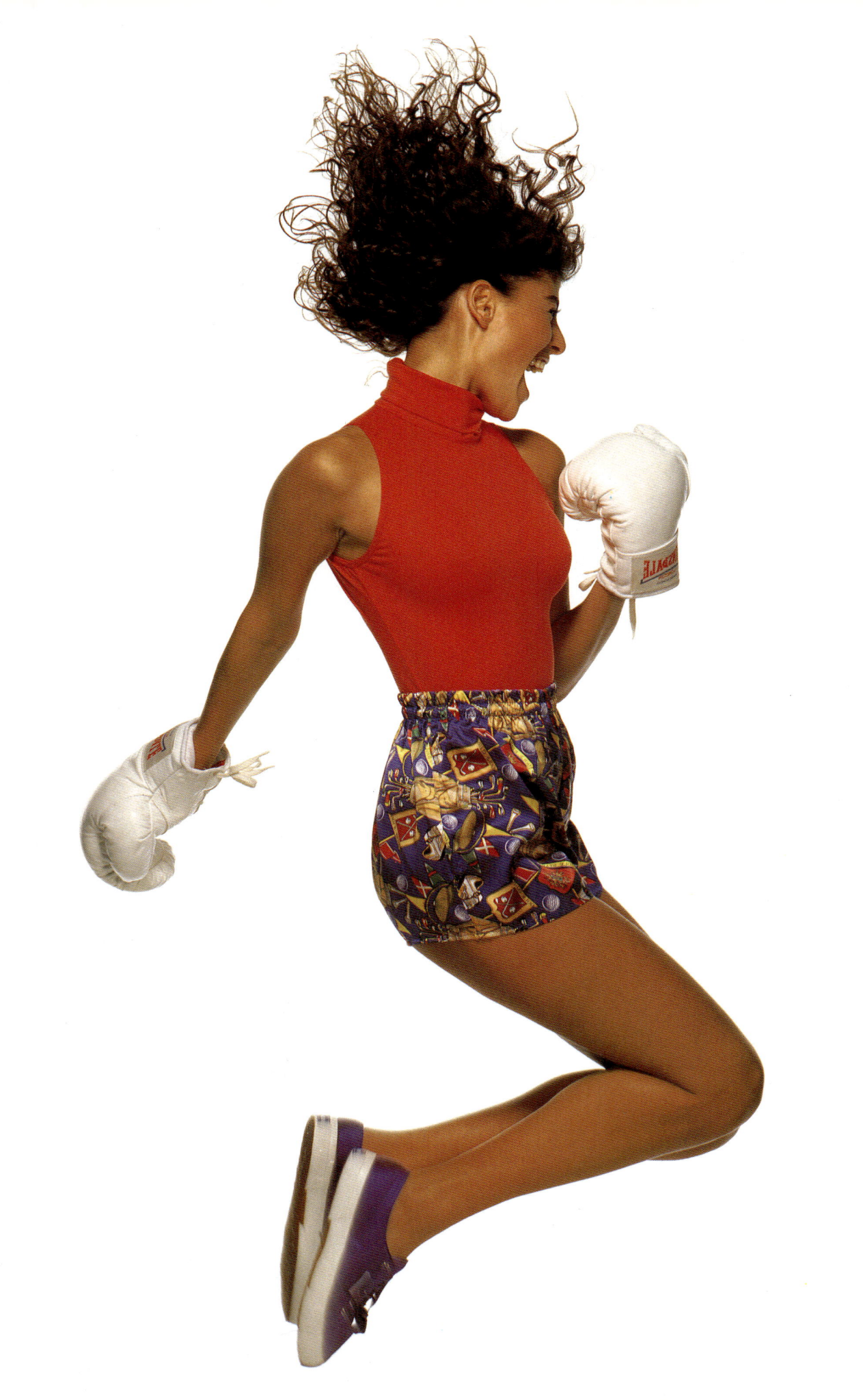

COSMOPOLITAN
SHORT CUTS TO
LOOKING GOOD
& FEELING GREAT

EVE CAMERON & CHRISSIE PAINELL

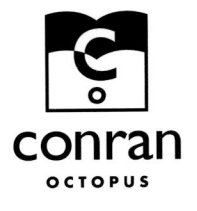

conran
OCTOPUS

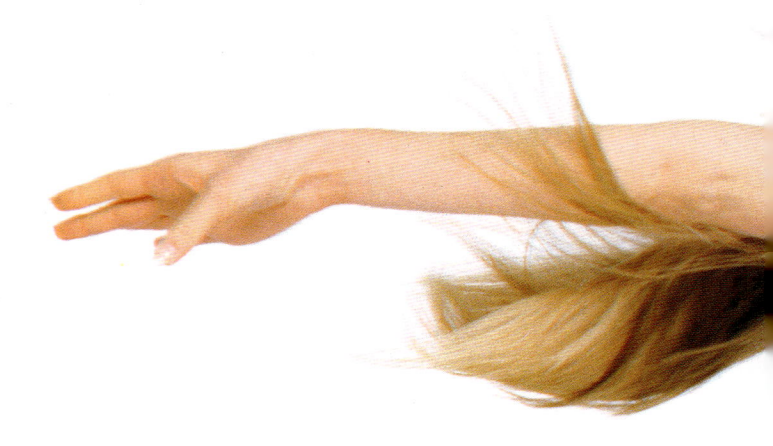

For Brenda and Jill
and Renate and Gilly

First published in 1989 by
Conran Octopus Limited
37 Shelton Street
London WC2H 9HN

Reprinted 1990
This revised paperback edition first published in 1994 by Conran Octopus Limited

Copyright © 1989 and 1994 Eve Cameron and Chrissie Painell

Cosmopolitan is published in the UK by
The National Magazine Company Limited.
Cosmopolitan copyright © 1994 The Hearst Corporation.
Cosmopolitan is a trademark of The Hearst Corporation.
Reproduction in whole in in part without written permission
of the copyright owner is prohibited.

All rights reserved. No part of this book may be reproduced,
stored in a retrieval system, or transmitted in any form
or by any means, electronic, electrostatic, magnetic tape, mechanical,
photocopying, recording or otherwise, without permission in writing
from the publishers.

ISBN 1 85029 594 8

Art Editor Karen Bowen
Picture Research Jessica Walton, Abigail Ahern, Joan Tinney
Production Jill Macey
Editorial Assistant Jane Chapman
Illustrators Lynne Robinson, Barbara Mullarney Wright

Printed in Hong Kong

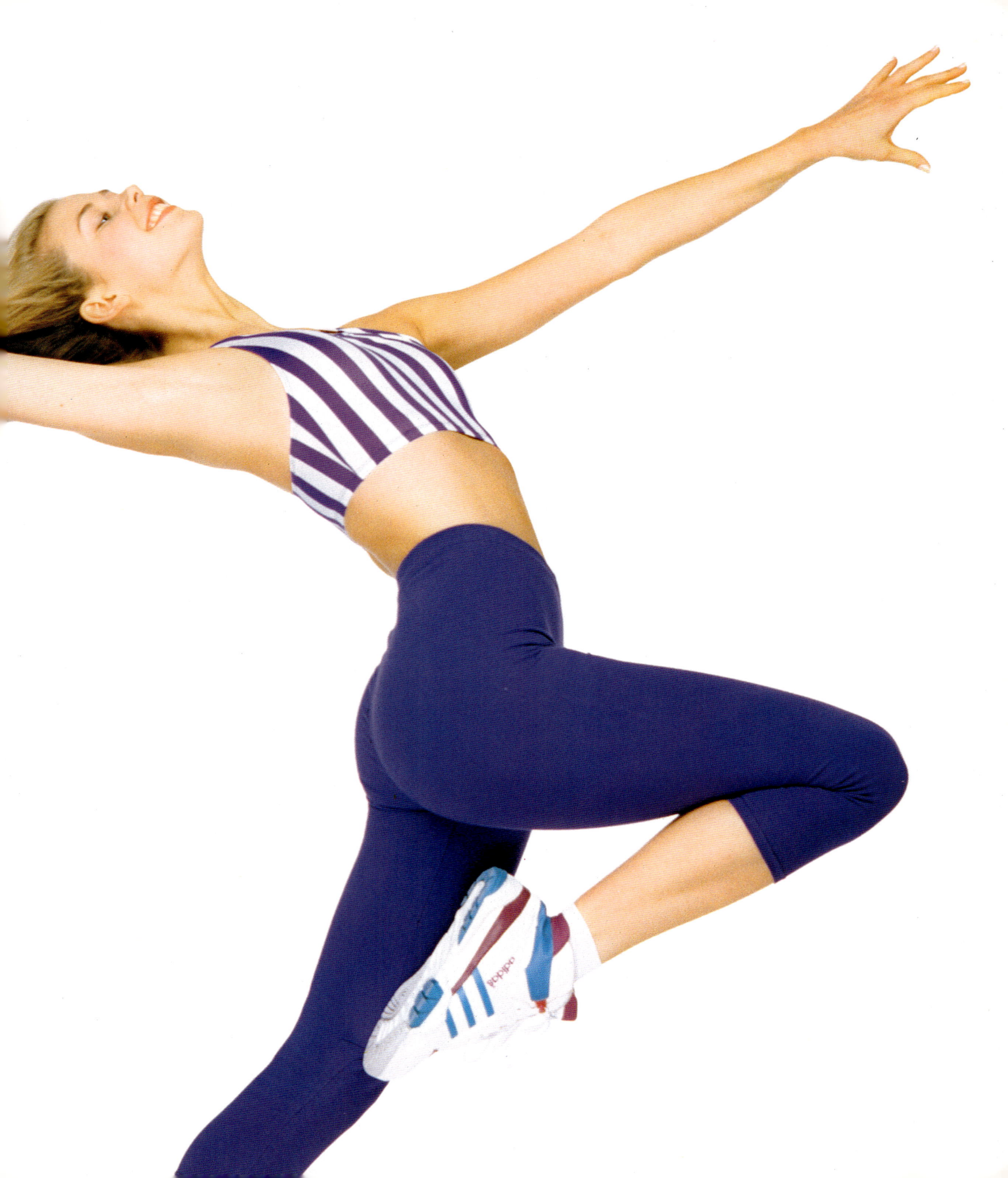

CONTENTS

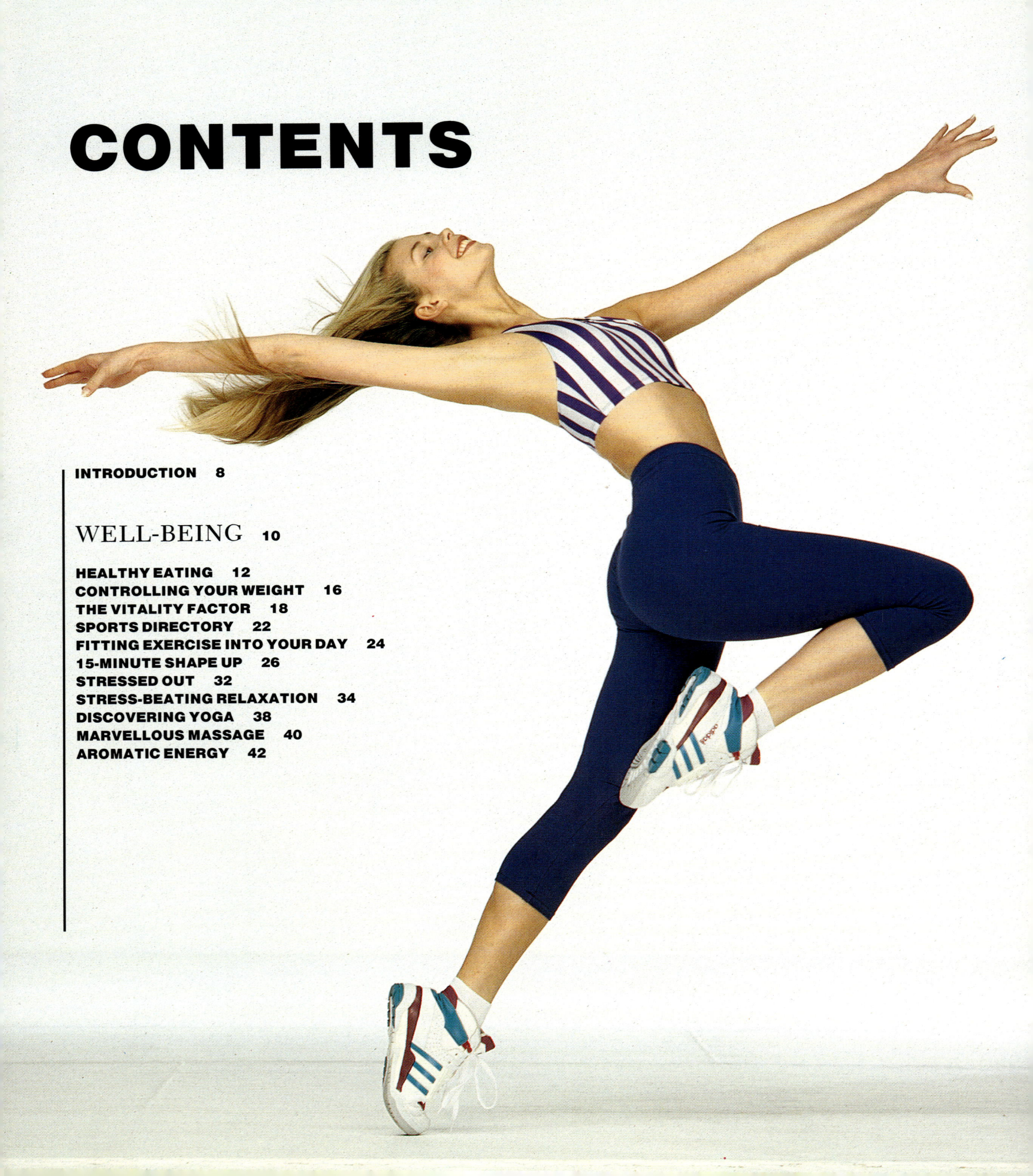

INTRODUCTION 8

WELL-BEING 10

HEALTHY EATING 12
CONTROLLING YOUR WEIGHT 16
THE VITALITY FACTOR 18
SPORTS DIRECTORY 22
FITTING EXERCISE INTO YOUR DAY 24
15-MINUTE SHAPE UP 26
STRESSED OUT 32
STRESS-BEATING RELAXATION 34
DISCOVERING YOGA 38
MARVELLOUS MASSAGE 40
AROMATIC ENERGY 42

SKINCARE 46

SKIN TYPING 48
PERFECT YOUR SKIN 50
QUICK SKINCARE SYSTEMS 52
FAST SKIN BOOSTERS 54
FABULOUS FACIALS 56
ANTI-AGEING STRATEGIES 58
ENVIRONMENT 60
SUN AND TANNING 64
YOUR SKIN PROBLEMS SOLVED 70

MASTERING MAKE-UP 72

COMPLEXION PERFECTION 74
EYES RIGHT 78
LIP SERVICE 82
THE 5-MINUTE MAKE-UP 84
THE NATURAL LOOK 86
THE CLASSIC FACE 88
MODERN GLAMOUR 90
WORKING GIRL 92
COSMOPOLITAN COLOURS 94
PARTY TIME 96

HAIRCARE 98

HAIR BASICS 100
HAIR TYPING 102
HAIR PROBLEMS 104
CUTTING CLEVER 106
COLOUR SENSE 108
PERMANENT SOLUTIONS 112
SHAPE AND STYLE 114
TWISTS, PLAITS AND ROLLS 116

THE BODY BEAUTIFUL 118

ARM AND SHOULDER SHAPERS 120
BACK STRENGTHENERS 122
BUST BEAUTY 124
STOMACH AND WAIST FLATTENERS 126
HIP, THIGH AND BOTTOM TONERS 130
LEGS WORKOUT 134
HAND AND NAIL SAVERS 136
FEET FIRST 138
SMOOTH HAIR REMOVAL 140

INDEX AND ACKNOWLEDGMENTS 142

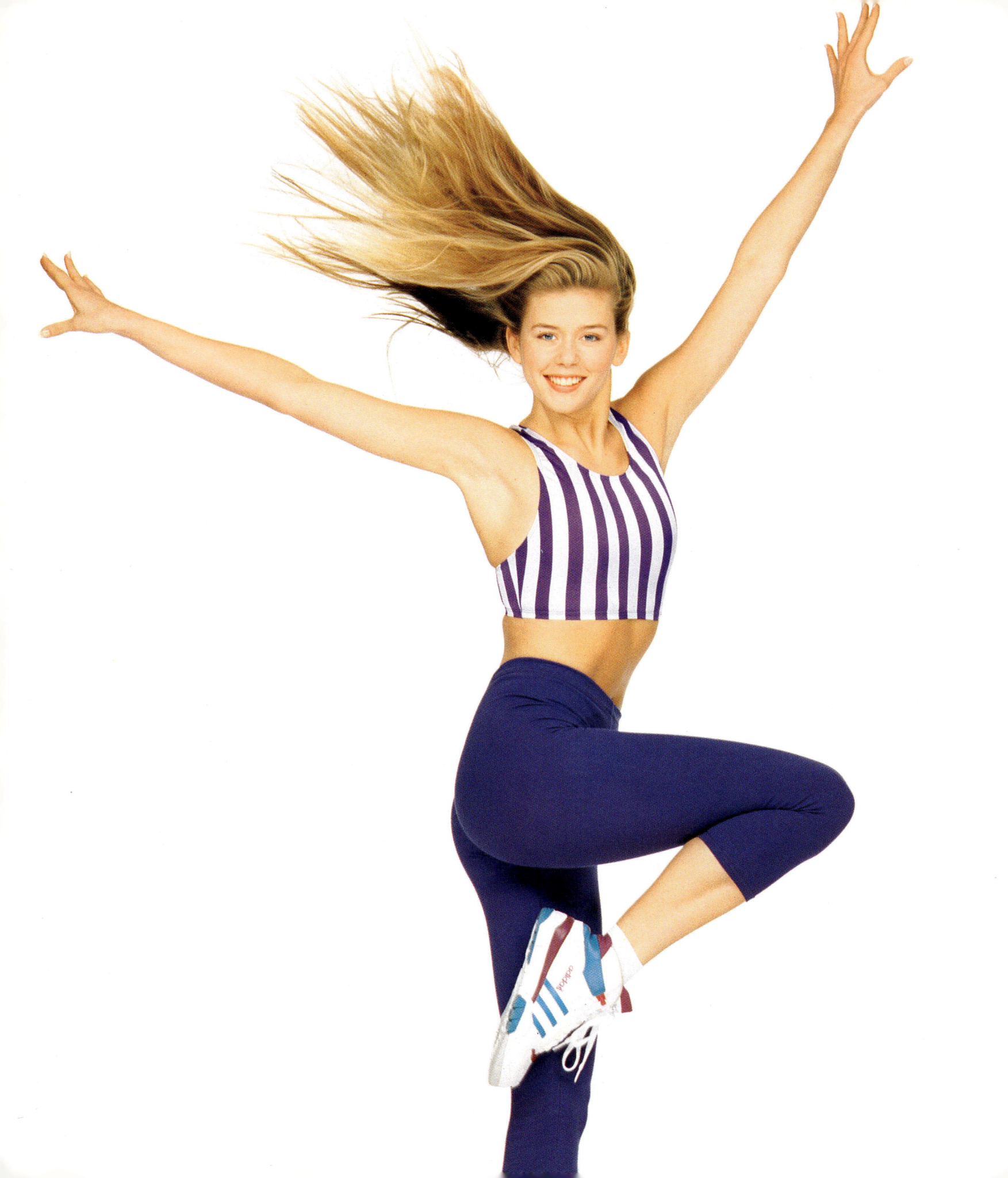

INTRODUCTION

'Why not be oneself? That is the whole secret of a successful appearance.' Edith Sitwell

Beauty today no longer means conforming to ideals. Although we all care about our appearance, we are also allowed to be very individual. Modern women come in all shapes and sizes, with widely differing features.

Perhaps the most important change in our concept of beauty in recent years is an emphasis on health, vitality and confidence. These ageless qualities are probably the greatest beauty secrets of all! Taking care of your well-being on a daily basis not only boosts your energy levels and your self-esteem, but will also be reflected in a fit body, glossy hair and great skin. Equally, looking and feeling your personal best should be seen, we feel, as your right. It's about self-respect, not vanity.

Yet as the pace of our lives accelerates, it has become essential that beauty and fitness should be fitted into our schedules with the minimum of fuss and in the shortest time possible. And, after all, who would want them to be a full-time occupation?

As health and beauty writers, we believe that beauty, health and vitality-boosting routines should take the short-cut route – that wherever possible they should be fast, and also fun to do. As well as general advice that is simple, honest and easy to put into practise, we've tried in this book to show you how to cut down on lengthy routines. For example, key beauty systems are tailored to your skin type and the environment you live in. We've quizzed make-up artists for the fastest make-up hints and gathered together all the haircare wisdom you need. The fitness moves will firm you up quicker than you thought possible, while the dietary hints will speed you towards eating for optimum health, as well as losing a few extra pounds if you wish.

We hope you enjoy *Cosmopolitan's Short Cuts to Looking Good and Feeling Great*. You'll soon wonder how you ever managed without it!

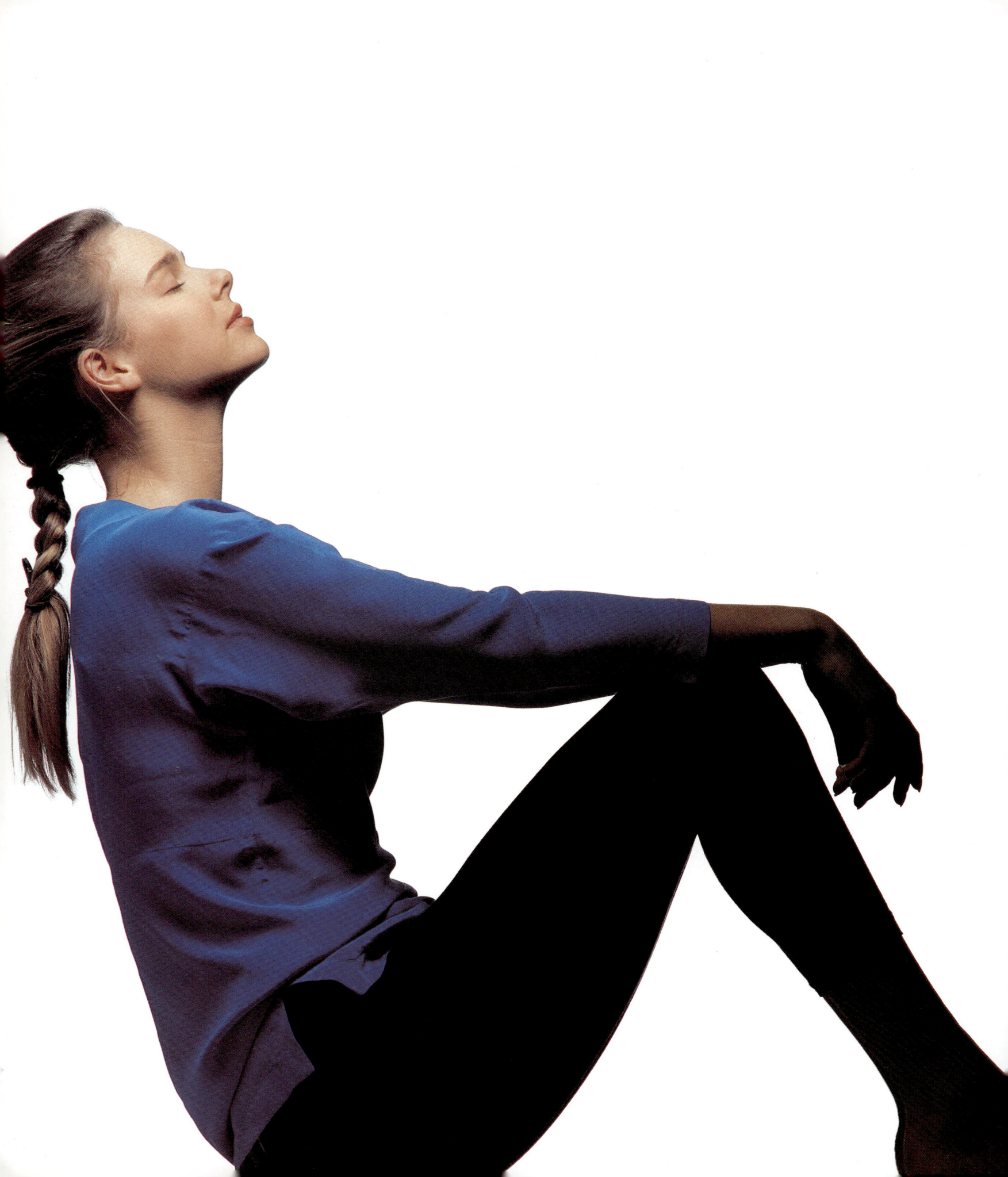

WELL-BEING

What are the vital elements that keep your well-being high? First a varied and nutritious diet. Next, regular exercise to increase energy levels and build a stronger body. And last, but definitely not least, stress-beating strategies to help you relax and enjoy life. Use our health secrets and you'll feel better than ever in just a few days!

HEALTHY EATING   12
CONTROLLING YOUR WEIGHT   16
THE VITALITY FACTOR   18
SPORTS DIRECTORY   22
FITTING EXERCISE INTO YOUR DAY   24
15-MINUTE SHAPE UP   26
STRESSED OUT   32
STRESS-BEATING RELAXATION   34
DISCOVERING YOGA   38
MARVELLOUS MASSAGE   40
AROMATIC ENERGY   42

HEALTHY EATING

Natural, nutritious food is a vital ingredient in a healthy life-style. Here are easy ways to develop good food habits.

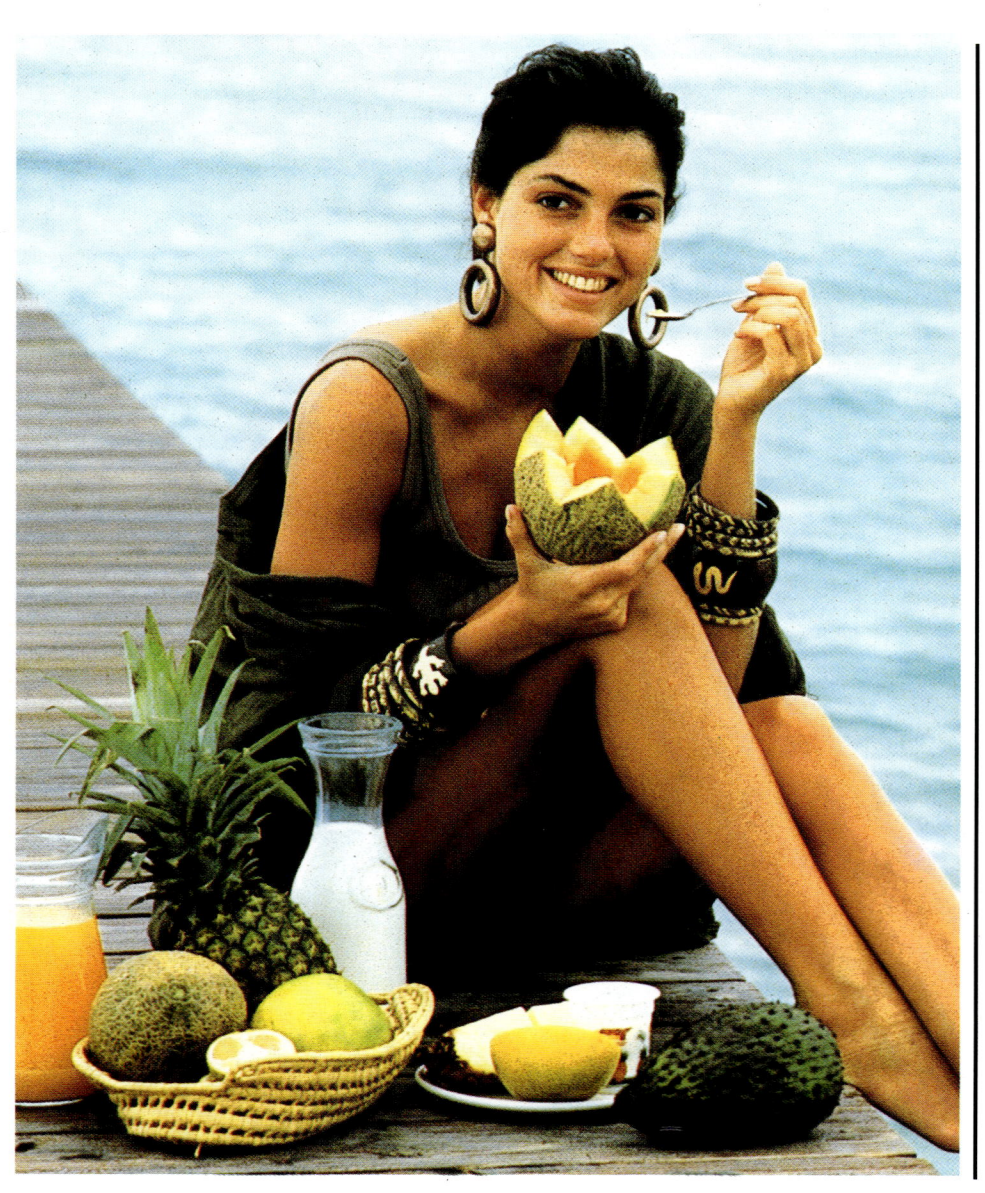

Eating junk food won't harm you, provided it is not the staple of your daily diet. However, the foundation of healthy eating lies in supplying your body with all the nutritious items it needs, and at the same time cutting down on the extras that are less good for you.

Here are some healthy guidelines:

Eat fresh fruit, vegetables and salads daily
They are storehouses of vitamins and minerals and also supply vital fibre. The latest guidelines suggest you should have 3–5 servings daily from the vegetable group and 2–4 servings from the fruit group.

Ensure you get your daily A, C and E vitamins
Research is showing that these vitamins play a major role in protecting against cancers, heart disease and age-related damage. Vitamin E is particularly important and the latest Suggested Optional Nutrient Allowance (SONA) is 400 international units (i.u.). Good natural sources of vitamin E include sunflower and wheatgerm oils, egg yolk and almonds. Up your vitamin C intake with baked potatoes, oranges, blackcurrants, Brussel sprouts and parsley. For beta-carotene (which

your body converts to vitamin A) choose spinach, carrots, broccoli, tomatoes, apricots and prunes.

Eat fish at least twice a week
Fish is low in fat and high in protein. Grilling, poaching and baking, say with vegetable juices or purées, are fast, healthy ways to prepare fish. Flavour it with herbs and spices. Oily fish, such as mackerel and salmon, is important too as it contains Omega-3 oil, which helps to protect against heart disease.

If you eat meat, make sure it's the smallest proportion of your meal
Aim for a meat content of about 20 per cent, with grains or pasta and vegetables making up the rest of your main course. Limit your intake of red meat and always choose lean meat. Chicken, turkey and rabbit are low-fat choices, but always remove the fatty skin from poultry.

Buy skimmed milk and low-fat yoghurt
Adding non-fat dried milk powder to skimmed milk will make it thicker if you find skimmed milk too thin for your taste.

ENERGY BREAKFAST
Kick off your day with a glass of hot water and lemon, adding a small amount of clear honey if you wish. It's refreshing and cleansing to your system.

Make your breakfast a combination of protein and complex carbohydrates. Cereals are a good source of fibre. Top them with seeds, such as delicious pumpkin seeds, and chopped nuts. Soak sugar-free muesli and some dried fruit in a little apple juice overnight for added sweetness. Low-fat yoghurt provides protein and calcium. Toast provides fibre and carbohydrates. Try it with sugar-free fruit spread (but not butter).

FAST MEAL TIPS
Healthy food does not have to be time-consuming to prepare – there are plenty of fast food options that also do you good.
- Steaming vegetables is just as fast as boiling and preserves more nutrients. They should be cooked to the point where they are tender but still crisp.
- Always keep frozen vegetables in the house. Many of them are just as nutritious as the fresh varieties.
- Eat 50 per cent of your vegetables raw. Serve some as crudités while the food is cooking.
- Quick-cook rice is slightly more processed than plain rice, but is much better for you than a pan of fried potatoes!
- Brown noodles are super-quick to cook and make a delicious base for many dishes.
- Fresh wholewheat spaghetti takes a minute to cook. Serve it with pesto and steamed courgettes.

EASY WAYS TO INCREASE FIBRE INTAKE
Since the beginning of the century, the amount of fibre in the Western diet has dropped by a staggering 75 per cent. At the same time, the incidence of constipation and bowel diseases has risen substantially.

We should be eating approximately 30 g (1 oz) of fibre per day for general health and to avoid diseases of the bowel. Here are some suggestions to help you increase the fibre in your diet.
New forms of fibre These are being introduced into the shops. Mixtures of soluble and insoluble fibre, they are very finely ground and can be mixed instantly into cereals, soups and casseroles.
Bread A slice of wholegrain bread provides 3 g of fibre.
Muesli 1 serving (3 tablespoons) of muesli provides 3 g of fibre.
Fruit Oranges contain 3 g; a pear with skin 3.4 g; apples 2 g.
Vegetables Broccoli contains 1.8 g per spear; spinach 6.3 g per tablespoon; ½ aubergine with the skin left on 3.2 g.

14 SHORT CUTS

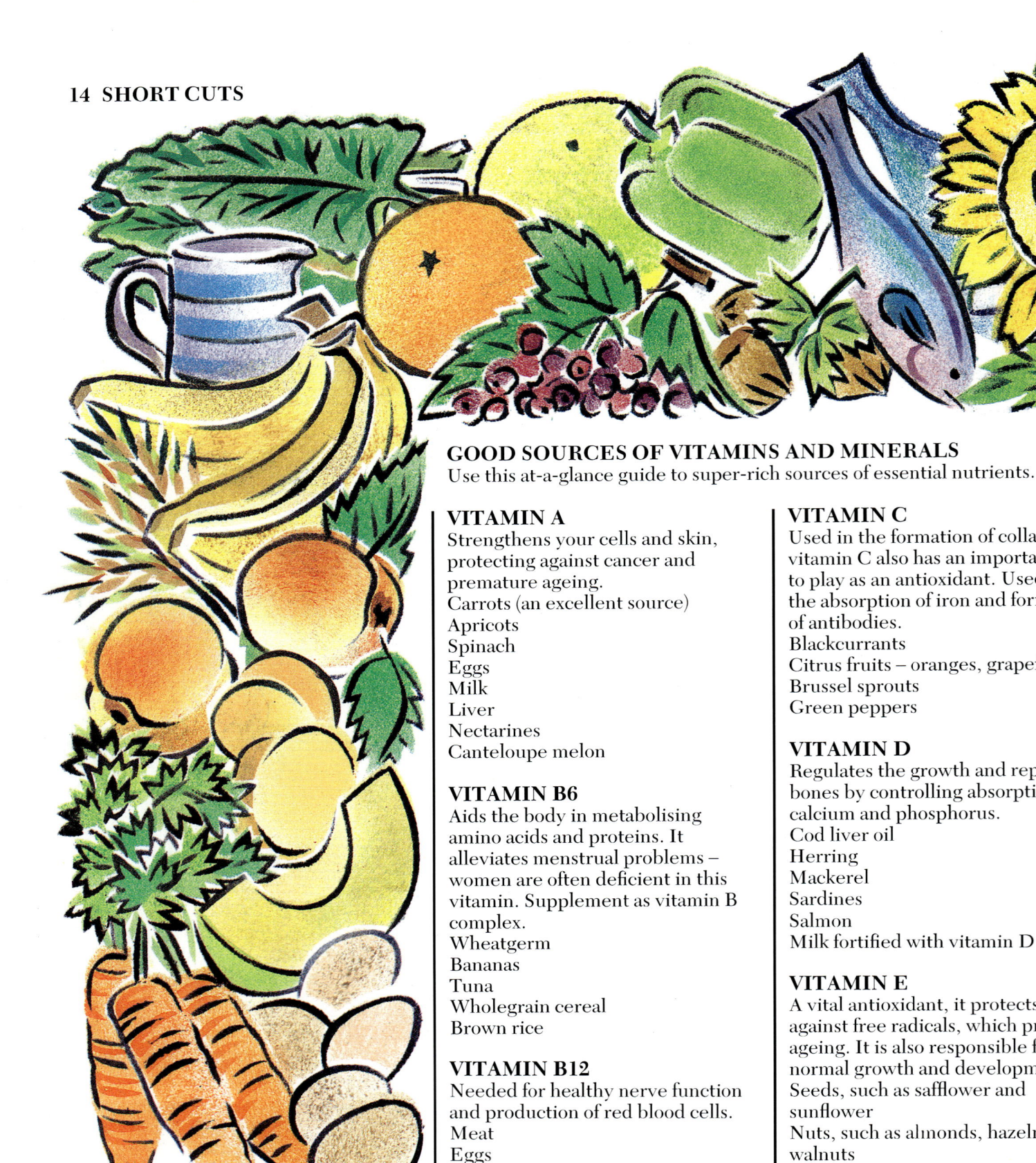

GOOD SOURCES OF VITAMINS AND MINERALS
Use this at-a-glance guide to super-rich sources of essential nutrients.

VITAMIN A
Strengthens your cells and skin, protecting against cancer and premature ageing.
Carrots (an excellent source)
Apricots
Spinach
Eggs
Milk
Liver
Nectarines
Canteloupe melon

VITAMIN B6
Aids the body in metabolising amino acids and proteins. It alleviates menstrual problems – women are often deficient in this vitamin. Supplement as vitamin B complex.
Wheatgerm
Bananas
Tuna
Wholegrain cereal
Brown rice

VITAMIN B12
Needed for healthy nerve function and production of red blood cells.
Meat
Eggs
Milk
(Vegetarians are advised to take supplements.)

VITAMIN C
Used in the formation of collagen, vitamin C also has an important part to play as an antioxidant. Used for the absorption of iron and formation of antibodies.
Blackcurrants
Citrus fruits – oranges, grapefruit
Brussel sprouts
Green peppers

VITAMIN D
Regulates the growth and repair of bones by controlling absorption of calcium and phosphorus.
Cod liver oil
Herring
Mackerel
Sardines
Salmon
Milk fortified with vitamin D

VITAMIN E
A vital antioxidant, it protects against free radicals, which promote ageing. It is also responsible for normal growth and development.
Seeds, such as safflower and sunflower
Nuts, such as almonds, hazelnuts, walnuts
Milk
Wheatgerm
Vegetable oils, such as corn oil

WELL-BEING 15

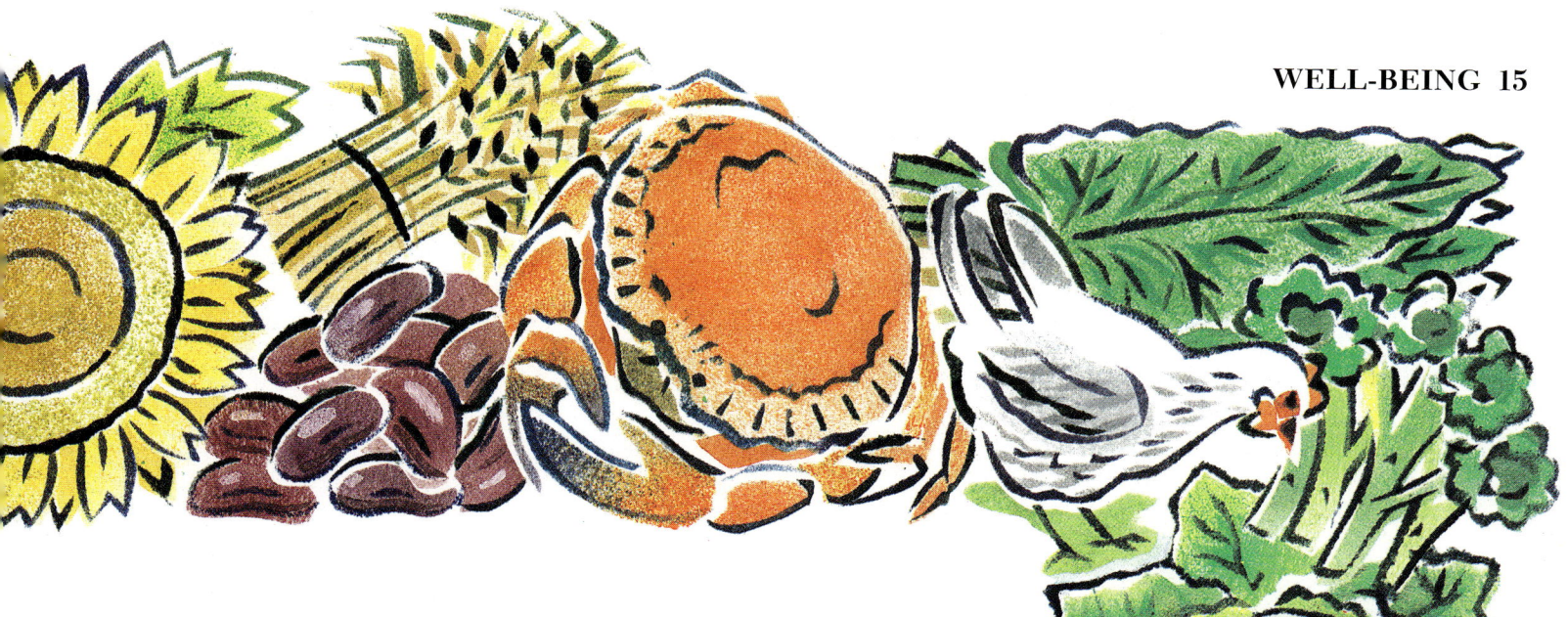

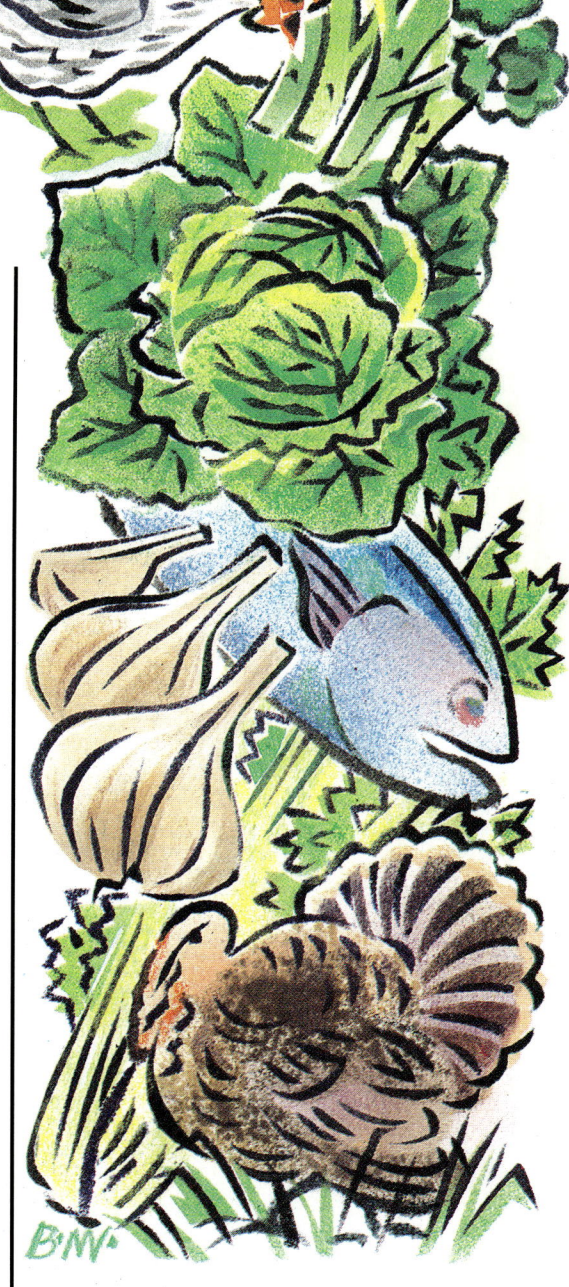

CALCIUM
Helps prevent osteoporosis (brittleness of the bones) which affects many women after the menopause. Builds bones and teeth and helps regulate heartbeat and blood clotting.
Milk
Yoghurt
Nuts
Seeds
Broccoli
Green vegetables
Pulses
Fish, particularly sardines, pilchards, whitebait, crab, cod
Rhubarb

IRON
Prevents anaemia, stimulates the production of haemoglobin, which carries oxygen to the cells.
Kidneys
Cane molasses
Tuna fish
Pulses, such as lentils
Seaweed
Wholegrain products
Egg yolk

MAGNESIUM
Aids bone growth and nerve and muscle function.
Cod
Mackerel
Leafy green vegetables
Sunflower seeds
Lemons

SELENIUM
Complements vitamin E as an antioxidant and promotes growth and development.
Seafood
Tuna
Wheatgerm
Milk
Liver
Chicken
Broccoli
Cabbage
Celery
Garlic
Onions

ZINC
Aids wound-healing and promotes cell growth and repair.
Sesame, pumpkin and sunflower seeds
Fish
Milk
Oysters
Pilchards
Wholegrain products
Turkey
Soya beans
Egg yolk

CONTROLLING YOUR WEIGHT

Forget faddy diets. Instead switch to a balanced eating plan to maintain your ideal weight.

It is an established fact that the great majority of diets claiming to make you lose weight *don't work*. When you diet, your body automatically adjusts to the reduction in calories, slowing down the metabolism and therefore burning calories less efficiently. When you resume your usual eating patterns, the weight goes right back on. In addition, when you deprive your body of food, it prefers to derive the energy it needs from your *muscle* instead of using up fat stores, so the weight reduction you see on the scales is actually loss of lean muscle and not just fat.

The good news is that there is an answer. Forget fad diets and don't use very low calorie diets. All of these deplete your energy levels and may even be harmful to your health. Instead you should switch to a *long-term*, sensible, balanced eating plan that is low in fats and sugar. Research at American universities has shown that women who were put on a low-fat diet lost weight even though other foods were not restricted.

It is easy to make a low-fat diet a way of life and, as well as helping weight loss, it is the road to a healthy heart.

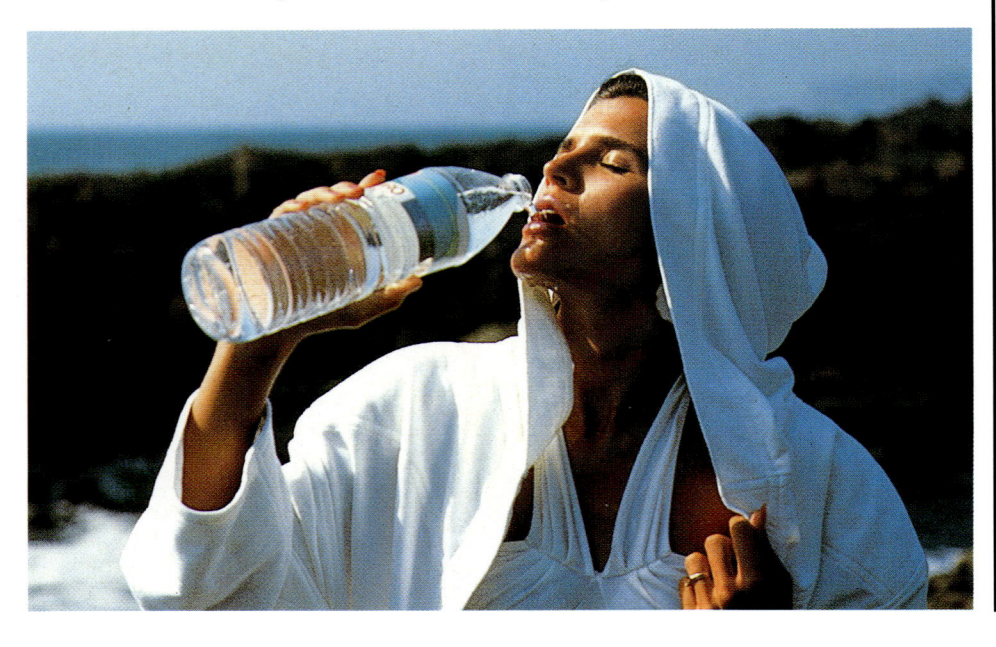

CUTTING DOWN THE FAT CONTENT IN YOUR DIET

Fat is not all bad. Small amounts are needed to help process vitamins A, D, E and K, for example. However, controlling the types and quantity of fat in your diet can aid your health and your waistline. Nutritionists recommend that fat makes up no more than 30 per cent of your daily diet. Below, fat types, what they do and where to find them in the foods you eat:

Saturated fats
These raise cholesterol levels and cause plaque (fibrous lesions) to build up in the arteries. You should avoid these whenever possible. Saturated fats include all fats from meat and poultry, dairy fats and coconut oil.

Hydrogenated fats
The process of hydrogenating turns polyunsaturated fats into saturated fats, making them more solid. They are often included in prepared foods such as ice cream, baked products, some vegetable shortenings and cereals. Check food labels.

Polyunsaturated fats
This type of fat may help to lower cholesterol levels. Use them, in small amounts, instead of saturated

fats. Polyunsaturated fats are found in sunflower, safflower and corn oils, and oily fish such as tuna, salmon and mackerel.

Mono-unsaturated fats
Thought to help lower cholesterol levels in general and, in particular, LDL, or 'bad' cholesterol. They are found in olive oil and peanut oil.

HEALTHY SLIMMING TIPS
- Skip butter or margarine on toast and in sandwiches.
- Add extra (low-fat) filling to a jacket potato such as sugar-reduced baked beans or sweet corn and peppers, instead of butter or margarine.
- Use lemon or low-fat yoghurt as a dressing on salad rather than salad cream or mayonnaise.
- Try to limit the number of ready-prepared dishes you eat – they are often a source of hidden fat – or look for low-fat versions.
- Non-dairy frozen desserts, such as sorbets, are a better choice than ice cream. You could also try freezing grapes and sliced banana for sweet, but healthy, snacks.
- If trying to lose weight don't take appetite suppressants. They can be addictive and they mess up your system. Long-term sensible eating is a far better way to slim down and stay slim.
- Aerobic exercise boosts weight loss, burning up calories and toning your muscles.

If you are undereating rather than overeating, or eating unhealthily, seek expert advice in order to solve any underlying psychological problems you may be experiencing. Your family doctor will be able to refer you to a specialist.

The most important thing to bear in mind is not to become obsessed with food or body shape.

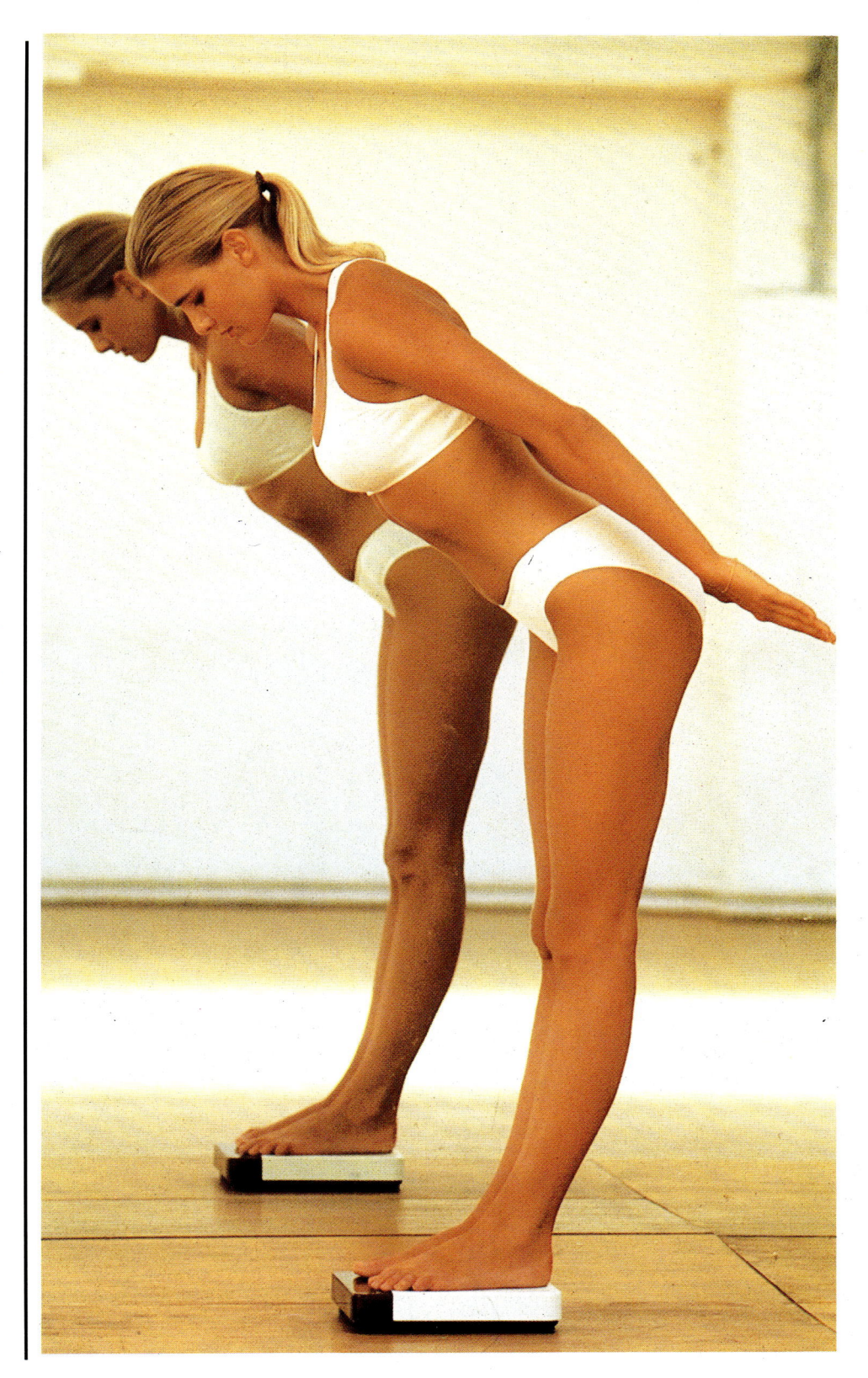

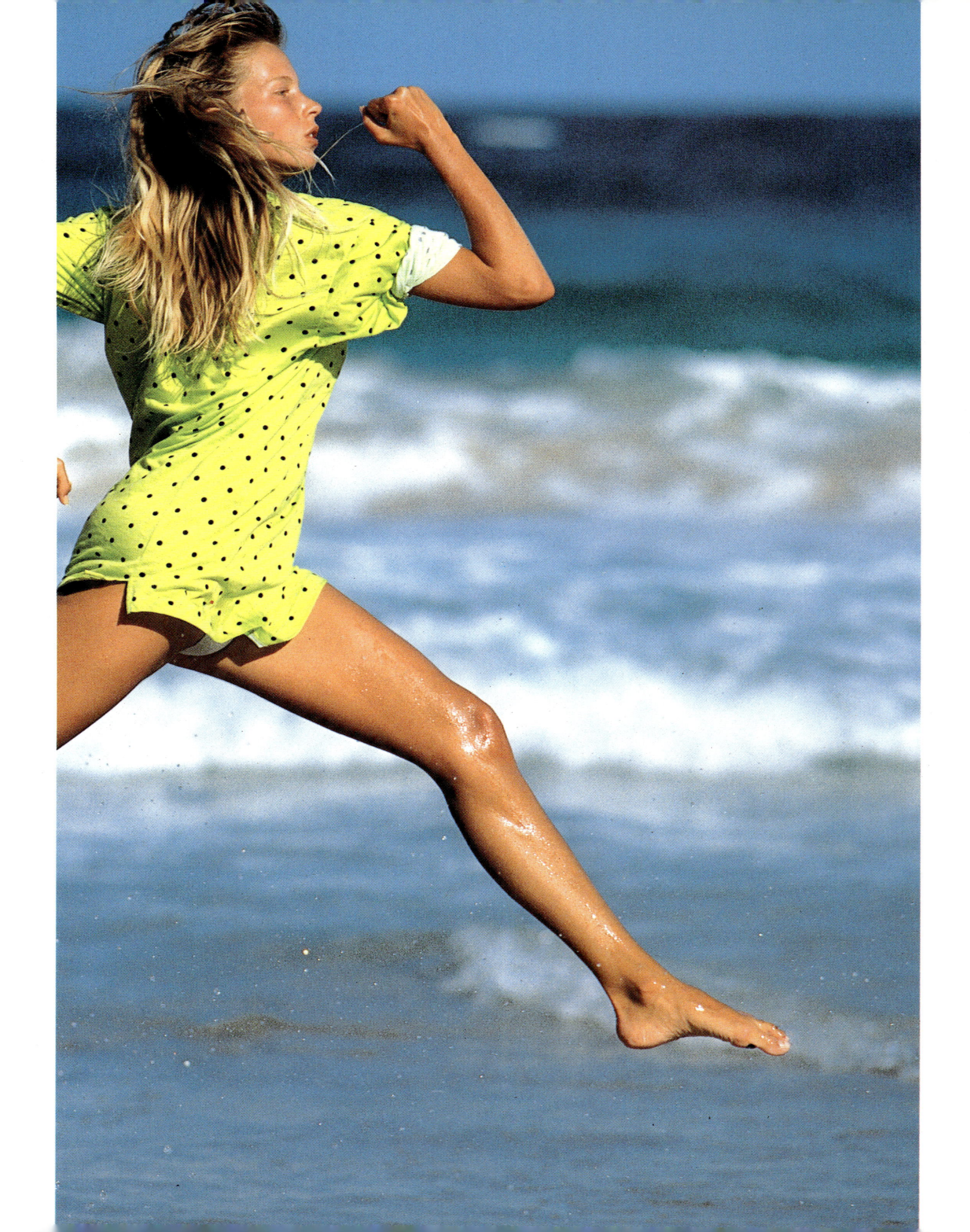

THE VITALITY FACTOR

Exercise gives us the energy to speed through life. Increase your energy resources today!

Exercising regularly can make a huge difference to your energy levels. Without exercise, we feel sluggish and slow, but when we exercise vigorously the benefits are wide-ranging. Exercise:
- actually gives you more energy than you had before
- helps nutrients to be absorbed more efficiently
- tones and shapes your body
- curbs high blood-pressure and reduces the risk of heart disease
- relaxes you and produces hormones that improve your mood
- burns calories
- improves your circulation
- helps prevent osteoporosis (brittleness of the bones) if weight-bearing

In order to be truly fit, we need to ensure that our exercise routine includes all the elements in the exercise equation:
- Aerobic exercise to work our heart and lungs, improve stamina and get our circulation moving faster
- Strengthening exercises to improve muscle tone and power
- Stretching exercises to develop flexibility, to balance our strength, and to protect against injury

For cardiovascular fitness (heart and lungs), aim to work out aerobically for 20 to 30 minutes three times a week. Variety of exercise, i.e. as in the exercise equation, is important for overall conditioning, plus it ensures you don't get bored. Do remember, however, to have rest days as over-exercising can be counter-productive, leading to strain and possible injuries.

AEROBIC EXERCISE

This raises the heart rate, increasing the flow of oxygen to the muscles and internal organs, most importantly, the heart. When exercising aerobically you should be comfortably out of breath. You can judge this by seeing how well you can keep up a conversation – if you can't talk, you're overdoing it! Aerobic exercise comes in a number of forms – there are the obvious 'aerobics' classes at gyms and dance studios, but swimming and walking can also be aerobic if done fast enough.

Motivation tips
- Re-read and learn by heart the benefits of exercise. After every workout spend a few minutes reminding yourself of them.
- Work out with a friend or invest in a personal trainer.
- Schedule exercise into your diary just like other appointments.
- Set yourself goals, but try to be realistic with them.

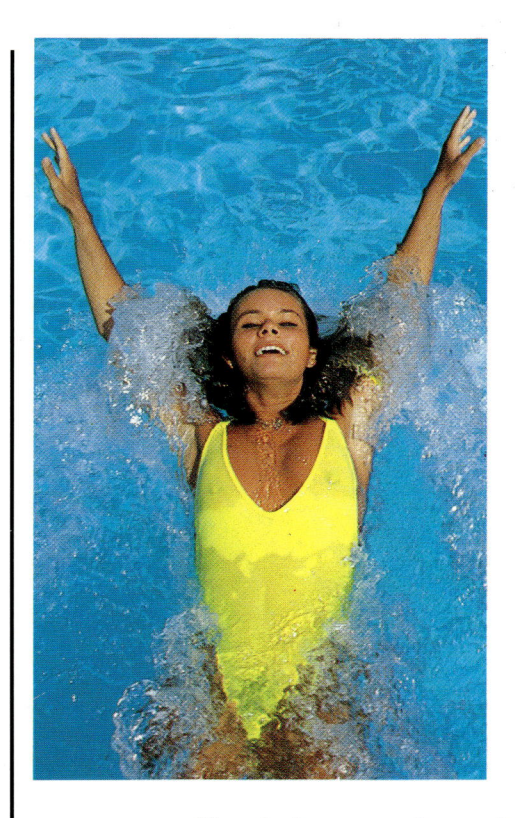

Here's a brief run-down of some of the different types of exercise you could try:

Exercise bikes
You'll find them at just about every gym. Equally, if you enjoy using them and have the space, you could invest in one for home use. It will

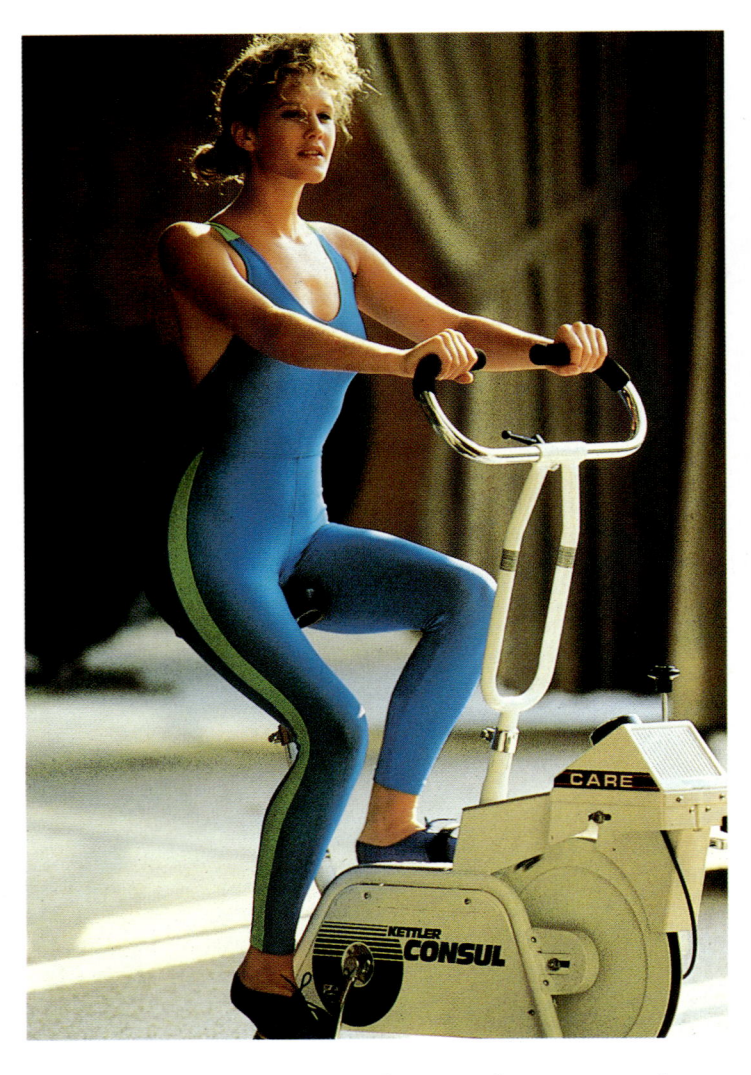

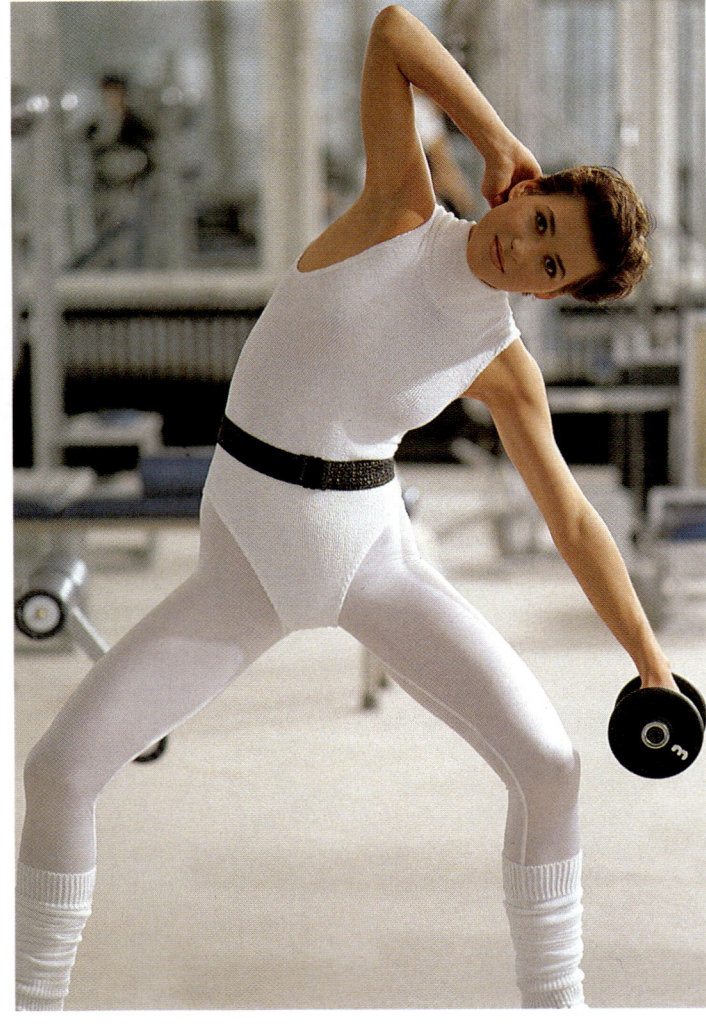

strengthen and tone up your legs, and will give you a cardiovascular workout, too, if a good pace is maintained for 20 minutes or so.

Rebounding
A rebounder is a mini-trampoline. Many gyms have them and they're not expensive, so they're ideal for home use, too. Just put on some music, dance and jump!

Gym circuits
Many gyms and health clubs offer circuits which are a combination of cardiovascular work and weight-training moves. They're fast, intensive, but very effective.

Rowing and rowing machines
Very effective, all-round exercise.

Swimming
You need to have good technique in order to make this an aerobic workout – a slow breaststroke is unlikely to get your heart rate up, unless you are very unfit. However, it's a good overall toning exercise as the water provides resistance to work against.

Aerobic dance
If you haven't exercised for some time, don't head straight for an aerobics class. Go to body conditioning classes first, where you'll be taught body control and good posture. You can then progress to aerobic dance classes and you'll perform the movements more effectively. An exercise video for beginners can also help to get you started.

Jogging and running
Good for cardiovascular fitness and shaping up your lower body. It is, however, high-impact and can place stress on the joints. Walking is a good way to get started.

Step workouts
Popular in health clubs and possible to do at home with a specially

WELL-BEING 21

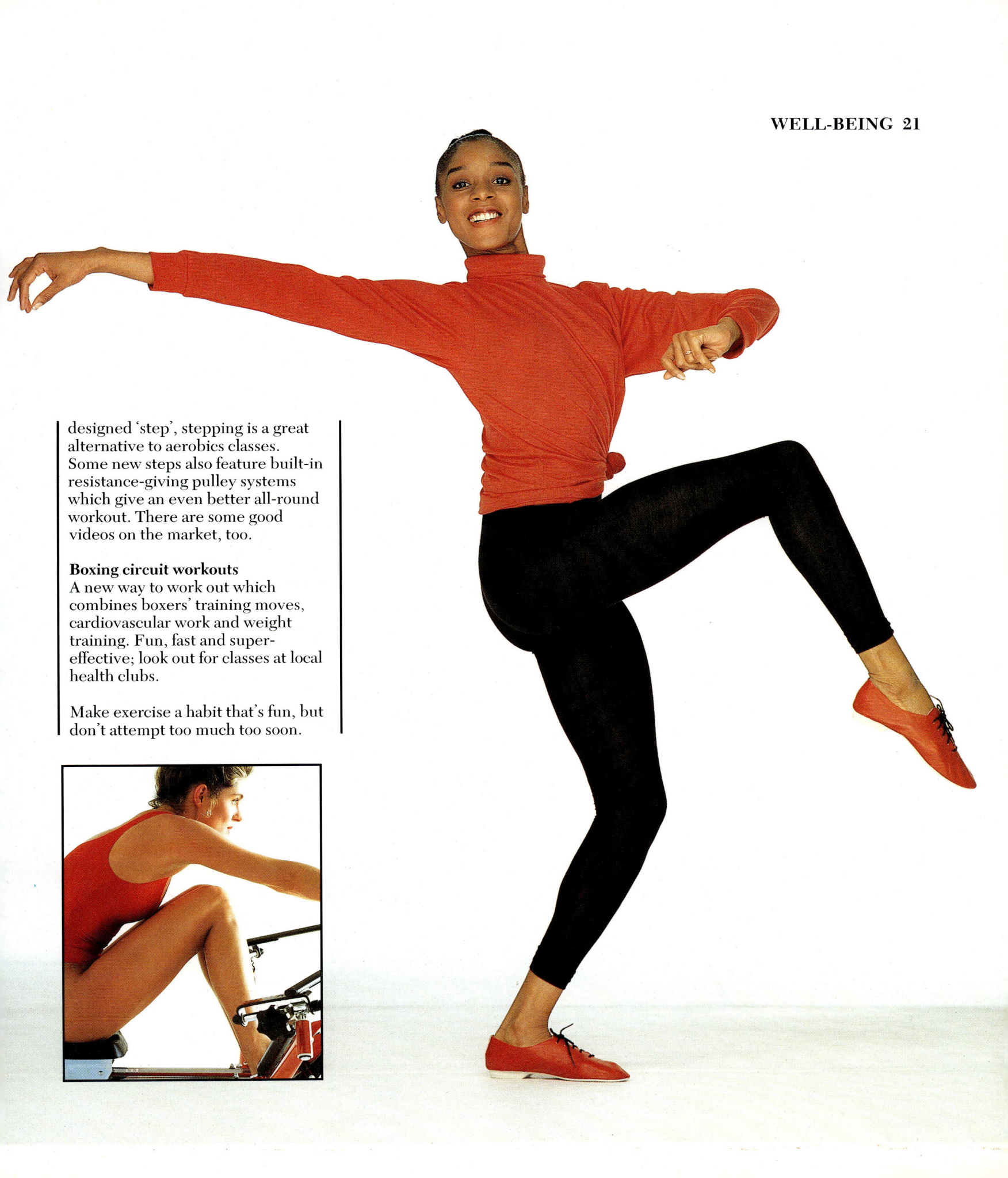

designed 'step', stepping is a great alternative to aerobics classes. Some new steps also feature built-in resistance-giving pulley systems which give an even better all-round workout. There are some good videos on the market, too.

Boxing circuit workouts
A new way to work out which combines boxers' training moves, cardiovascular work and weight training. Fun, fast and super-effective; look out for classes at local health clubs.

Make exercise a habit that's fun, but don't attempt too much too soon.

SPORTS DIRECTORY

Sporting activities are a fast, fun way to fitness.

Many people prefer to shape up and increase their fitness level through sport instead of doing workout classes. For optimum fitness, the ideal is to incorporate sport into a total fitness programme.

Here you'll find a brief guide to popular sports, their benefits and some easy-to-remember tips. Many provide good aerobic workouts, if played fast enough, and all have body-conditioning advantages. Most importantly, sport is fun, great for de-stressing and a sociable activity offering opportunities to make new friends.

BADMINTON
Badminton is excellent for developing flexibility and eye-hand co-ordination. Strength is not so important for this sport initially, though it will develop as you advance and skills and tricks are usually picked up with practice.

As with tennis and basketball, remember to wear shock-absorbing shoes (for the jumps and lunges).

BASEBALL, SOFTBALL and ROUNDERS
All three are bat and ball games and so throwing and catching are important skills. They help to firm and tone the legs and strengthen the upper body and back. They are not a key means of building stamina, since running tends to be in short bursts; when your team is batting, quick sprints from base to base are necessary to score runs. You will need to develop flexibility, however, in order to react quickly.

Coaching sessions and team practices usually start with batting, throwing and catching exercises, so you have a chance to improve your technique.

Unless you already have an accurate, long throw, leave deep fielding for a while, as it's easy to overdo it and pull arm muscles.

You'll need to equip yourself with a good pair of running shoes and protective gloves and pads.

BASKETBALL
Basketball is a physically demanding team game, involving quick sprints up and down the court, dribbling and throwing the ball, dodging opponents and shooting to try and score a 'basket'. It provides a good aerobic workout and you will improve co-ordination and flexibility as you practise.

With all the jumping and running, you must wear ankle-supporting, shock-absorbing shoes.

RIDING
Horse-riding does not simply mean sitting there, letting the horse do all the work! You have to give

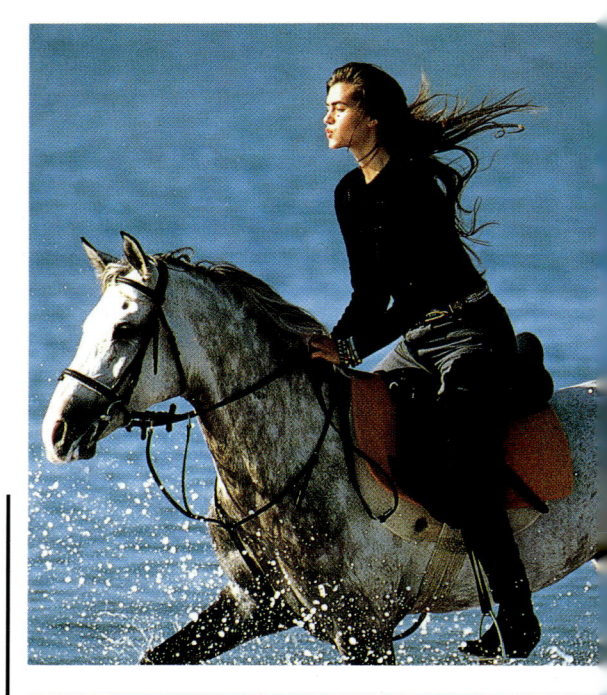

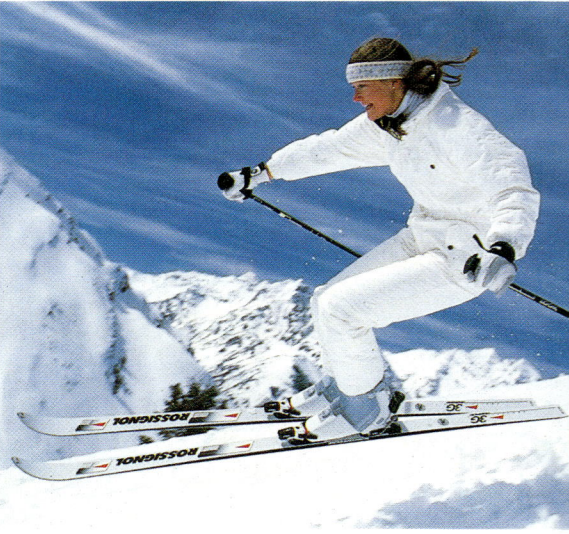

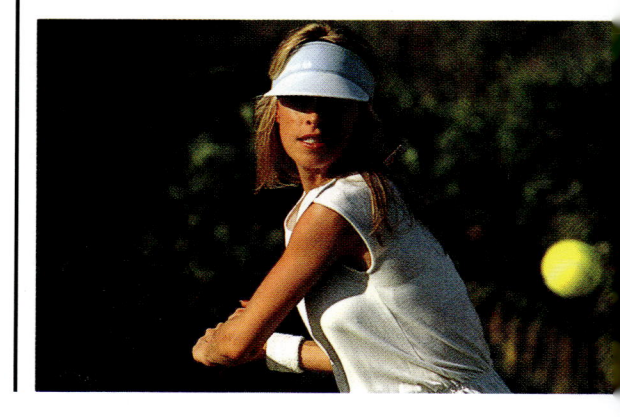

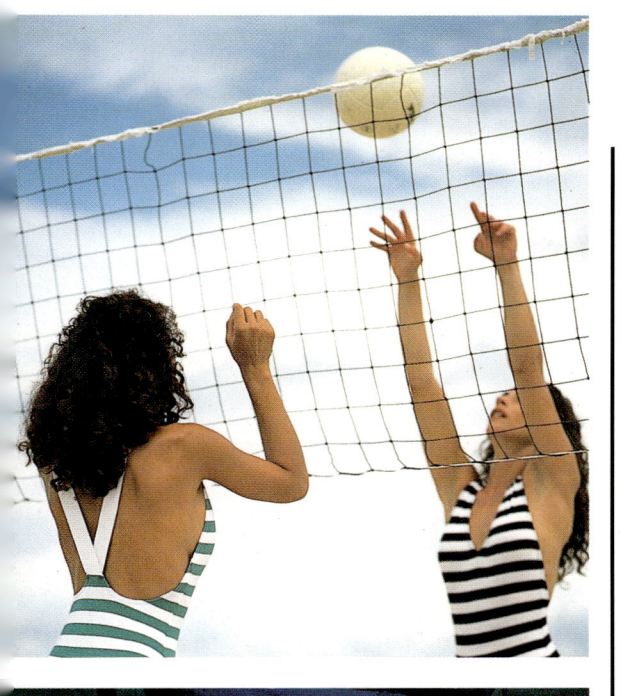

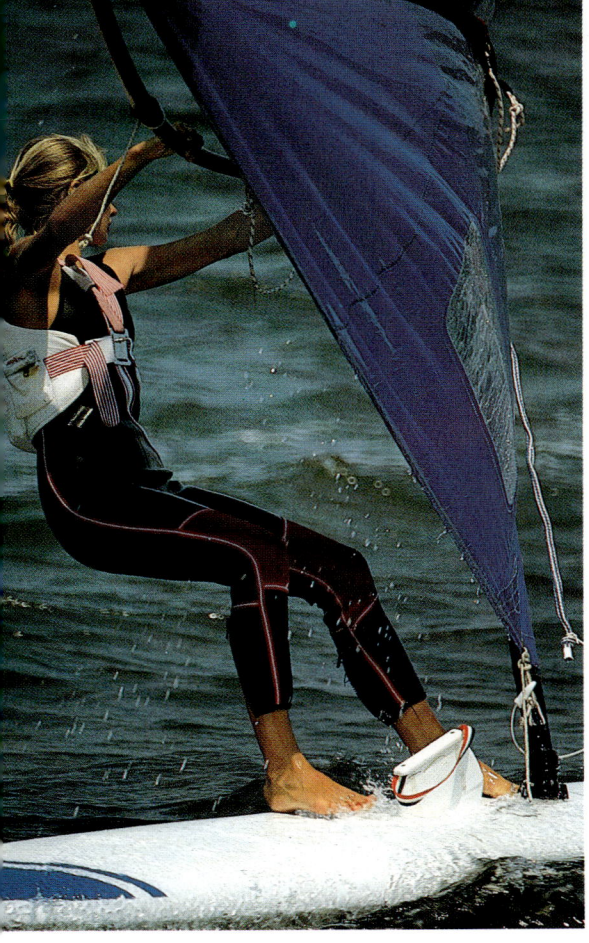

commands, your posture is vital and you need to develop good abdominal control to move with the horse. You will find that it helps to strengthen your back and also strengthens and stretches your thigh and calf muscles.

SAILING
Sailing can be very relaxing, when cruising, for example, or it can be physically challenging, as when yachting in the open seas.

Pulling ropes will strengthen the muscles in your upper back and arms. As you lean out to balance the boat, your abdominal muscles and legs take the strain. Good flexibility is needed to handle a boat when you are changing direction.

SKIING
Skiing is invigorating and exhausting! The fitter you are, though, the less taxing it is. It is necessary to learn correct technique to avoid strains and breaks, and it is wise to do leg-strengthening and stamina-building exercises before you head off for the slopes.

At beginner's level, you need strength and co-ordination between arms/sticks and legs/skis. As you get more advanced, flexibility becomes increasingly important, particularly if you attempt slalom or jumps.

MOUNTAIN-BIKING
An increasingly popular sport, mountain-biking can take you off-road into picturesque country but with physically demanding terrain. It's challenging and as fast as you want it to be, plus a potentially very sociable activity, too. Plenty of mountain-biking clubs and teams now exist.

TENNIS
With tennis, the level of your game relates directly to its fitness value. A gentle game of doubles is less taxing than a hard-fought singles match, for example.

It is good for developing general fitness and flexibility. You will develop a strong wrist and grip in your racquet arm and footwork is important too. Practise side steps and moving for the ball with backhand and forehand strokes.

Stretch your calf and thigh muscles regularly (see page 135) so that they are less at risk of being pulled.

Before starting a game, warm up your shoulders (see page 123) to reduce the risk of pulled muscles, and wear shock-absorbing shoes.

VOLLEYBALL
Volleyball strengthens the hands and wrists and the pectoral muscles in the chest. You can increase the strength in those areas by hitting the ball with a partner or against the wall. Volleyball also firms and strengthens the legs, particularly the front of the thighs, because of all the jumping, but make sure you've got good shock-absorbing shoes.

WINDSURFING
Windsurfing is good for improving co-ordination and a strong upper body and back is an advantage. It also firms and strengthens your leg muscles.

It is important to have some lessons to learn good techniques in windsurfing or else you will probably never enjoy it. When you have become competent, there are plenty of advanced techniques to learn which will enable you to race and jump waves.

24 SHORT CUTS

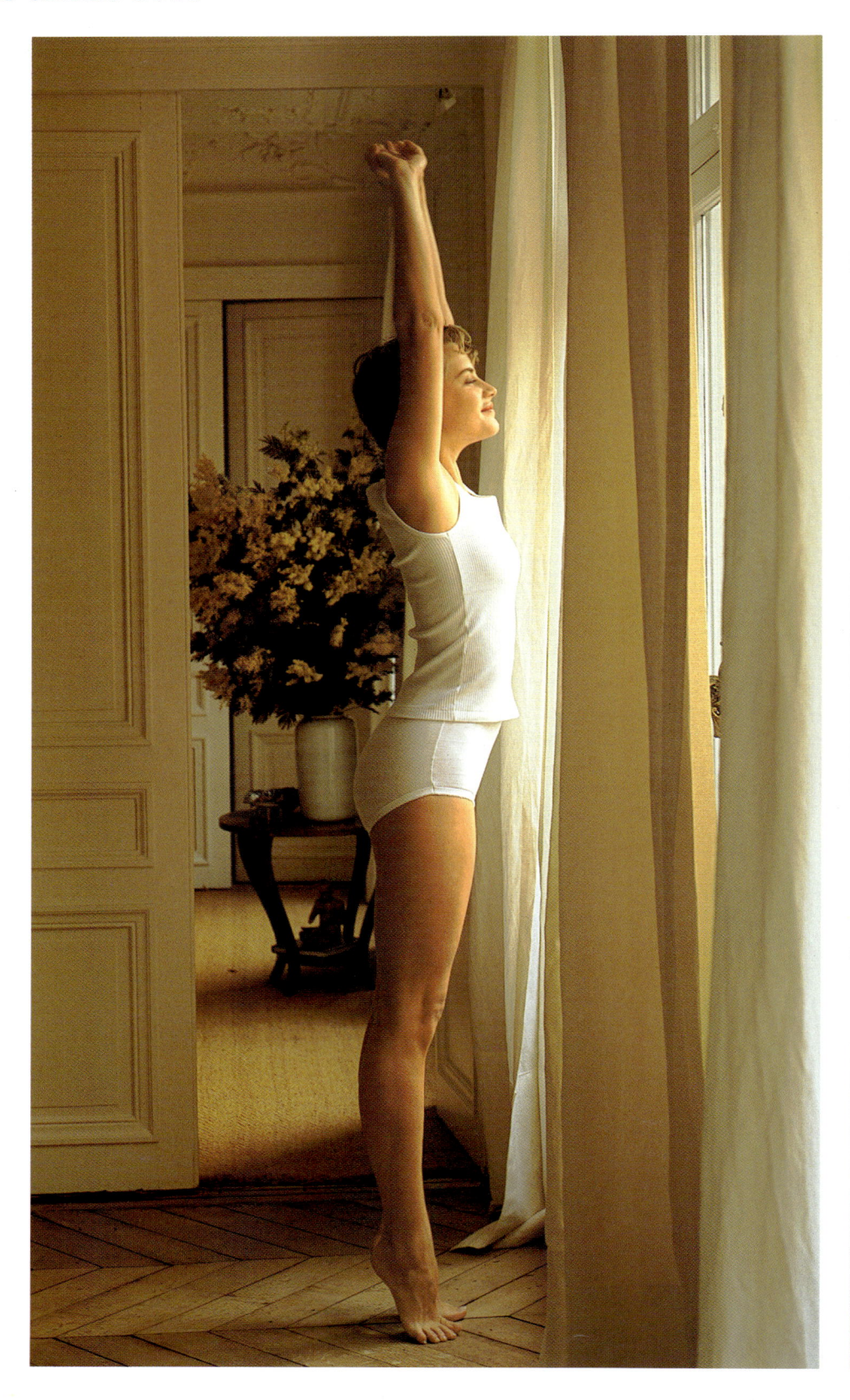

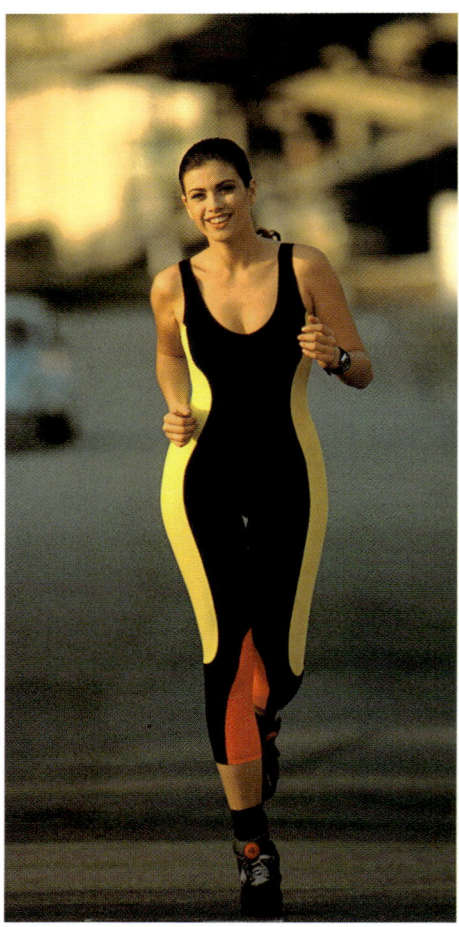

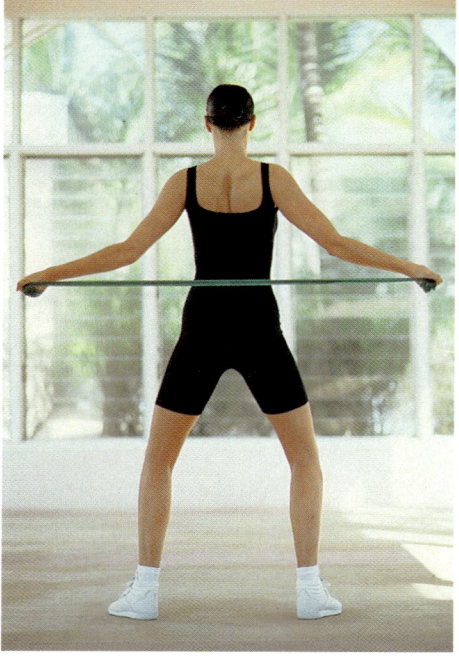

FITTING EXERCISE INTO YOUR DAY

If you are too busy to get to an exercise class, these simple tips will keep you fit while you are on the move.

It can be difficult to schedule exercise sessions when you have a hectic lifestyle. It's a good idea, therefore, to squeeze fitness moves into your day whenever and wherever you have the opportunity! That way you'll maintain your health and increase your energy levels. Here are some ideas.

Try a good morning stretch
It will get the circulation moving on waking up and only takes a few minutes.
- Stand with your feet wide apart and slightly turned out.
- Bend your knees and tuck your buttocks under, pulling your stomach in.
- Now raise your arms slowly and breathe in, stretching up so your legs straighten as you do so.
    Remember to s-t-r-e-t-c-h your arms and whole body up towards the ceiling.
- Lower your arms as you breathe out and bend your knees (check that your knees bend over your feet and do not roll in).
- Breathe in. Repeat the stretch 10 times.

Exercise in the morning
This will ensure that you've slotted it into your day. Get up 20 minutes early a couple of times a week and go for a brisk walk or a gentle jog.

Walk, don't ride
Park the car a few streets away or jump off the bus two stops early. Always climb the stairs.

Keep moving
If you are sitting at a desk for long periods of time, get up frequently and walk around to keep your circulation moving.

Avoid neck strain
- Tip your chin forwards and swing your head very slowly around to your right.
- Bring your head back to the centre and then sweep around to your left.
- Repeat as often as you wish.
Note: avoid tipping your head backwards.

Relax your shoulders
Circle your shoulders backwards, lifting them up to your ears and then pulling down so that you can really feel the movement.
    You can also try this shoulder and upper back stretch.
- Bend one arm up behind you and bring your other hand over your shoulder from the front.
- Clasp your hands if you can and gently stretch up. If your hands don't meet, use a scarf to help you.
- Hold for 30 seconds and then swap hands.

Get some fresh air
Go out for a walk *every* lunch-time. A stuffy environment will sap your energy and leave you feeling headachey and lethargic at the end of the day.

Tone your legs and knees
Try the leg-strengthening and knee-toning exercise on page 135.

Keep ankles and wrists supple
Do ankle and wrist circling whenever you remember – while watching television for instance.

Exercise at home
Buy an exercise video to use at home, if you have a video cassette recorder. If you don't have time to do the whole programme, just do the stretching as this is wonderfully relaxing. Warm up for a few minutes first by walking around the room briskly, circling your arms.

Loosen up your back
Use this lower back stretch whenever the muscles feel tight. It's especially relaxing at the end of a long day.
- Lie on the floor and bend your knees up to your chest.
- Bring your hands round to clasp your legs and rock very gently.
- Relax for a few moments afterwards and then get up slowly.

26 SHORT CUTS

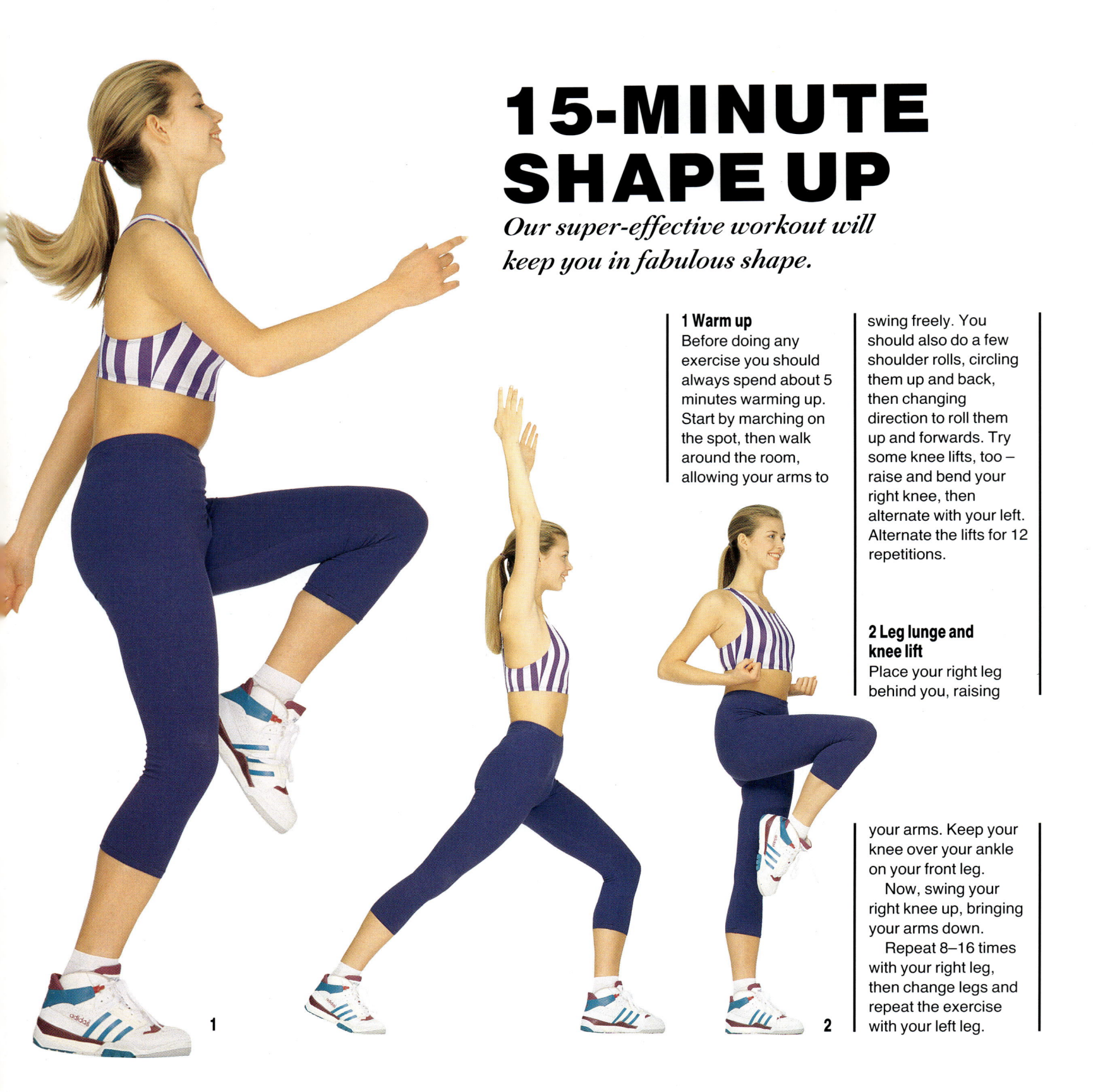

15-MINUTE SHAPE UP

Our super-effective workout will keep you in fabulous shape.

1 Warm up
Before doing any exercise you should always spend about 5 minutes warming up. Start by marching on the spot, then walk around the room, allowing your arms to swing freely. You should also do a few shoulder rolls, circling them up and back, then changing direction to roll them up and forwards. Try some knee lifts, too – raise and bend your right knee, then alternate with your left. Alternate the lifts for 12 repetitions.

2 Leg lunge and knee lift
Place your right leg behind you, raising your arms. Keep your knee over your ankle on your front leg.
  Now, swing your right knee up, bringing your arms down.
  Repeat 8–16 times with your right leg, then change legs and repeat the exercise with your left leg.

WELL-BEING 27

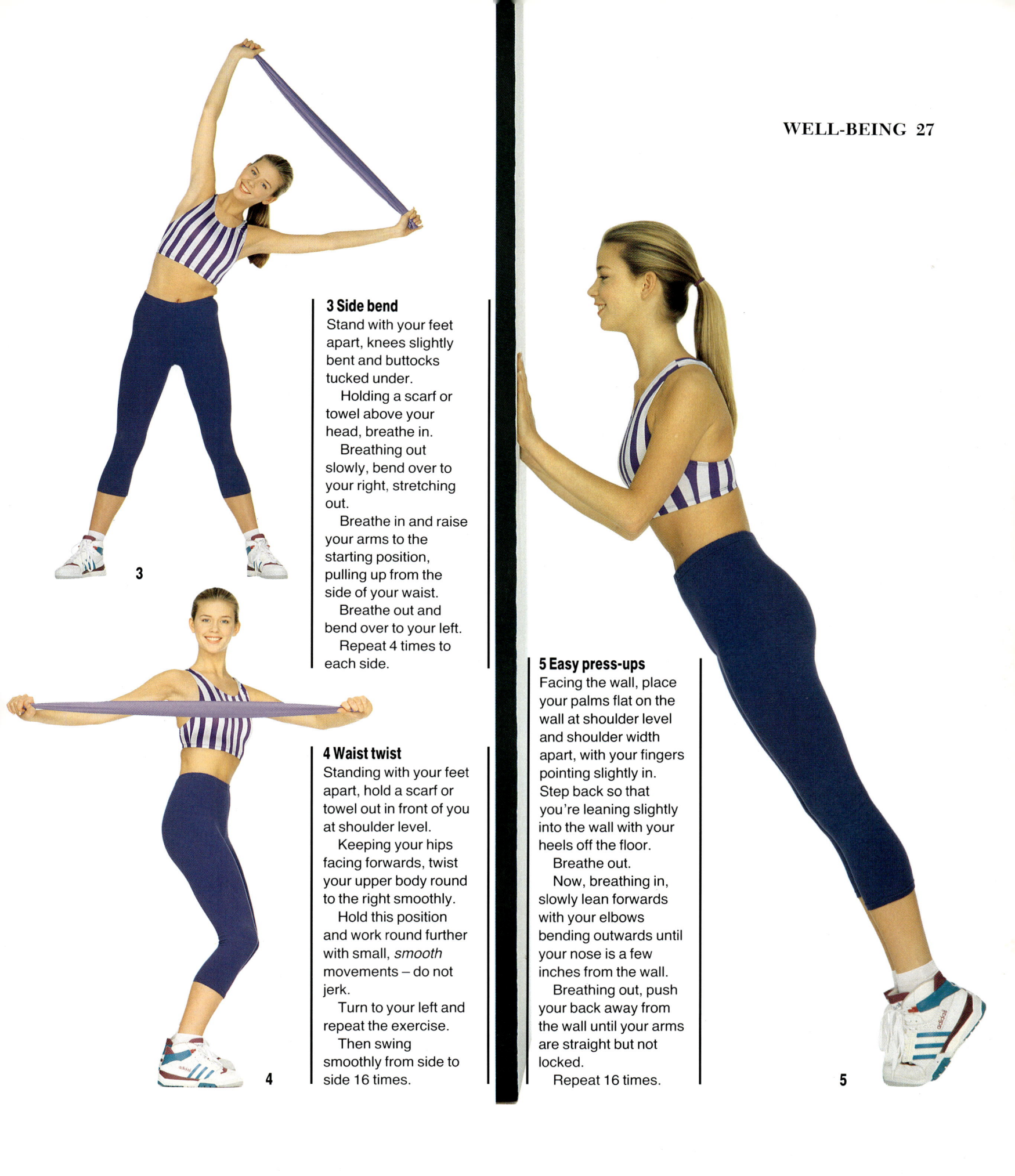

3 Side bend
Stand with your feet apart, knees slightly bent and buttocks tucked under.
　Holding a scarf or towel above your head, breathe in.
　Breathing out slowly, bend over to your right, stretching out.
　Breathe in and raise your arms to the starting position, pulling up from the side of your waist.
　Breathe out and bend over to your left.
　Repeat 4 times to each side.

4 Waist twist
Standing with your feet apart, hold a scarf or towel out in front of you at shoulder level.
　Keeping your hips facing forwards, twist your upper body round to the right smoothly.
　Hold this position and work round further with small, *smooth* movements – do not jerk.
　Turn to your left and repeat the exercise.
　Then swing smoothly from side to side 16 times.

5 Easy press-ups
Facing the wall, place your palms flat on the wall at shoulder level and shoulder width apart, with your fingers pointing slightly in. Step back so that you're leaning slightly into the wall with your heels off the floor.
　Breathe out.
　Now, breathing in, slowly lean forwards with your elbows bending outwards until your nose is a few inches from the wall.
　Breathing out, push your back away from the wall until your arms are straight but not locked.
　Repeat 16 times.

28 SHORT CUTS

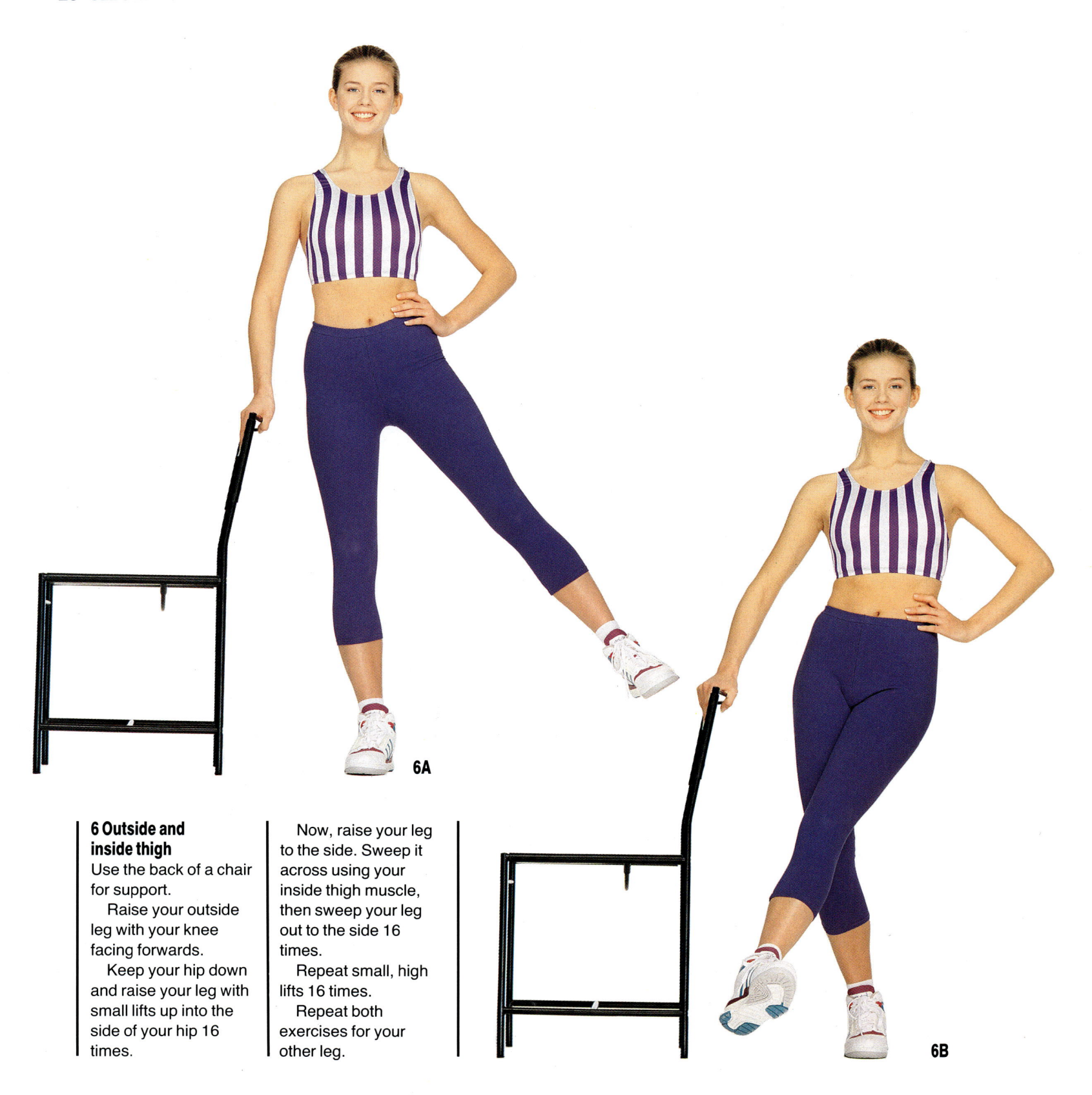

6A

6B

6 Outside and inside thigh
Use the back of a chair for support.

Raise your outside leg with your knee facing forwards.

Keep your hip down and raise your leg with small lifts up into the side of your hip 16 times.

Now, raise your leg to the side. Sweep it across using your inside thigh muscle, then sweep your leg out to the side 16 times.

Repeat small, high lifts 16 times.

Repeat both exercises for your other leg.

7 Buttocks and backs of thighs

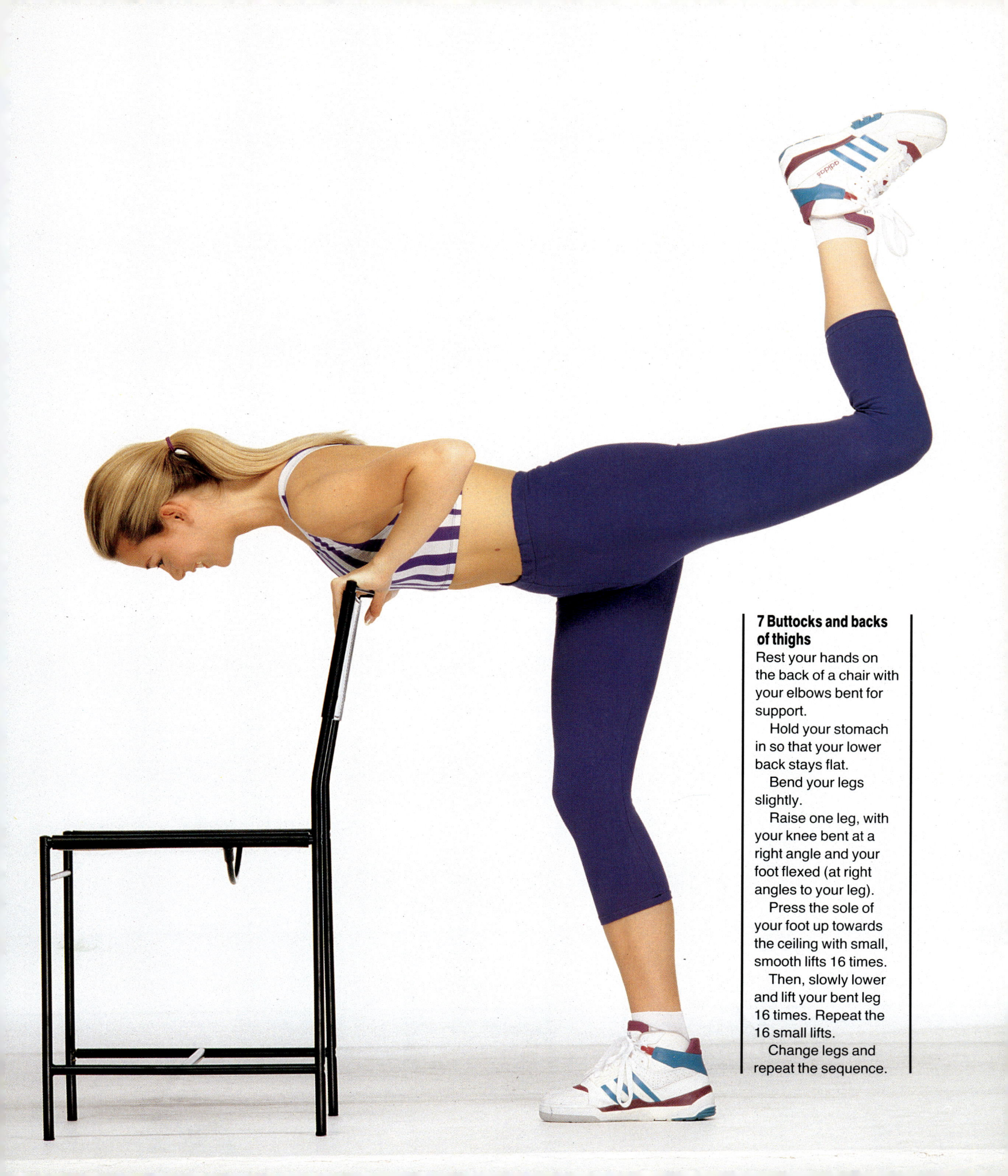

Rest your hands on the back of a chair with your elbows bent for support.

Hold your stomach in so that your lower back stays flat.

Bend your legs slightly.

Raise one leg, with your knee bent at a right angle and your foot flexed (at right angles to your leg).

Press the sole of your foot up towards the ceiling with small, smooth lifts 16 times.

Then, slowly lower and lift your bent leg 16 times. Repeat the 16 small lifts.

Change legs and repeat the sequence.

30 SHORT CUTS

8 Backs of arms
Place your hands on either side of the front of a chair seat, with your back facing the seat.

Place your feet forward so that your bottom drops comfortably and your body-weight is held by your arms.

Bend your elbows, lowering your body, then straighten your arms smoothly, keeping your shoulders down.

Repeat 16 times.
Note: do not try to push up using your thighs or your bottom – only your arms should be working.

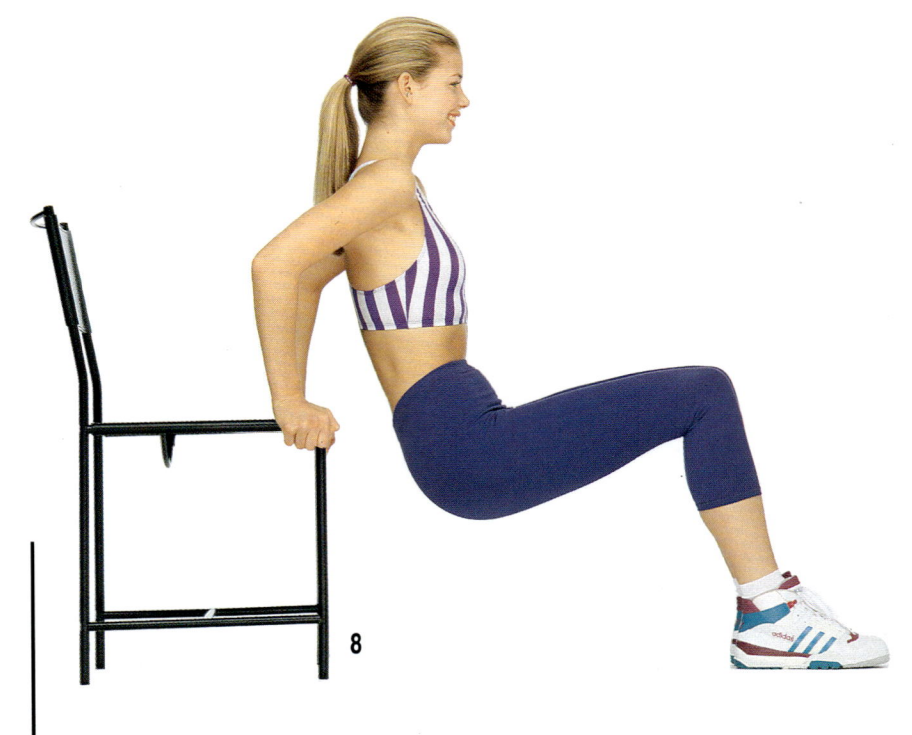

9 Stomach
Sit in the middle of a chair with your hands placed on either side of the front of the seat.

Pull your stomach in so that your lower back rounds slightly.

Breathe normally. Holding your stomach in, draw your right knee up to your chest, then lower it with control. Then draw your left knee up and lower it.

Repeat 8 times with each leg.

To increase the resistance, draw both your knees up to your chest.
Note: make sure that your stomach muscles are taking the weight of your legs – you should not feel *any* pull in your lower back.

Now, lie on the floor with legs bent up at right angles, supported by a chair seat.

Pull your stomach in so that your lower back presses into the floor.

Place your hands lightly under your head with your elbows dropped out to each side.

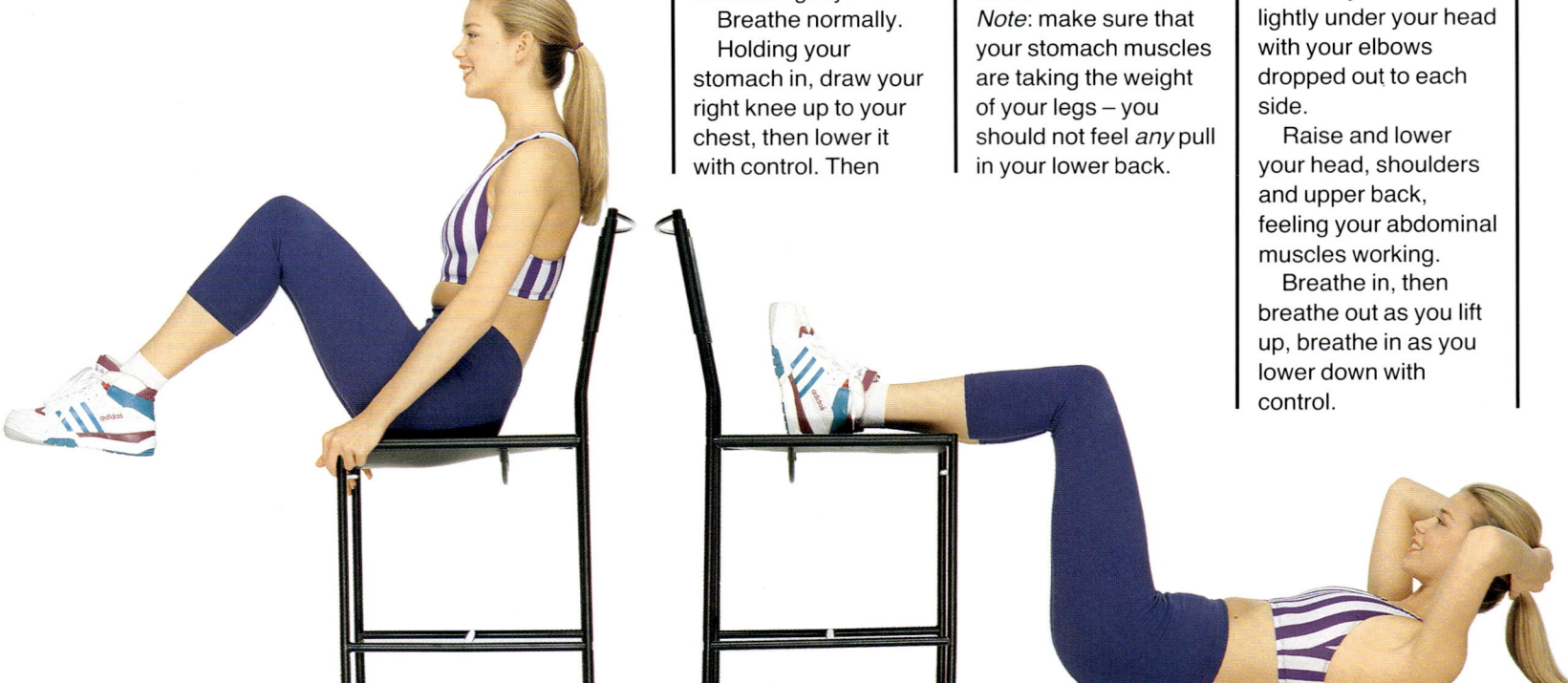

Raise and lower your head, shoulders and upper back, feeling your abdominal muscles working.

Breathe in, then breathe out as you lift up, breathe in as you lower down with control.

8

9A

9B

WELL-BEING 31

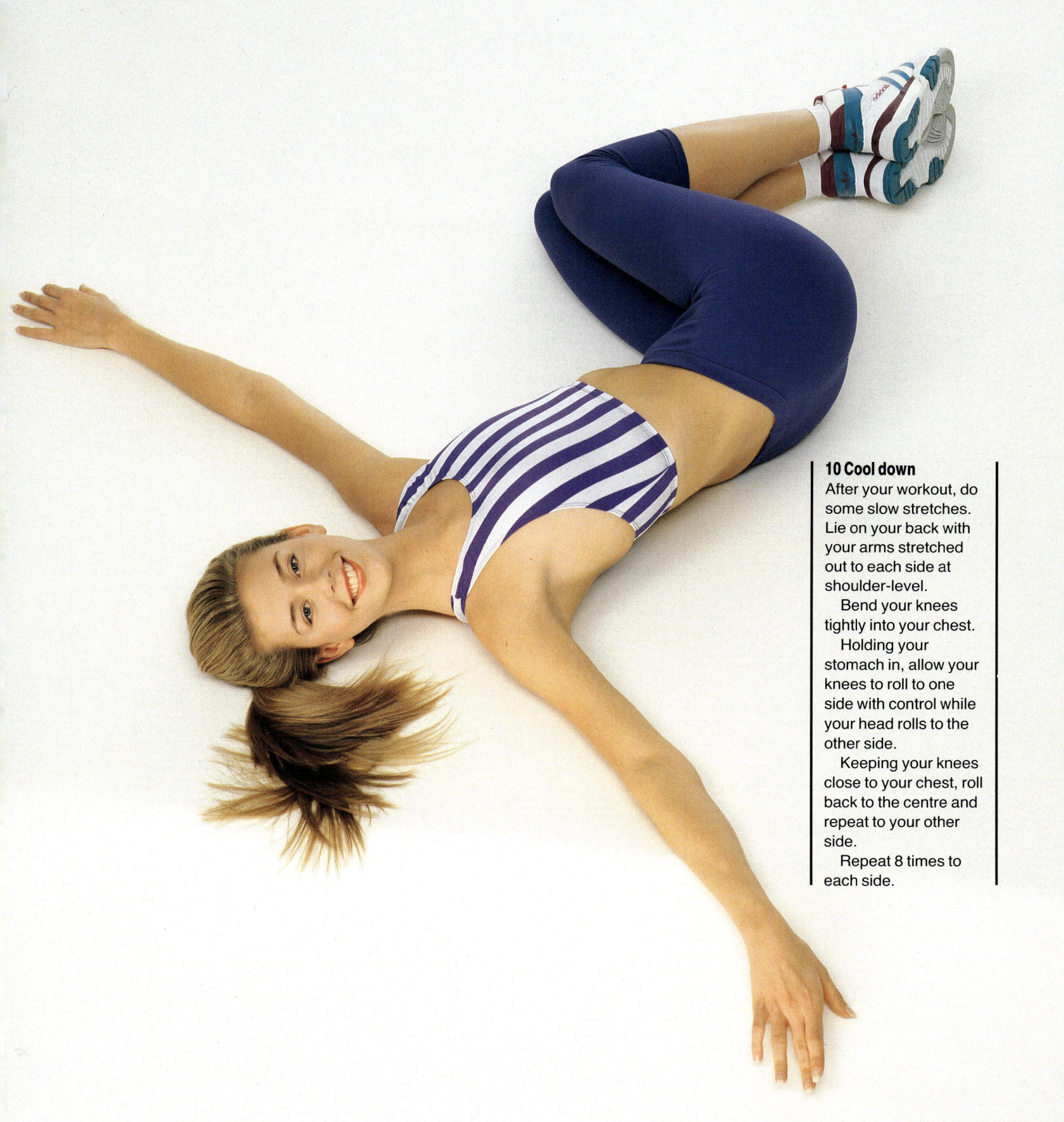

10 Cool down
After your workout, do some slow stretches. Lie on your back with your arms stretched out to each side at shoulder-level.
 Bend your knees tightly into your chest.
 Holding your stomach in, allow your knees to roll to one side with control while your head rolls to the other side.
 Keeping your knees close to your chest, roll back to the centre and repeat to your other side.
 Repeat 8 times to each side.

STRESSED OUT

Identify the sources of stress in your daily life and then stress-proof your environment with these easy tricks.

Stress – that feeling of pressure – sets off a chain reaction of disturbances in the body. Extra adrenalin rushes round (this is part of the body's defence system to give you energy in a crisis). The nervous system is stimulated, hormone production altered, muscles tense up, white blood cells produce fewer antibodies and acid production is increased in the digestive organs. These internal changes give us outward signs of stress.

Stress signals
- irritability, headaches, anxiety
- fatigue, coupled with difficulty in actually getting to sleep
- mood swings, sudden outbursts, indecision
- loss of libido, lack of interest or enjoyment in life
- increased incidence of spots – adult acne has been linked to stress
- vulnerability to illness and flare-ups of existing conditions such as eczema and herpes
- digestive problems
- undereating, overeating, binge-eating
- hair loss – stress is a major cause of female hair loss
- trembling and other nervous reflexes.

Everyone is vulnerable to stress. Its causes are manifold and include relationship problems, bereavement, moving house and a high-pressure job, but we all have different tolerance levels.

One theory psychologists have put forward to explain why people react differently to stress is that stress is related to personality type.
- The 'type A' personality is typically impatient, speaks fast and loudly, is ambitious and always in a hurry, with a tendency to try and do a number of things at the same time, such as working and eating.
- The 'type B' personality is altogether much calmer, taking life at a slower pace with a more relaxed and easy-going approach.

While we are mostly a *mixture* of the two types, we tend to exhibit more characteristics of one or the other. Type A is more stress-prone and thus more at risk of stress-related disease, such as a heart attack, than type B.

Protecting yourself from stress
There are certain steps you can take to guard against stress.
- Make time for relaxation and leave work at work.
- Keep rhythm in your life, as the body responds well to routine. Try, particularly to establish sleep patterns, that is, go to bed and wake up at the same time each day.
- Be aware of what may be causing your stress and try to sort out the problem, or at least anticipate it. Get support from others – suffering in silence doesn't help.
- Prioritize and do only what is important. What wouldn't bother you in a few months or years really isn't worth worrying about.
- Eat a healthy, balanced diet.
- Take some form of exercise three times a week and make it a habit. Exercise is a great antidote to stress, because it lowers your blood pressure and releases endorphins, the body's own natural mood-enhancing chemicals.

DAILY DE-STRESSORS
There are many recurring sources of stress that are part of the regular pattern of your life. It helps to be aware of them when you are aiming to reduce your stress levels.

Stress at the desk
Often, it is at work that you feel at your most 'stressed out'. Colleagues' demands, the constant ringing of telephones and a heavy workload can add up to pressure that at times may seem too much.

Don't panic! Close your eyes and count slowly back from 50. You should be feeling calmer already.

Read on and discover other ways to stress-proof your workspace.

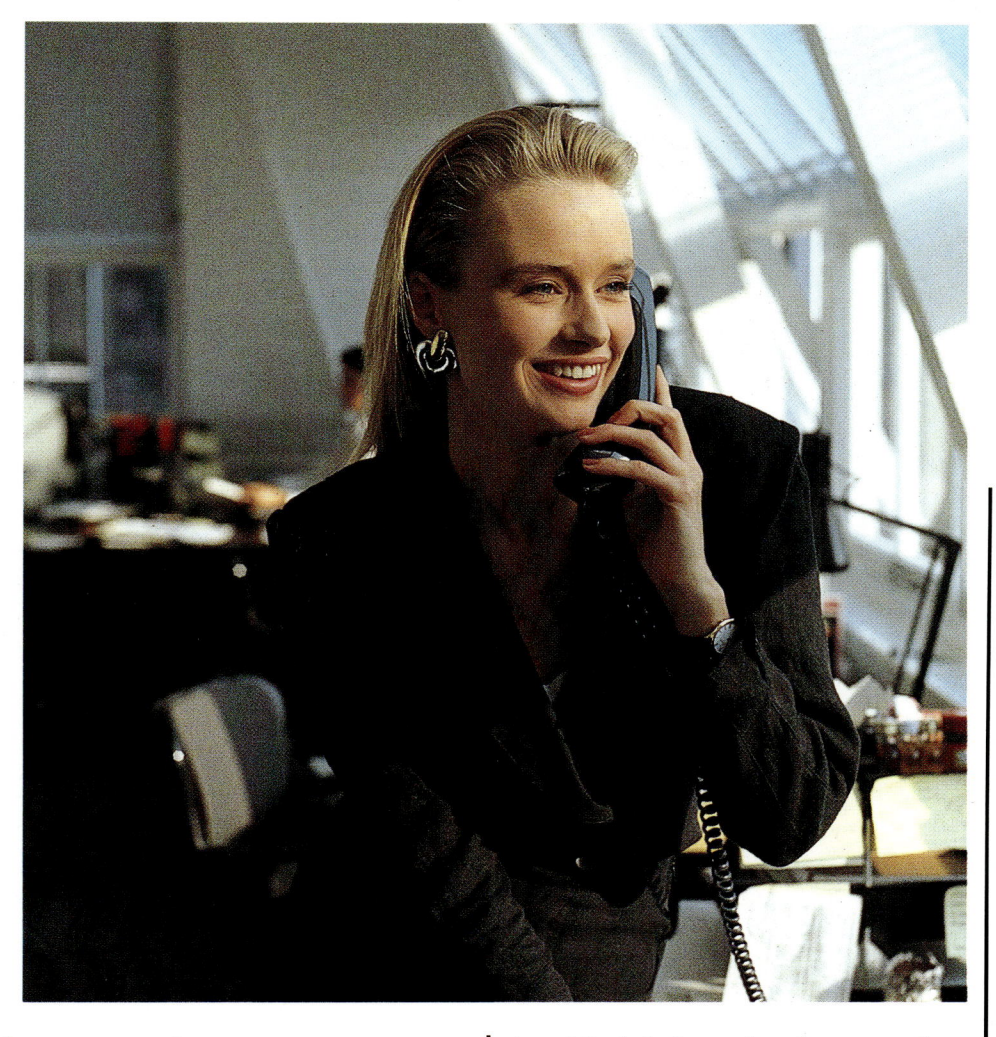

Stress-proofing tips
● Check your posture while you are sitting at your desk. You should be sitting up straight, with your bottom into the back of the chair, with your shoulders down and back, and your chest forward.

It is a natural reaction to let your posture go when you are under stress, so that your shoulders are slumped forward and your head sinks into your neck. In this position, you're setting yourself up for aches and pains and will also be breathing incorrectly.

Try sitting up straight with your head facing forwards – place two fingers on your chin and 'push' back in towards your neck until your head feels balanced and your neck long instead of curved.
● When working at a VDU or reading lots of small print, look into the distance or close your eyes for a few minutes from time to time to avoid or ease eye strain.
● Don't cradle the phone between your shoulder and chin. It will lead to headaches, neck and upper back pain and possibly 'telephone acne' on the chin.

Use your hands to hold the receiver and switch it from ear to ear and, as a preventive measure against spots, clean the mouthpiece daily.
● Do quick exercises during the day to avoid neck strain and relax your shoulders (see page 24).

STRESS AND YOUR DIET
A regular, balanced diet keeps your body in optimum health. During times of stress – whether short-term or prolonged – it is even more important to watch what you eat, as stress is a nutrient robber. See page 12 for general advice, but bear in mind the following points.
● Vitamin C is used at a faster rate when you are under stress, so increase your fruit and vegetable intake, especially raw fruit and vegetables as some vitamin C is lost during cooking.
● When you are under stress you may find yourself craving sugar as a comforter. Carbohydrates have actually been found to trigger a calming chemical in the brain, soothing negative feelings, anxiety and anger. Although you may want refined carbohydrates such as chocolate, choose complex carbohydrates such as pasta, crackers and grains instead. These will give you a more prolonged feeling of calm, rather than the quick 'up', followed by a deep low that refined carbohydrates induce.
● Avoid drinking lots of stimulating tea and coffee, which, like refined carbohydrates will make you go faster temporarily, but bring you down with a thud a little later. Opt for mineral water, juice and herb teas instead.

STRESS-BEATING RELAXATION

Calm your mind and revitalize your body with our instant stress-reducing strategies.

If, in spite of all your efforts to eliminate sources of stress from your life, you still become tense and anxious, there are many ways to deal with it.

SLEEPING IT OFF
Restful sleep is one of the best reliefs for stress. However, you may find that your stress is causing disturbed sleep patterns or creating problems with actually getting to sleep. Try these tips.

Before bed-time . . .
- Avoid stimulants such as tea, coffee and nicotine.
- Beware alcohol – it may make you *feel* sleepy at first, but it tends to create a fitful sleep, making you wake up at frequent intervals.
- Try a relaxing bath, listening to soothing music.
- Gentle stretching exercises are good before bedtime, but don't undertake aerobic activity as it stimulates the cardio-vascular and nervous systems for up to six hours afterwards.
- If you've got a problem, try to solve it *before* going to bed or leave it and vow you'll sort it out in the morning.

In bed . . . and still not asleep?
Concentrate on how heavy, sleepy and warm your body feels,

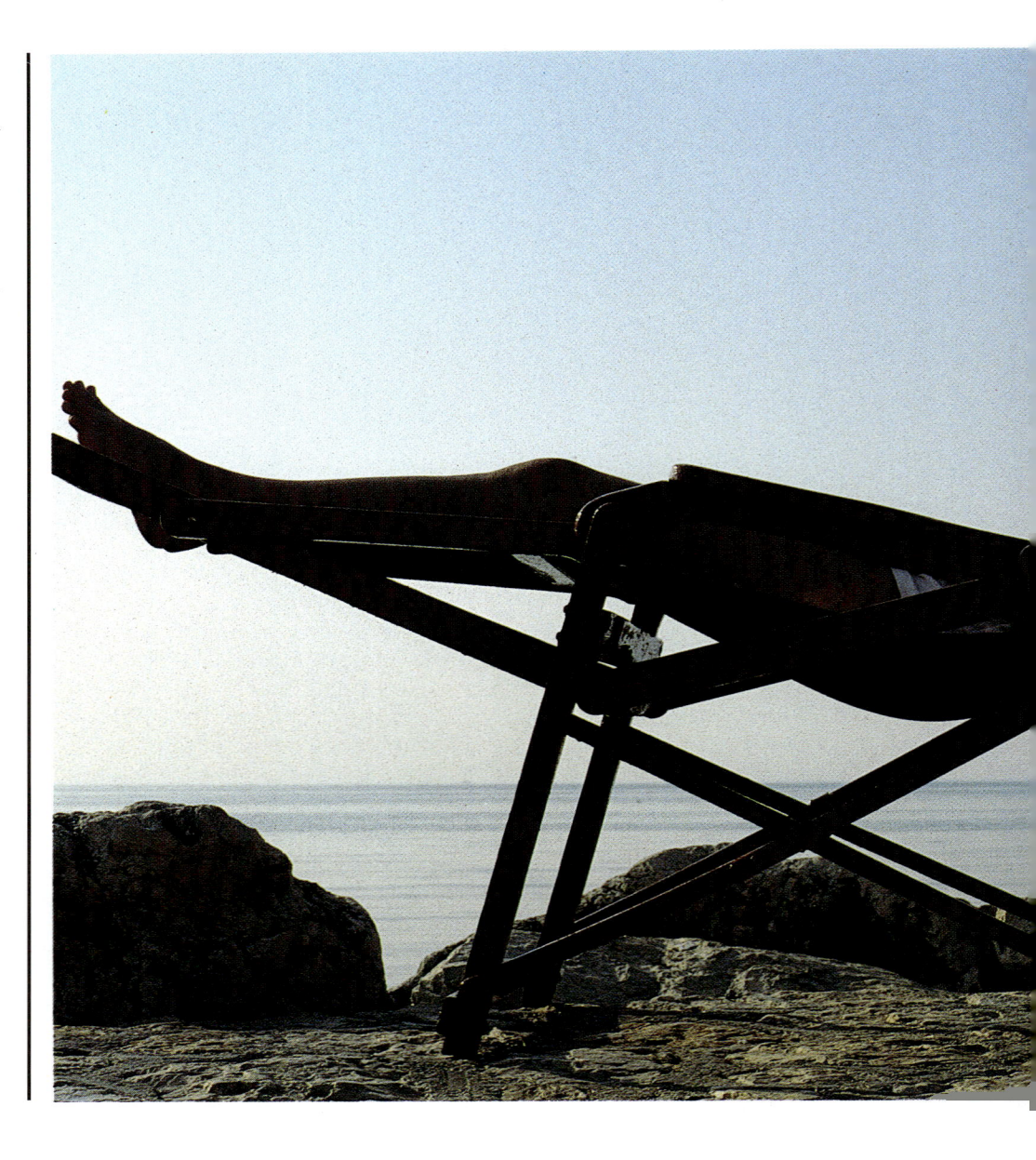

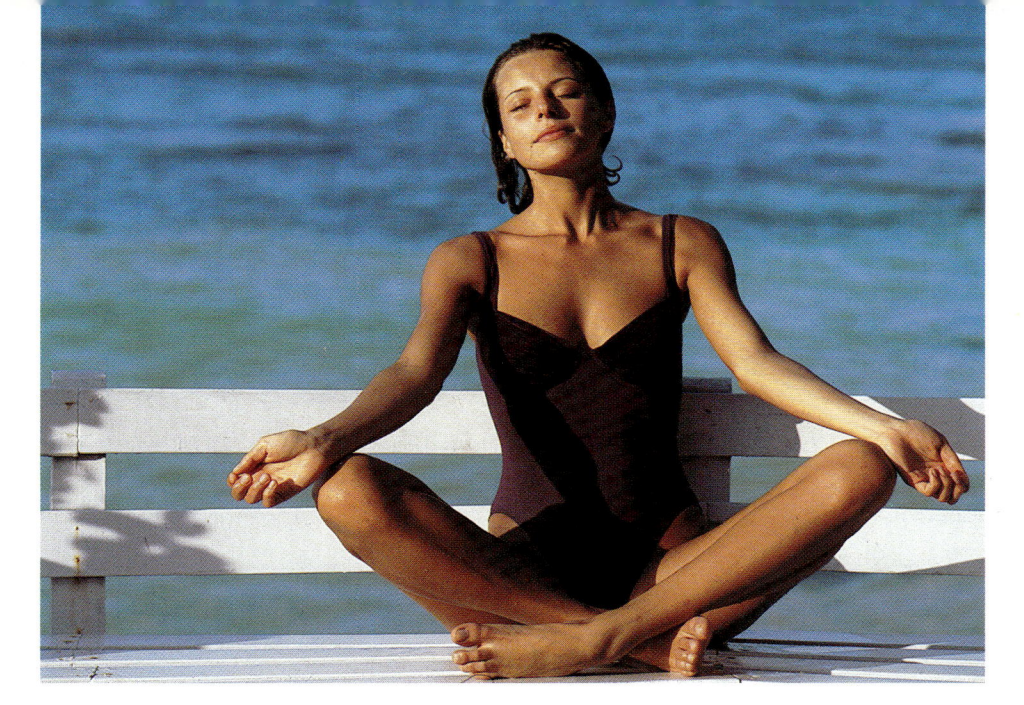

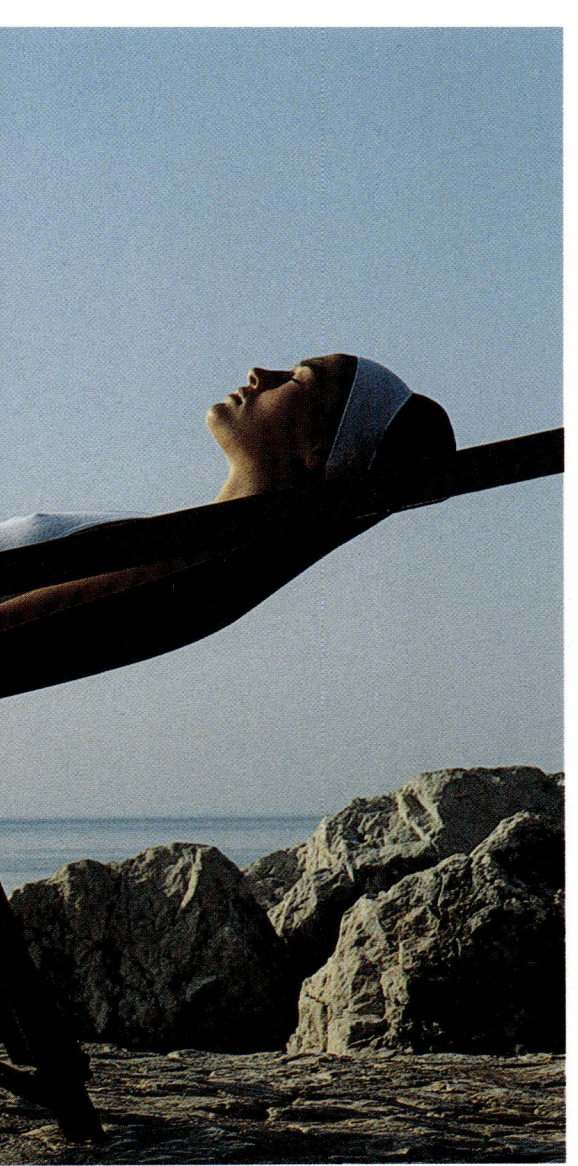

imagining all the muscles and limbs from head to toe.
- Counting sheep or visualizing a black space helps because it is meaningless and diverts your mind from your troubles.
- As a last resort, try a diversionary tactic like getting up and reading or watching TV.

MEDITATING

When your mind is racing you need specific techniques to turn off the 'flight or fight' stress response that is in play.

You can slow your mind with a number of techniques. Try sitting quietly for 5 minutes with your eyes closed, and repeat a word you have positive associations with, either out loud or in your head.

Relaxation tapes use creative visualization to wind you down in a pleasant and easy way. You will quickly notice that your breathing becomes slower and deeper and your body feels warmer as you relax.

By becoming aware of where you are storing tension you can help to release it. Sit or lie quietly, eyes closed, and starting at your feet become aware of how they feel. Now tense and relax the muscles in that area and repeat, moving slowly up the body, finishing with the face and neck.

BREATHING

We rarely think about how we breathe. Yet we often breathe incorrectly – too shallowly and irregularly. Poor breathing habits can cause tension, lack of concentration and even panic attacks.

To breathe correctly, lift up from the waist, bring your shoulder blades together to open up the chest, and relax your stomach. Inhale deeply, drawing the diaphragm down, and exhale with the same control.

FLOATING

Floatation therapy is increasingly available. You lie in darkness or semi-darkness in a tank or pool filled with warm water that contains high concentrations of Epsom and other mineral salts. By taking away the effects of gravity and reducing sensory stimulation your mind produces brain waves like those produced by deep meditation.

Sessions last around 40–60 minutes. Some floatation centres have tanks that are fitted with video screens or speaker systems so that you can receive hypnotherapy or meditation training whilst in a state of relaxation.

The door is easily opened so that you don't feel shut in. Most people emerge feeling on top of the world!

36 SHORT CUTS

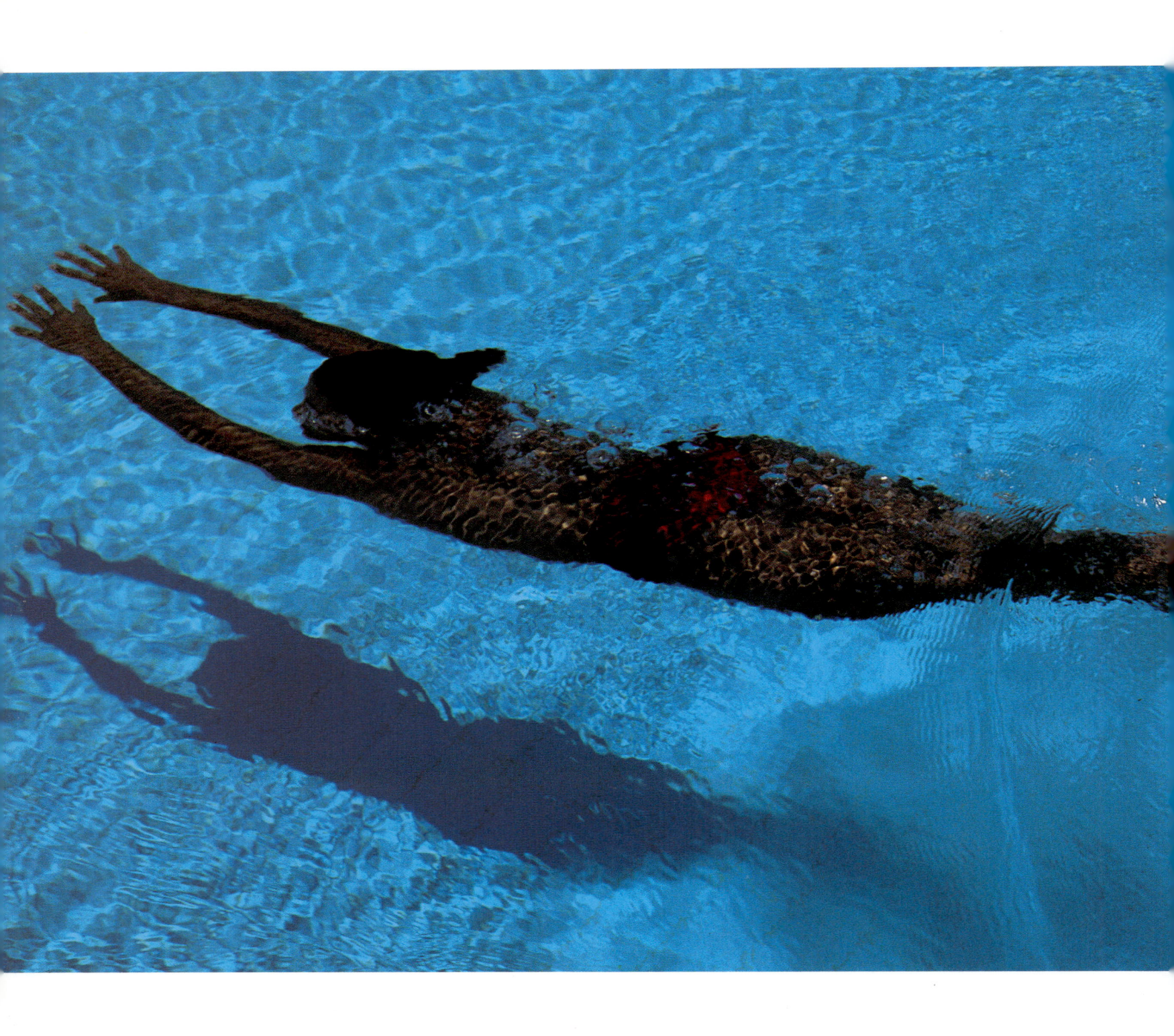

BIOFEEDBACK

Biofeedback proves that the human brain influences, and can control, the body's automatic nervous system. This is the involuntary system that regulates heartbeat and many other processes.

By willing your body to produce a certain response you can alter your brain waves, your blood pressure, relaxation levels and even the amount of acid produced by the stomach.

With biofeedback, electrodes are connected to, for instance, the palm of your hand and a machine registers your level of relaxation by producing different tones or through visual displays. A whining high-pitched tone indicates that stress levels are high.

Once you can lower the tone yourself to a satisfactory level, you can then practice controlling your stress levels without the equipment.

Biofeedback training is available in specialist centres countrywide; machines are also available for use at home.

NATUROPATHY

Also known as the 'nature cure', this form of complementary medicine was developed during the nineteenth century. Its principles centre around fresh air, exposure to light, pure water and simple food to prevent disease and where necessary to help the body heal itself.

Naturopaths believe that disease is the result of an accumulation of toxins and waste products in the body and an upset in the balance of the body or mind, caused by stress.

Fasting, nutritional therapy, hydrotherapy, exercise, cleanliness and psychotherapy are all used by trained naturopaths.

You can apply the naturopathic methods yourself to help control stress. Gradually increase the number of healthy habits in your lifestyle over one week and evaluate how you feel at the end of this time.

1 Assess your stress levels by writing down all the sources of tension that may be affecting you. Everyone reacts differently to stress so changes in your routine or pressures at work or in your personal relationships do not *necessarily* present a problem.

2 Work out a lifestyle for you that will create a balance between rest and work and that features fresh air, exercise and good eating habits.

3 Make sure you get outside into the air and daylight for at least half an hour everyday. Why not go for a brisk walk at lunchtime? You should also schedule some time for daily exercise.

4 Drink at least eight glasses of water every day. If you feel at all anxious and nervous and are a coffee, tea or cola drinker, it is very likely that you are susceptible to the effects of caffeine on your nervous system. Cut down the amount you consume gradually to avoid withdrawal headaches which can be severe, and consider giving up caffeine (also found in chocolate) altogether. Check, too, that you are eating at regular intervals and try eating complex – not refined – carbohydrates at least every three hours to keep your blood sugar balanced. If your intake of alcohol has been increasing or is already high, then consider whether you can reduce it or whether you need an expert's advice on addiction. Food allergies or a candida (yeast) overgrowth should also be suspected if you crave sugar or alcohol.

5 Consider having a mini-fast to give your digestive system a break. Try eating, for instance, lamb, rice and pears or just fresh juices for one to two days. You should not use a cleansing diet like this for more than two days.

6 Swim at least three times a week and go to the health club for a spa session in the steam room and jacuzzi, and book a full body massage, aromatherapy or reflexology treatment.

7 Use a natural bristle brush very firmly over your whole body every day before you bathe or shower, moving up towards the heart, to improve lymph drainage (the body's waste disposal system). Apply lots of body lotion afterwards.

8 Set aside private time every day when you can sit quietly on your own. Use this time to reflect, to read or to do something that encourages artistic expression.

DISCOVERING YOGA

Face the day feeling refreshed and ready for anything with energizing yoga exercises.

Yoga originated in India at least 3,000 years ago. Today it offers a great deal to the beginner and the advanced expert alike, and is becoming one of the most popular of exercise systems. Hatha yoga is a commonly practised form in the West today.

Just 10 to 15 minutes of yoga stretching and breathing each day will bring you a wide range of health and beauty benefits, and will help to put you in touch with your inner self.

Yoga is not difficult to learn, even for a beginner. It isn't necessary to wrap your legs behind your head – or to stand on it – to do yoga. In fact, the more advanced classical postures should be attempted only when you are very experienced.

Yoga exercises stretch and tone your muscles and greatly improve flexibility. By stimulating the nervous system, and improving breathing and circulation, yoga gives you strength and stamina, and resistance to stress and illness. And that's just on the physical level.

Practising yoga also develops emotional balance. It gives you a feeling of being centred and encourages a positive attitude to life. In time it will improve your powers of concentration and your creativity. Yoga classes are the best place to begin. A teacher will be able to guide you towards performing the postures correctly and effectively.

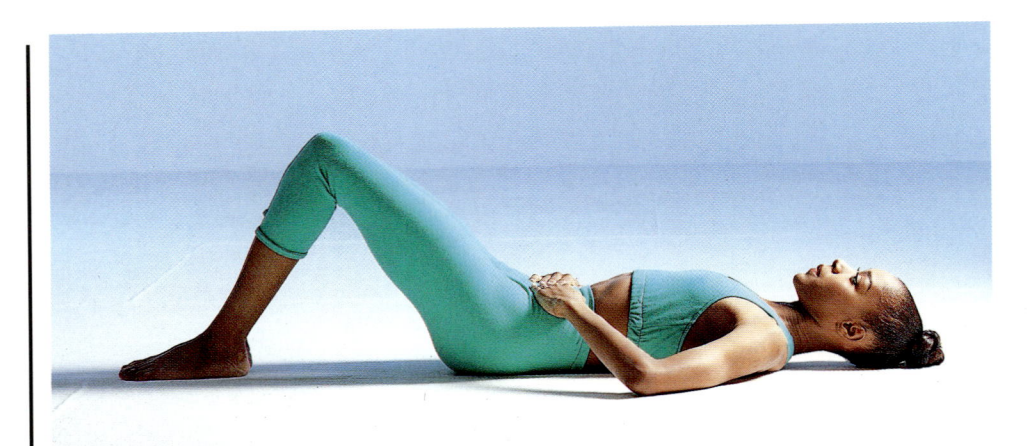

You should wear clothes that are warm and comfortable, giving you complete freedom of movement, preferably in natural fibres such as cotton. Wearing a leotard and footless tights will help you and the teacher to see how well aligned your body is. Yoga is always done in bare feet, but take a pair of socks and a sweatshirt to keep you warm during the relaxation at the end of the session.

Try to avoid eating anything for at least 2 hours before practising.

It is important to focus on a gentle releasing of the body during the postures. You shouldn't strain. Think all the time about how your body is feeling, rather than how your body looks, and be aware of areas of stiffness and flexibility during each posture.

After just one class, you will find that you feel calm and relaxed and that locked-in tensions are being eased out. You will probably enjoy it so much that you will want to make yoga part of your daily life!

THE YOGA STRETCH

The stretch you do at the start of a class is also the ideal way to start the day, to relax and gently revitalize yourself when you feel fatigued or stressed. Inhale and exhale deeply and regularly throughout.

The exercise can also be done standing up.

Lie on the floor on your back. Now spread right out, moving slowly about and feeling the contact

WELL-BEING 39

your body makes with the floor. Imagine you are a child again, and try to move without inhibitions.

Flattening your back towards the floor, slowly bring your arms up over your head and very gently stretch up. Concentrate on stretching up and out from the waist, all the way to your wrist and fingertips.

While continuing the upward stretch, and still pressing down with the back of your waist, bring your focus of attention downwards. Stretch down through the thighs, knees, ankles and toes.

Circle your feet and wiggle your toes and stretch them out.

Now let go. Simply let your whole body flop. Repeat the exercise a couple of times.

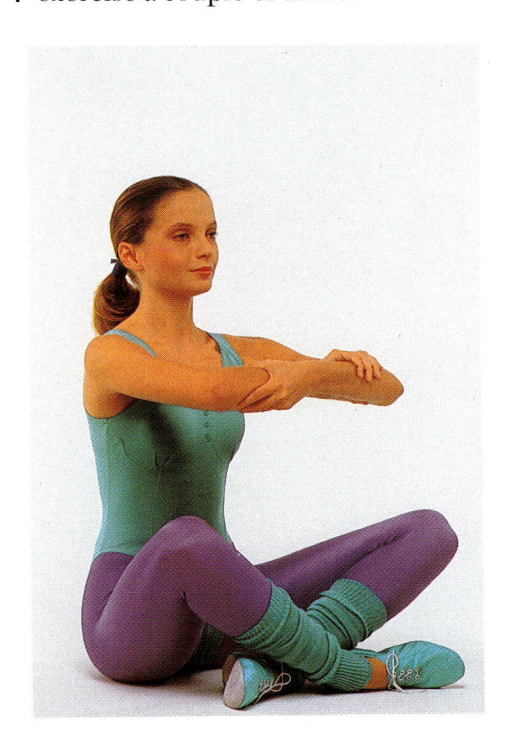

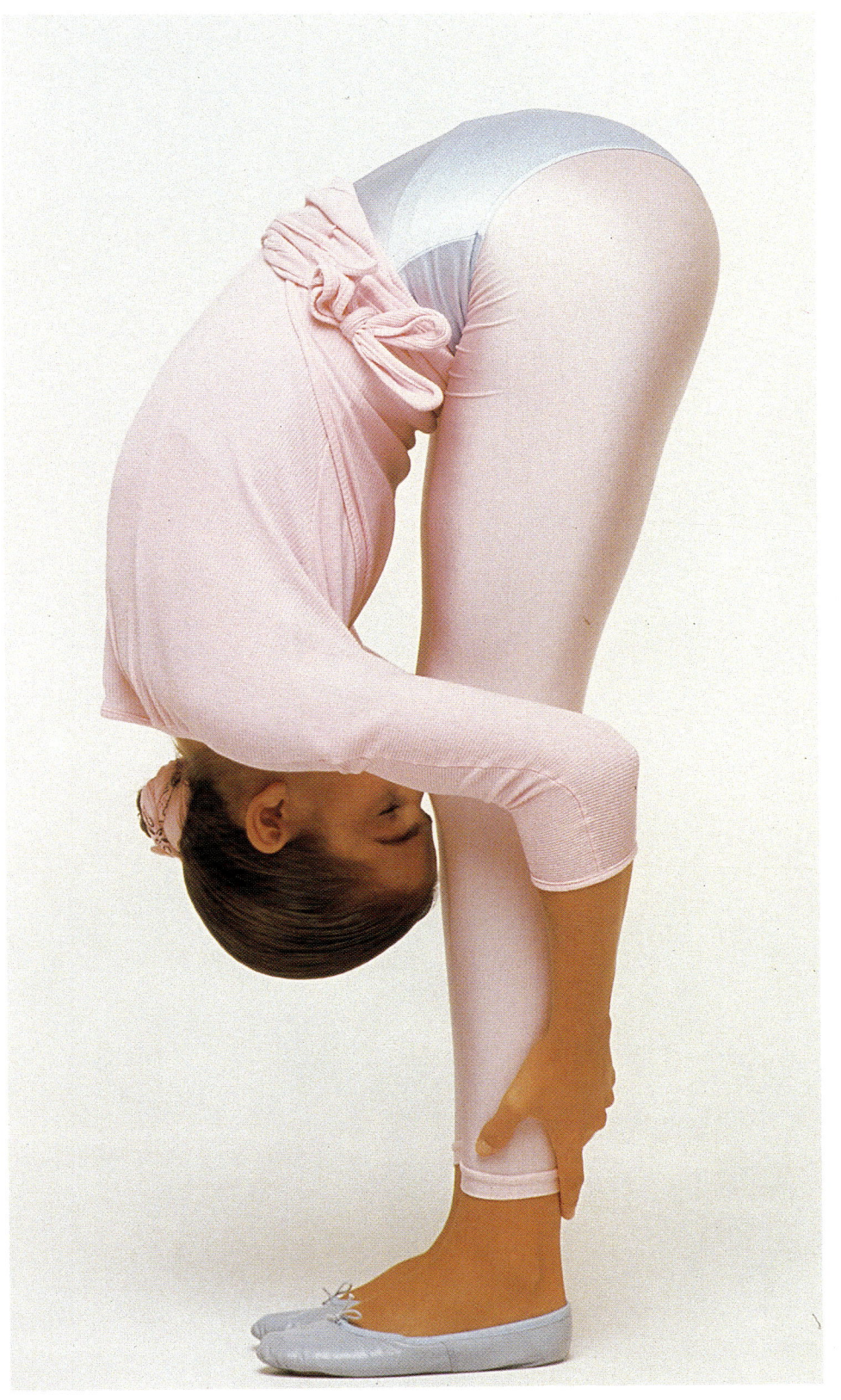

40 SHORT CUTS

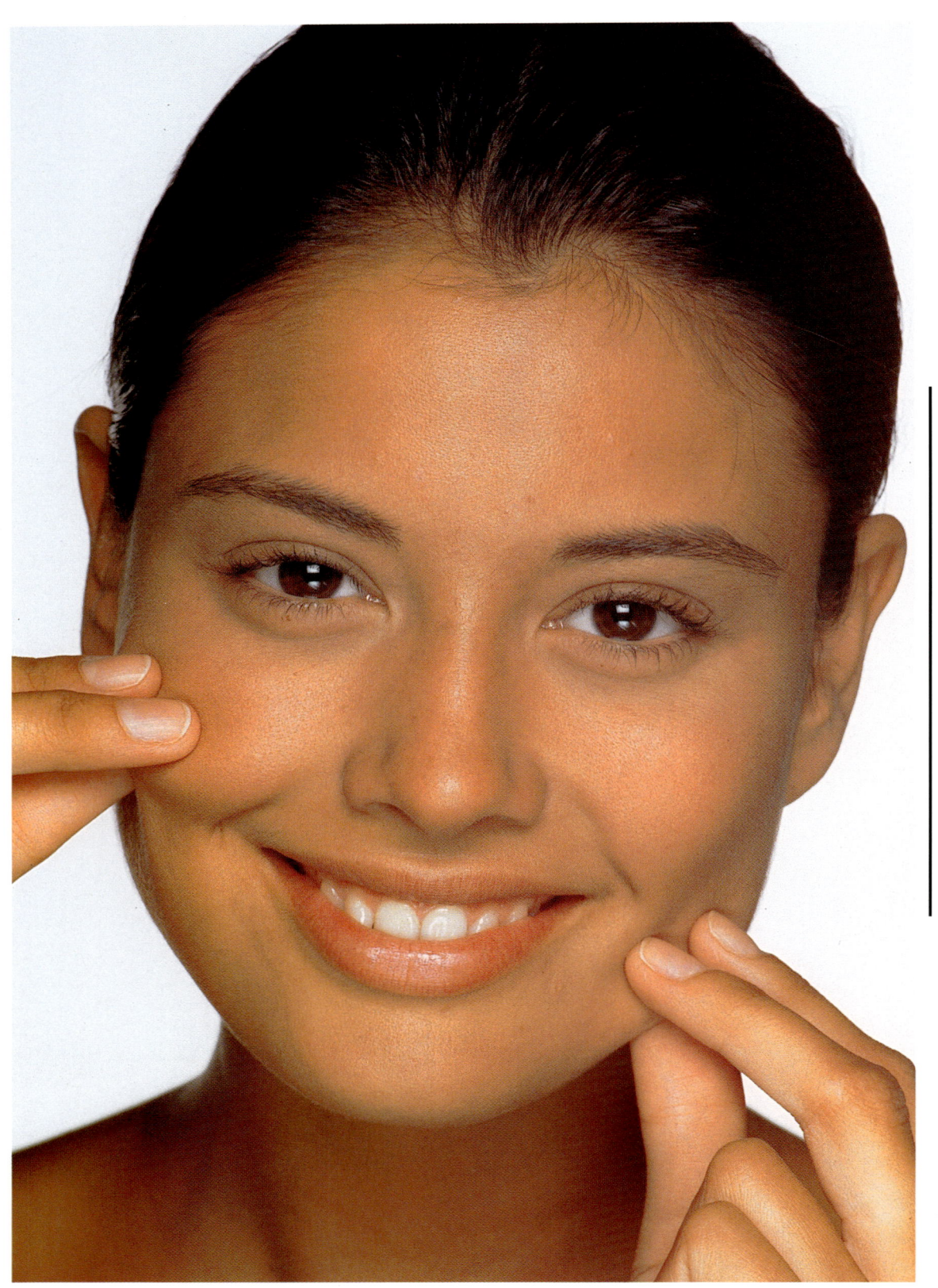

1 Apply the moisturizer or oil all over your face and neck using upward sweeping strokes.

2 Morning: gently pinch the area from cheek-bones to jawline.
 Evening (not shown): replace the pinching action with circular movements using your index fingers. Press for a few seconds on tension zones – the inner and outer corners of your eyes and beginning of brows.

MARVELLOUS MASSAGE

You can ease away tension, revive your skin and increase circulation by using the simplest massage techniques.

Massage has been practised for centuries to relax the body and soothe the mind. It's almost as enjoyable for the masseur as it is for the recipient.

You can also practise DIY massage. For example, simply massaging your upper arms and shoulders when you feel fatigued and tense will help to keep circulation moving and prevent problems. Squeeze and release the skin firmly, moving up the arm and across the shoulders using the hand of the opposite arm. Concentrate on areas where you feel tight.

FACIAL MASSAGE
This is another fast way to ease a stressed and tired-looking complexion. It increases the colour and condition of your skin. The routine shown here takes just a few minutes. The moves will be easier if you use moisturizer or facial oil.

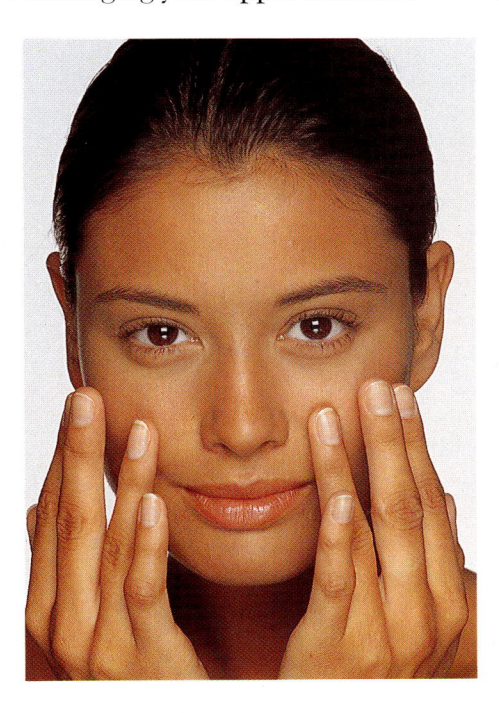

3 Rhythmically tap your fingers all over your face. Start with your chin and move gently over the jaw line and the cheeks, working your way up to and under your eyes. Avoid the actual eye area.

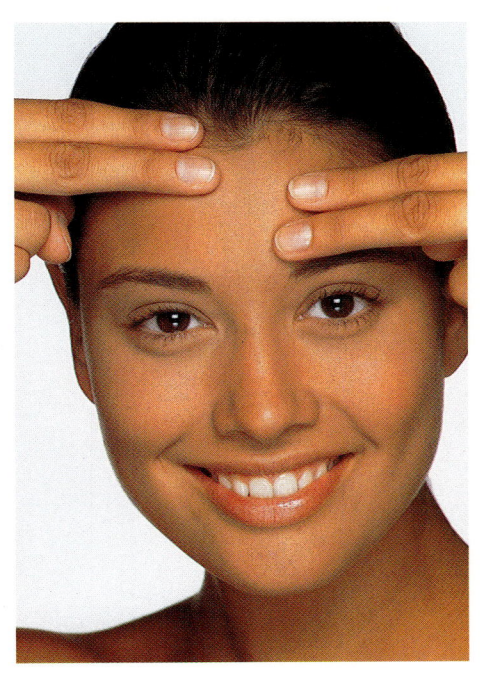

4 Use two fingers to stroke from your brows up to your hairline. Use rapid movements in the morning to feel wide awake. Slower movements are more relaxing and soothing in the evening.

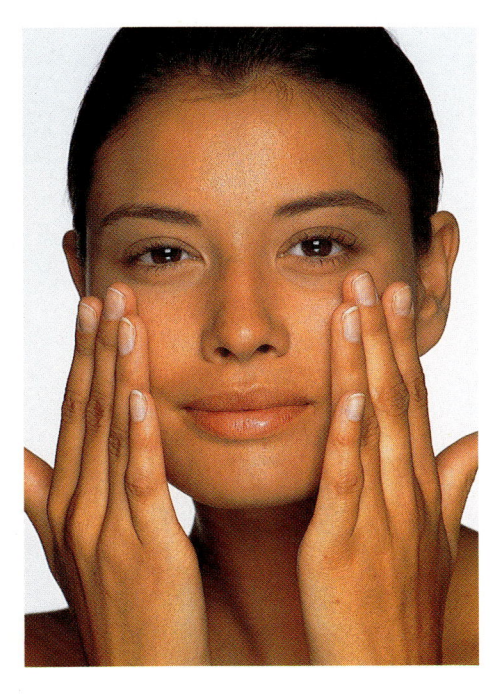

5 Finally, place both your hands together over your nose and mouth and gently smooth them out over your face several times. Do this quickly to revive the skin, or slowly to relax.

AROMATIC ENERGY

Aromatherapy oils bring immediate improvement to everyday health and beauty problems. Discover the power of these potent plant remedies.

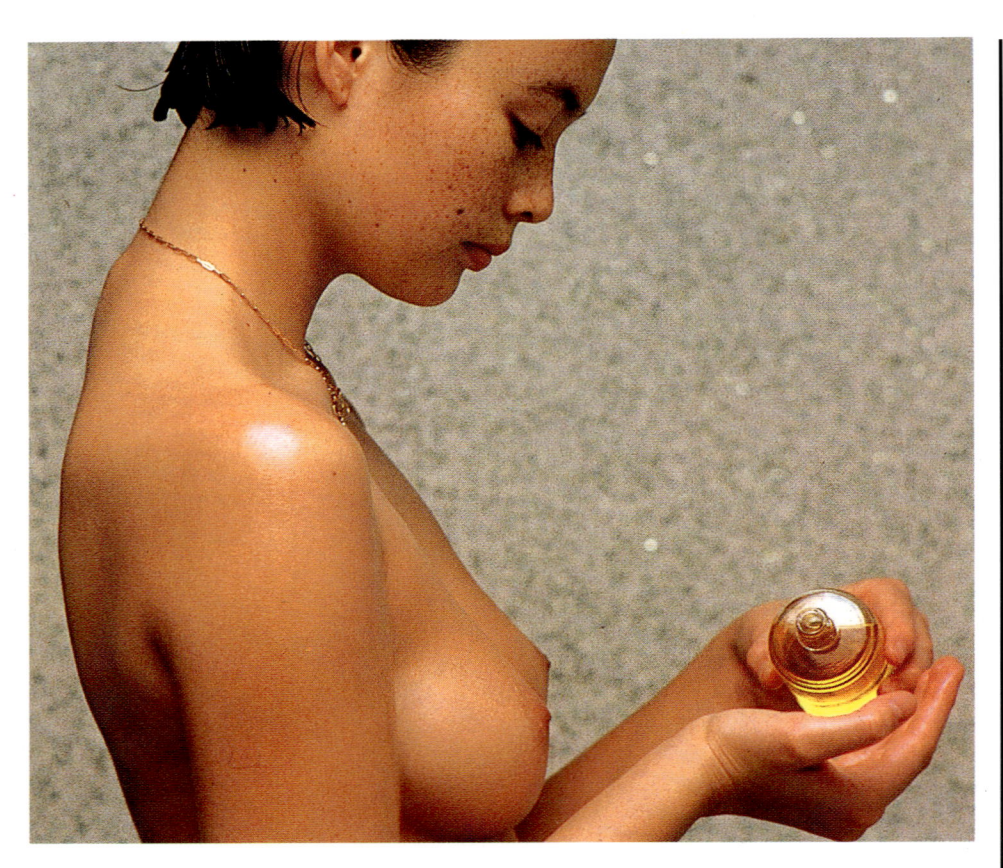

Aromatherapy is a natural and powerful way to treat a wide variety of everyday health problems and to maintain your well-being. In fact, essential oils, distilled from plants and herbs, have been used for medicinal purposes since 2000 BC.

These potent remedies can be stimulating or relaxing. Some oils are able to lift depression, others are reputed to be aphrodisiacs, while some will heal and balance the skin.

The majority of oils have antiseptic, anti-viral, and in some instances, antibiotic properties (although they should never be taken internally).

Aromatherapy works on two levels. Firstly, it can revive you emotionally and psychologically. This is because aromatic molecules have a direct pathway, via the olfactory system, to the limbic area of the brain which is your emotional centre. Secondly, aromatherapy performs at a physical level, the molecules entering the skin and travelling through the bloodstream.

The quality of the essential oils you use is vital. It is the complex molecular structure of the individual oils that gives them their therapeutic properties. It is advisable to buy oils that are distributed by professional aromatherapists through clinics, chemists or health food shops.

As well as being able to choose from a wide range of individual oils, ready-blended formulations that combine a number of oils are readily available. These have been prepared by an aromatherapist and are designed to treat a specific ailment or condition, such as PMT.

Aromatherapy oils may be potentially toxic if used to excess. They are best used with the advice of a trained aromatherapist. You should not use them every day and you should not use more than the recommended amount at any one time. They are very concentrated and the majority of them should not be applied directly to the skin without diluting them first.

Some oils should NOT be used in pregnancy. If you are pregnant, epileptic or have high blood pressure you must only use aromatherapy oils with the guidance of a trained aromatherapist.

Remember to keep essential oils tightly sealed in amber glass or metal bottles and store in a cool place out of the way of children. Essential oils are highly flammable.

There are a number of enjoyable and simple ways in which you can use essential oils:

In the bath
Add 6–8 drops to a warm bath (not hot, as this may damage the oil) and swirl around to disperse. Soak for at least 10 minutes with the door closed and breathe deeply.

Massage
You will need a 'carrier' oil such as grapeseed, almond oil or jojoba oil, available at the pharmacy counter or health food store. For a facial massage, add 2 drops to 5ml (one teaspoon) of the base oil. For a full body massage, use 15 drops to 50ml of the carrier oil.

Environment
You can surround yourself with the therapeutic molecules by dispersing them into the atmosphere. They will also scent your home or office and have an antiseptic and anti-viral action. The short-cut way is to place a drop or two of oil in a plant spray filled with warm water and spritz the rooms. Electric and candle vaporizers, which release the oils into the atmosphere, are available from health food stores. Some specialists prefer the electric versions, which use an airstream to spread the oils within the atmosphere, as extreme heat can damage them.

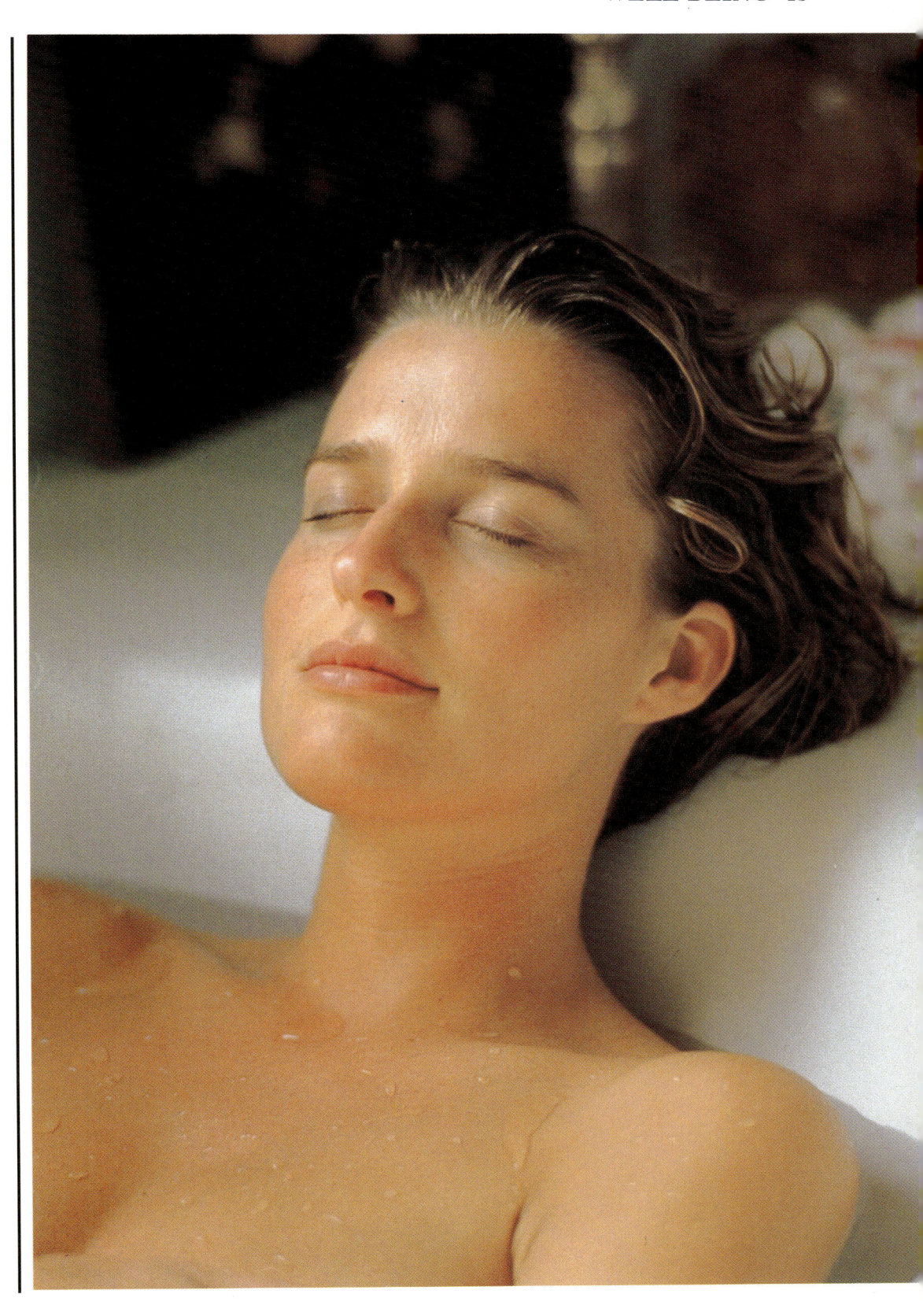

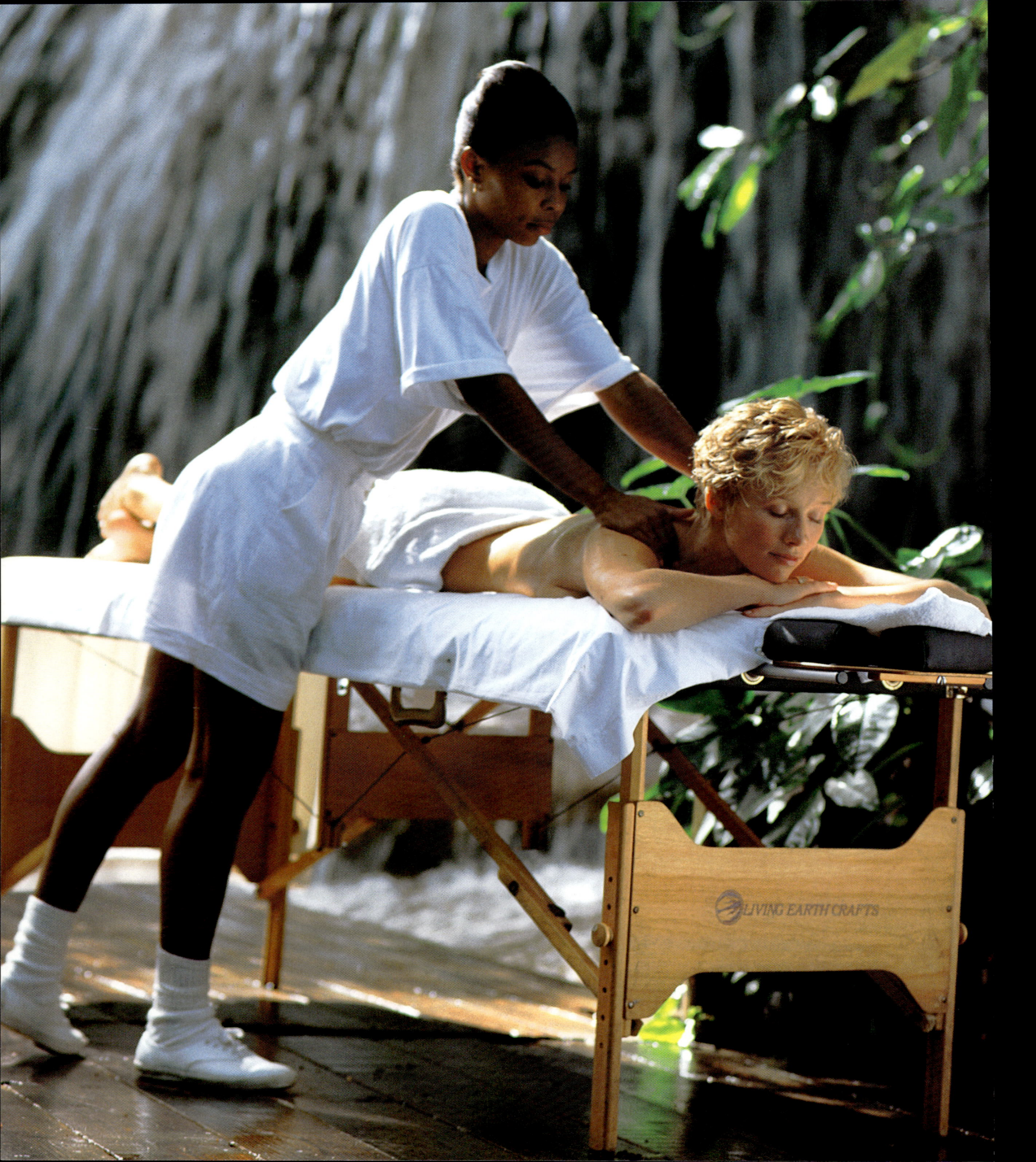

WELL-BEING

Inhalation
Put 3–4 drops onto a tissue and inhale deeply.

These are some of the most popular oils and their uses:

Cedarwood
This oil gives a warm, comforting scent to a room. With antiseptic qualities, it is useful for catarrh and can relieve aching muscles. Tones the skin and is useful for cellulite. Good for oily and combination skins and acne.

Camomile
Anti-inflammatory, antibiotic and very calming, camomile soothes nerves, insomnia, menstrual disorders and irritated skin.

Citronella
From the lemon grass plant, this invigorating oil works well in vaporizers. Discourages mosquitos. Citrus oils such as citronella should not be used on the skin before sunbathing.

Cypress
Good for massage, particularly where there is cellulite as it increases the circulation and helps to combat water retention. Also useful for stress.

Eucalyptus
Antibiotic, antiseptic and anti-inflammatory, eucalyptus is widely used to treat head colds. It can also ease rheumatism and arthritis.

Geranium
Good to use in massage and for the treatment of cellulite as it has diuretic properties. With an immediately uplifting floral scent, this anti-depressant can be added to the bath on cold winter mornings. Widely used by aromatherapists in massage to treat hormonal and menstrual problems. Also eases eczema and psoriasis.

Jasmine
This energizing oil makes a wonderful aromatherapy bath and massage. Particularly suitable for sensitive skins.

Juniper
A cleansing diuretic oil, juniper is used by aromatherapists to treat hormonal, digestive and urinary problems. Use in the bath to ease aching joints and in massage to treat cellulite.

Lavender
A calming oil which treats headaches and insomnia, aches and pains. Good for facial massage. Antiseptic, antibiotic, anti-viral and anti-fungal, lavender is also renowned for its ability to speed the healing of wounds.

Lemon
Stimulating, antiseptic and antibiotic, lemon oil is used by aromatherapists for digestive disorders, gallstones and anxiety. Added to massage oils, lemon will improve blood circulation and skin tone. Should not be used before sunbathing.

Neroli
Obtained from orange blossom, neroli is reported to be an aphrodisiac. It also eases PMT and hormonal disorders and calms the nerves. Makes a fragrant bath. Popular for facial massage as it boosts a tired, sluggish complexion.

Patchouli
Antiseptic, antibiotic and anti-fungal, patchouli is used to treat acne and scalp disorders. It also makes a sensual, fortifying bath and is helpful in massage for improving cellulite.

Peppermint
Stimulating and refreshing, peppermint will ease headaches and migraine. Best suited to massage for its invigorating action.

Pine
Antiseptic and antibiotic, pine eases the symptoms of colds and flu. Use it in a vaporizer or in the bath.

Rose
Soothing and an anti-depressant, rose otto eases PMT and fatigue. It is a wonderful facial and scalp massage in times of stress and will improve dry skin.

Rosemary
A very stimulating and antiseptic oil, rosemary is an all-round tonic. It relieves headaches and aids clear thinking. Good as a facial massage to treat problem skins. Excess can induce epilepsy if susceptible.

Sandalwood
With antiseptic and soothing qualities, sandalwood is also known as an aphrodisiac. It lends a sense of calm and can ease PMT. Use as a facial massage to treat flaky, irritated complexions or acne.

Tea tree oil
Antiseptic, antibiotic, anti-fungal and anti-viral, tea tree oil can be used in the bath to help treat thrush. It will provide protection from colds and flu. Effective against dandruff.

Ylang ylang
Antiseptic, uplifting and an anti-depressant, ylang ylang is also reputed to be an aphrodisiac. Ylang ylang relieves feelings of anxiety and stress and is also good for balancing combination skins. It should be used with caution initially as it can provoke an allergic reaction or headaches.

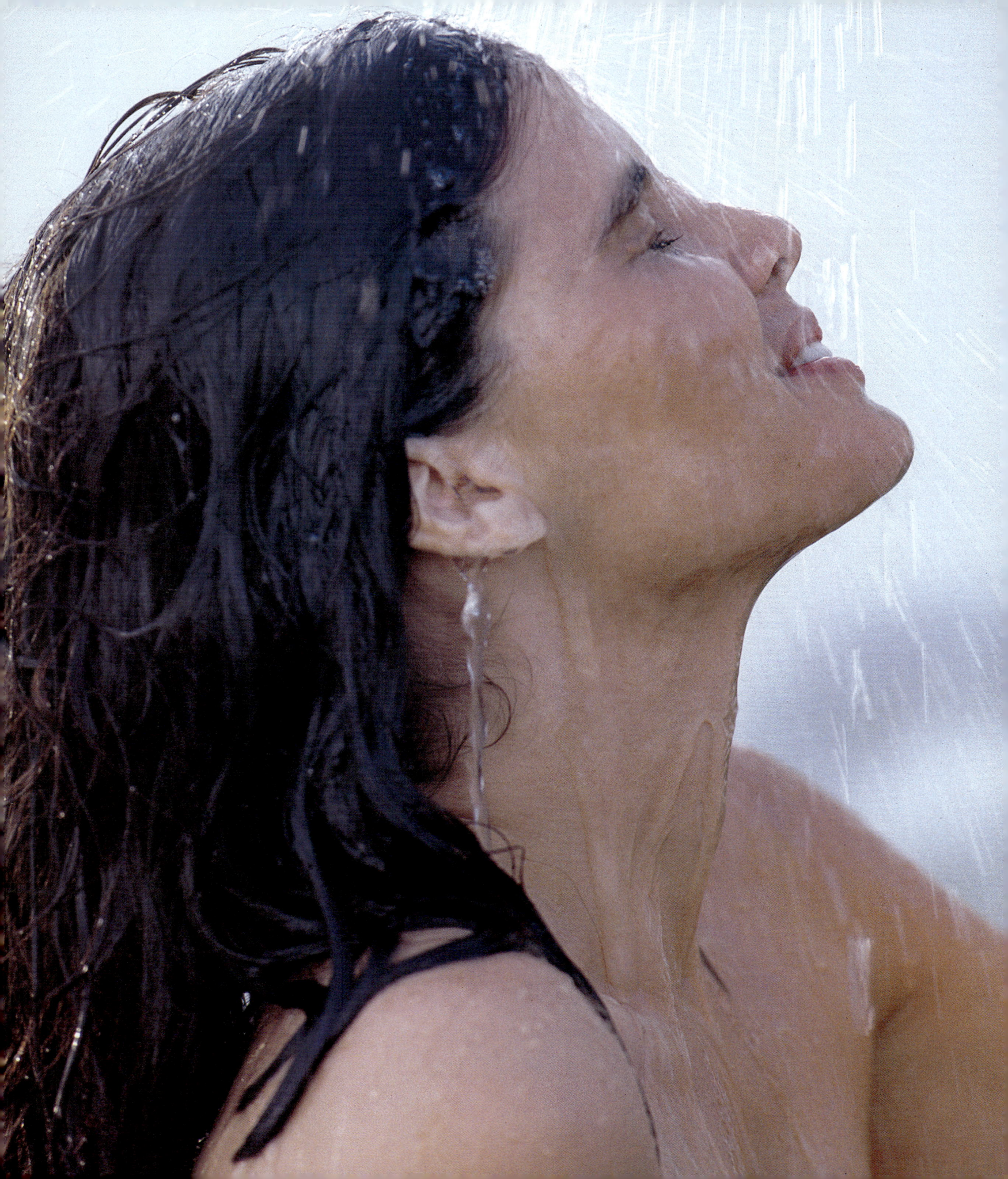

SKINCARE

What you do – or don't do – to your skin will be reflected in its condition today and in the years to come. It is not necessary to follow a complicated routine and, in fact, simple skincare is best. With our special quick-to-do programmes and vital tips, maintaining your skin in prime condition is easy – however short on time you may be.

SKIN TYPING 48
PERFECT YOUR SKIN 50
QUICK SKINCARE SYSTEMS 52
FAST SKIN BOOSTERS 54
FABULOUS FACIALS 56
ANTI-AGEING STRATEGIES 58
ENVIRONMENT 60
SUN AND TANNING 64
YOUR SKIN PROBLEMS SOLVED 70

SKIN TYPING

Finding your skin type is the key to developing an effective skincare programme.

Knowing a little about the structure of your skin will help you appreciate why certain things are good for it and others are not. Understand your skin and you are halfway to a glowing, healthy complexion.

The skin is formed from three main layers: the epidermis, dermis and hypodermis.

The epidermis is the outermost layer and is a microscopic 0.2 mm (8/1000 in) thick on the face. The surface consists of dead cells which are in the process of flaking away and new ones which are growing to take their place. Between the epidermis and dermis lies the basal layer, where new epidermal cells are formed and progress to the surface. It takes approximately twenty-eight days for a new cell to reach the top.

The dermis is usually 1.8 mm (7/100 in) thick. It is composed of a fibrous protein called collagen, elastin, which makes the skin supple, and a network of blood vessels, nerves, oil and sweat glands, pores and hair follicles.

The hypodermis is the tissue beneath both the epidermis and the dermis. It contains muscles, veins and fat cells and its thickness varies according to the part of the body.

The sebum and sweat produced by the oil and sweat glands in the dermis form a hydro-lipidic film on the skin. This film, known as the 'acid mantle', lubricates the skin's surface, helps to repel bacteria and protects against irritation. The acid mantle maintains the skin's slightly acid pH level. It takes one to two hours for the skin to return to its normal pH level after washing. Harsh cleansers, such as soaps, reduce the renewal process.

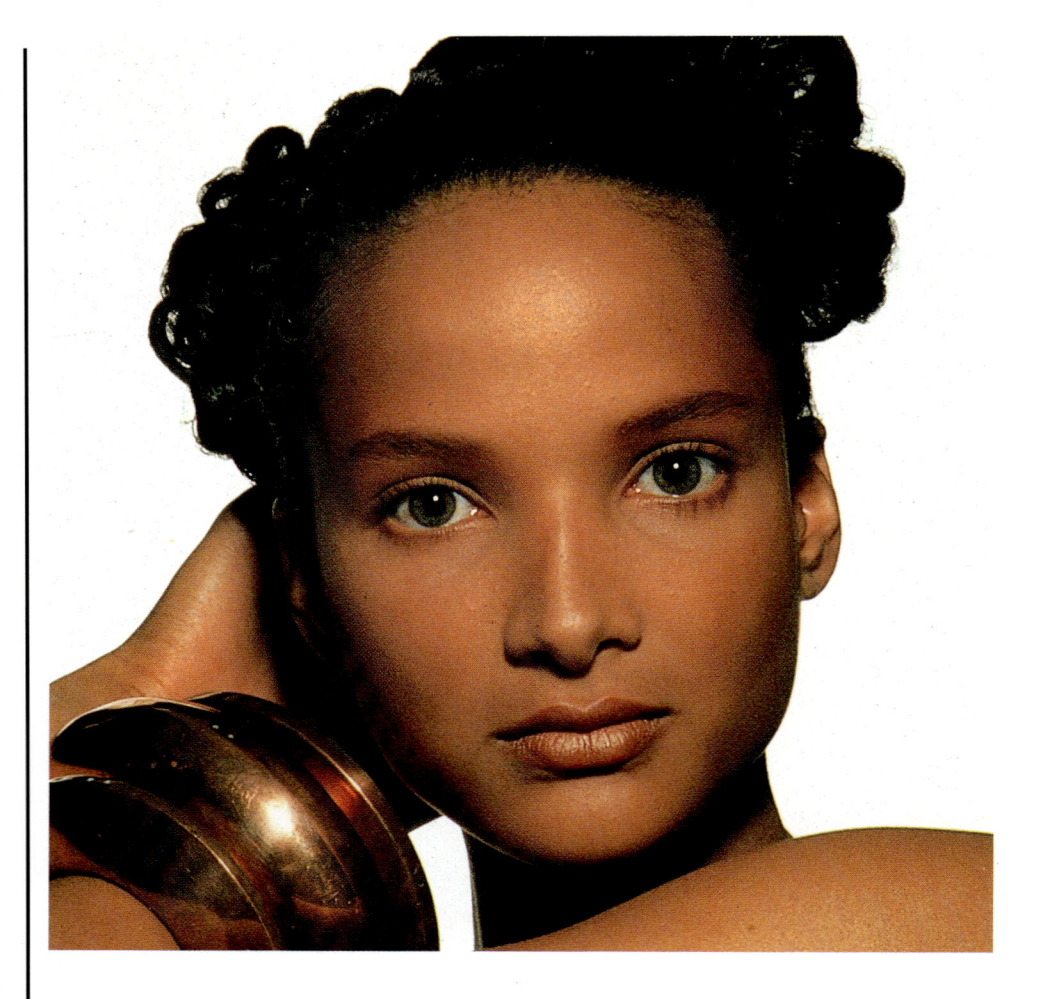

It is the activity of the sebaceous (oil-producing) glands that

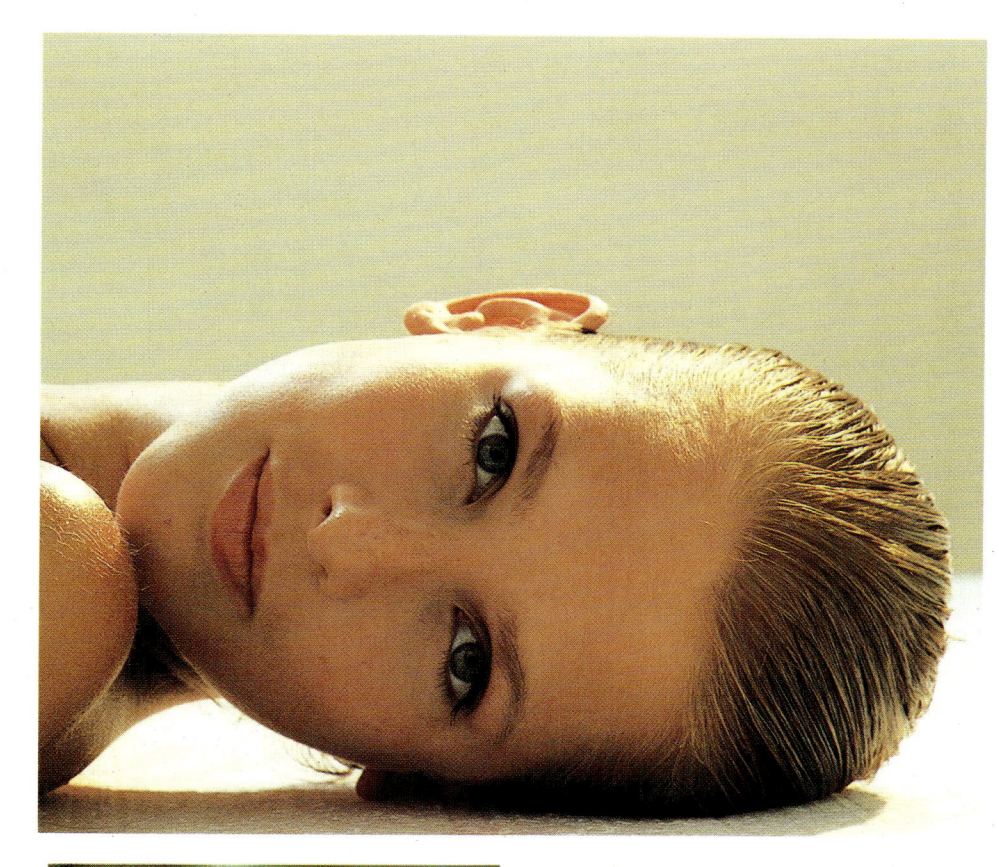

IDENTIFY YOUR SKIN TYPE

By answering the questions below you can find out what type of skin you have. Just tick the answer – a, b, c or d – that most closely applies to your skin.

1. **After cleansing, how does your skin feel?**
   a Tight and rough.
   b Smooth and supple.
   c Slightly oily.
   d Oily in some areas, tight in others.

2. **How often does your skin break out in spots?**
   a Almost never.
   b Rarely.
   c Often.
   d Only in the T-zone.

3. **Which of the following best describes your skin texture?**
   a Smooth and transparent.
   b Firm and even.
   c Slightly rough and uneven.
   d A mixture of the above.

4. **How does your skin look during the day?**
   a Flaky and chapped.
   b Clean and fresh-looking.
   c Shiny.
   d Shiny in the T-zone.

Now, add up how many a's, b's, c's and d's you scored.

If the majority of your answers are a's, your skin is dry.
If the majority of your answers are b's, your skin is normal.
If the majority of your answers are c's, your skin is oily.
If the majority of your answers are d's, your skin is combination.

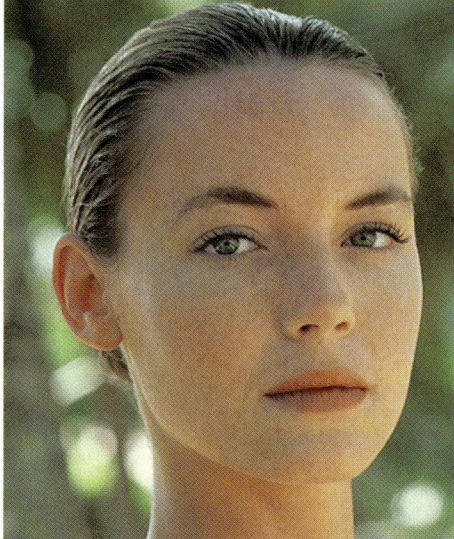

determine your skin type. Activity in the T-zone (across the forehead and down the nose and chin) may be greater than elsewhere.

There are four main skin types: dry, normal, oily and combination, although 'normal' skin often tends towards oily or dry.

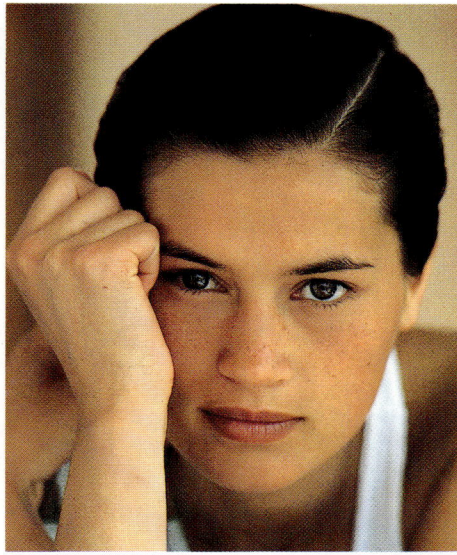

Within these four different groups there are skins that require special attention, such as sensitive or black skins.

PERFECT YOUR SKIN

Choosing the right type of cleanser, toner and moisturizer is the key to the healthiest, clearest skin.

The skin responds best to a regular routine, which can be quick but must be a discipline. Now that you have found out your skin type, learn the best cleansing and moisturizing system for you.

CLEANSING
This is a top priority if you want to have good skin. A quick cleanse in the morning (to remove toxins that have reached the surface via the sweat glands) and a thorough cleanse at night are important for every skin type. Soap doesn't remove make-up and can be drying, so use soap-free cleansing bars, or wash-off or wipe-off cleansing creams instead.

Toner, or freshener, removes the last traces of dirt and excess cleanser. Some toners contain alcohol to remove excess oil, but alcohol-free toners are a better choice. Toner containing alcohol can be drying and should be diluted even for oily skins.

Removing eye make-up
- Dab a little eye make-up remover on to two cotton wool pads. Never use tissue on eyes.
- Using one pad for each eye (to avoid the spread of infection), hold it against your lashes for a few seconds to dissolve the make-up.
- Supporting the skin by placing the fingers of your opposite hand on your brow, stroke in towards your nose and down from your eyebrow. Don't move the pad up and out as you will pull the skin in the wrong direction.

Using wipe-off cleanser
- Warm the cleanser in your hands so that it doesn't go on cold.
- Smooth it over your face with your whole hand, starting at the neck and working up and out.
- Place your thumbs under your chin and work the cleanser in little circles with your index fingers around your nose and chin.
- Remove the cleanser by wiping it off gently with a soft tissue or a piece of cotton wool.

Using wash-off cleanser
- Dampen the skin with warm water and use the same movements given above to apply the cleanser.
- Rinse the cleanser off very thoroughly with comfortably warm running water. Water that is too hot will dehydrate the skin and cause broken capillaries.
- Pat your face dry with a tissue or a clean towel.

Using toner
- Sweep the toner on to your face with a cotton wool pad, moving up and out, avoiding the eye area.
- Blot your skin dry with a tissue.

MOISTURIZING
Moisturizers are formulated to tackle different skin problems.

Creams help balance drier skin, while lotions and emulsions are designed for normal to oily complexions. Innovative, featherweight formulations are the latest trend – containing high-powered hydrating ingredients, they are suitable for every skin type except very dry.

Oil-free and gel moisturizers are perfect for oily complexions. Anti-ageing ingredients, such as ultraviolet filters, and nutrients, such as vitamins, are often added to moisturizers and serums to help protect the skin.

Night creams are useful from the age of twenty-five, especially for dry skins, but avoid very heavy creams as these can result in puffiness.

Moisturizing the very delicate skin surrounding the eyes calls for special products. Your usual moisturizer may cause puffiness and stretch the skin. Eye gel is refreshing in the morning, and a little eye cream will strengthen the tissues at night. Pat on either, using the third and fourth fingers, tapping quickly but gently.

Your usual moisturizer is fine for your neck.

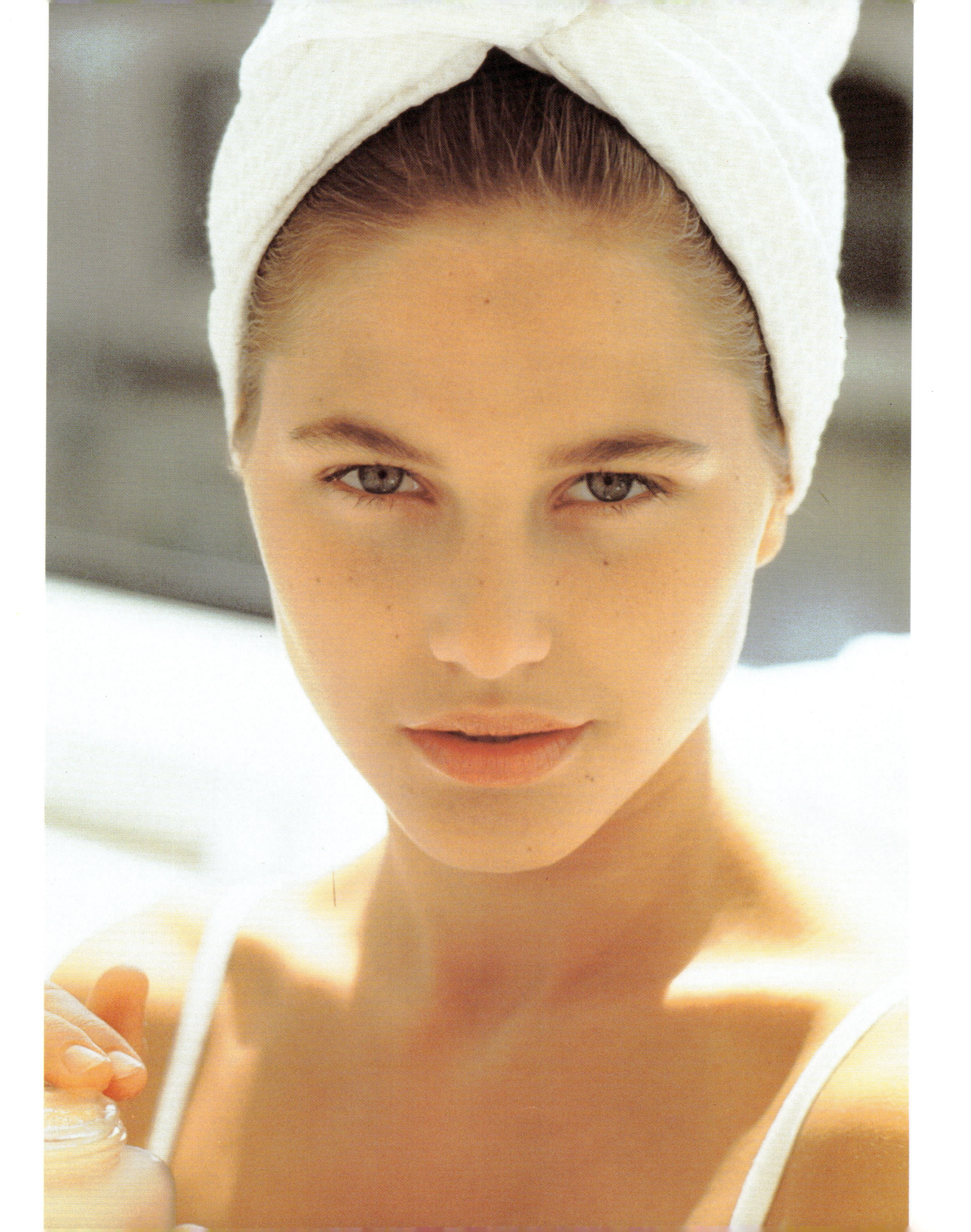

QUICK SKINCARE SYSTEMS

Customizing your skincare products to your skin type is easy with these 5-minute skincare programmes.

DRY SKIN
- It has a fine, matte texture.
- It may be on the sensitive side.
- There are usually no open pores.
- It is more prone to fine lines and wrinkles than other skin types.
- It is more vulnerable to the effects of central heating and sunlight.
- Very fair skin is often dry.

5-minute skincare

Morning
- Cleanse quickly, using a wipe-off cleanser for dry skin.
- Tone, using alcohol-free toner on water-moistened cotton ball.
- Hydrate with a moisturizer for dry skin, preferably one containing a broad-spectrum sunscreen. Avoid your eyes.

Evening
- Remove your eye make-up.
- Cleanse as above.
- Apply a night cream.

NORMAL SKIN
One hundred per cent normal skin is a rare blessing.
- It is smooth textured with no visible pores.
- It shows no signs of dryness in youth.
- It has an even tone that is not too pale, sallow or red.
- It will tend towards dryness with age and as a result of external influences.

5 minute skincare

Morning
- Cleanse using a wipe-off or wash-off cleanser for normal-to-dry skin.
- Tone using alcohol-free toner on a water-moistened cotton ball.
- Hydrate with a moisturizer for normal skin.

Evening
- Remove your eye make-up first, then cleanse as above, but more thoroughly.
- Apply moisturizer or a lightweight night lotion.

OILY SKIN
- It has open pores.
- It will shine an hour or so after washing.
- It may look oily on waking.
- It has a tendency to spots and blackheads.
- It is less susceptible to wrinkles than other skin types.

5-minute skincare

Morning
- Cleanse quickly using a wipe-off cleanser for normal-to-oily skin or a soap-free cleansing bar. Rinse very thoroughly.
- Tone using a toner that should be diluted if it contains alcohol so that it is not too drying. Moisten your cotton wool with water.
- Moisturize where needed using an oil-free or gel moisturizer.

Evening
- Remove eye make-up, then cleanse as above, but more thoroughly.
- Apply moisturizer just where needed.

COMBINATION SKIN
- The centre T-zone (across the forehead and down the nose and chin) is oily and coarser in texture than the rest of the skin, and may have a tendency to spots or blackheads.
- The cheeks are normal or even dry.

5 minute skincare

Morning
- Cleanse quickly using a wipe-off cleanser for normal-to-oily skins.
- Tone, using a toner without alcohol.
- Moisturize just where needed using an oil-free or gel moisturizer.

Evening
- Remove your eye make-up, then cleanse as above, but more thoroughly and concentrate on the T-zone.
- Use a moisturizer or night cream on dry areas only, particularly the cheeks.

SENSITIVE SKIN
- Looks fragile and translucent.
- It is generally dry.
- It may have freckles.
- It tends to become flushed, blotchy and irritated in extremes of temperature or through using harsh cleansing products.
- It may suffer from broken red veins, dermatitis, allergies.

5-minute skincare
Follow the programme for dry skin.

Special tips
- Look for hypo-allergenic products that are scent-free.
- Before trying a new product do a patch test. Rub a good amount on to your shoulder and leave it on overnight. If there is no sign of irritation, apply some to your neck and wait again. If there is no reaction then the product will probably be safe to use on your face.

SKINCARE 53

BLACK SKIN
- Tends towards extremes of oiliness or dryness which can be a real problem since these conditions are more visible against a darker complexion. Dry black skin may appear greyish in colour.
- It needs very gentle care as face scrubs, spots, ear piercing and hair removal can make the supply of melanin uneven, leading to skin that is darker or lighter in some places than others.

5-minute skincare
Follow the programme for dry or oily skins.

Special tips
- If your skin is sensitive use toners that do not contain alcohol, and choose fragrance-free products.
- If flaky, grey-looking skin is a problem, gently use a flannel to slough the skin, or use a peel-off mask.

OLIVE SKIN
- It tends towards oiliness and often has larger pores.
- Any sallowness is due to the lack of pink pigment.

5-minute skincare
Follow the programme for oily skins.

A MIXTURE OF SKIN TYPES
Skin may develop the characteristics of several skin types as a result of incorrect treatment and environmental skin hazards. For example:

- *An oily, spotty skin can also suffer from the dry skin problems of fine surface lines and flaking if you work in an over-heated office, perhaps smoke or eat a poor diet, or use harsh and abrasive cleaners (over-enthusiastic scrubbing with anti-bacterial products can aggravate oily skin and dry the surface).*
- *A skin that is usually dry can develop small bumps beneath the surface and spots as a result of a poor diet, insufficient cleansing or using a brand of face cream that is too rich for the skin.*

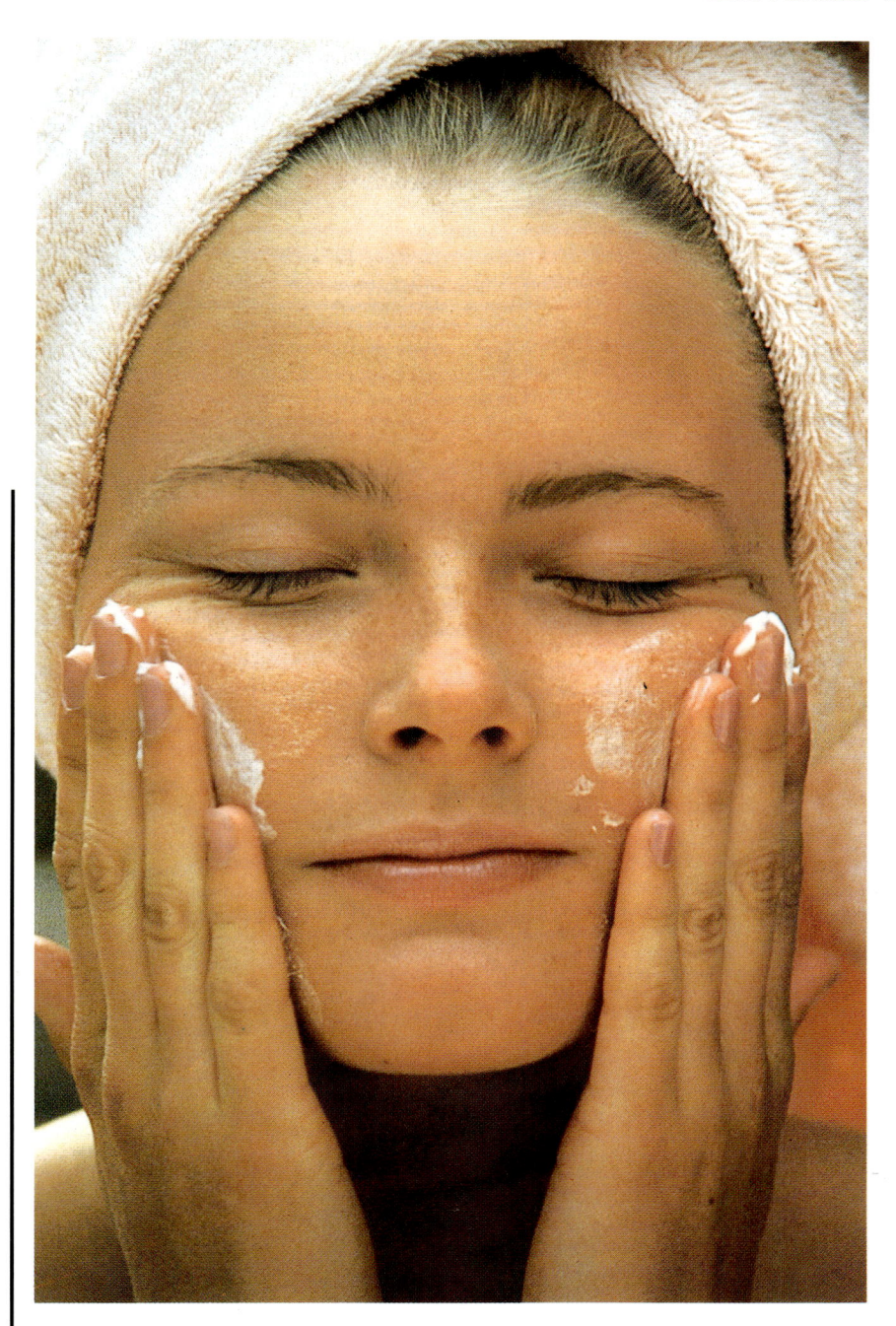

FAST SKIN BOOSTERS

Get your skin glowing with fast and easy treatments you can do at home.

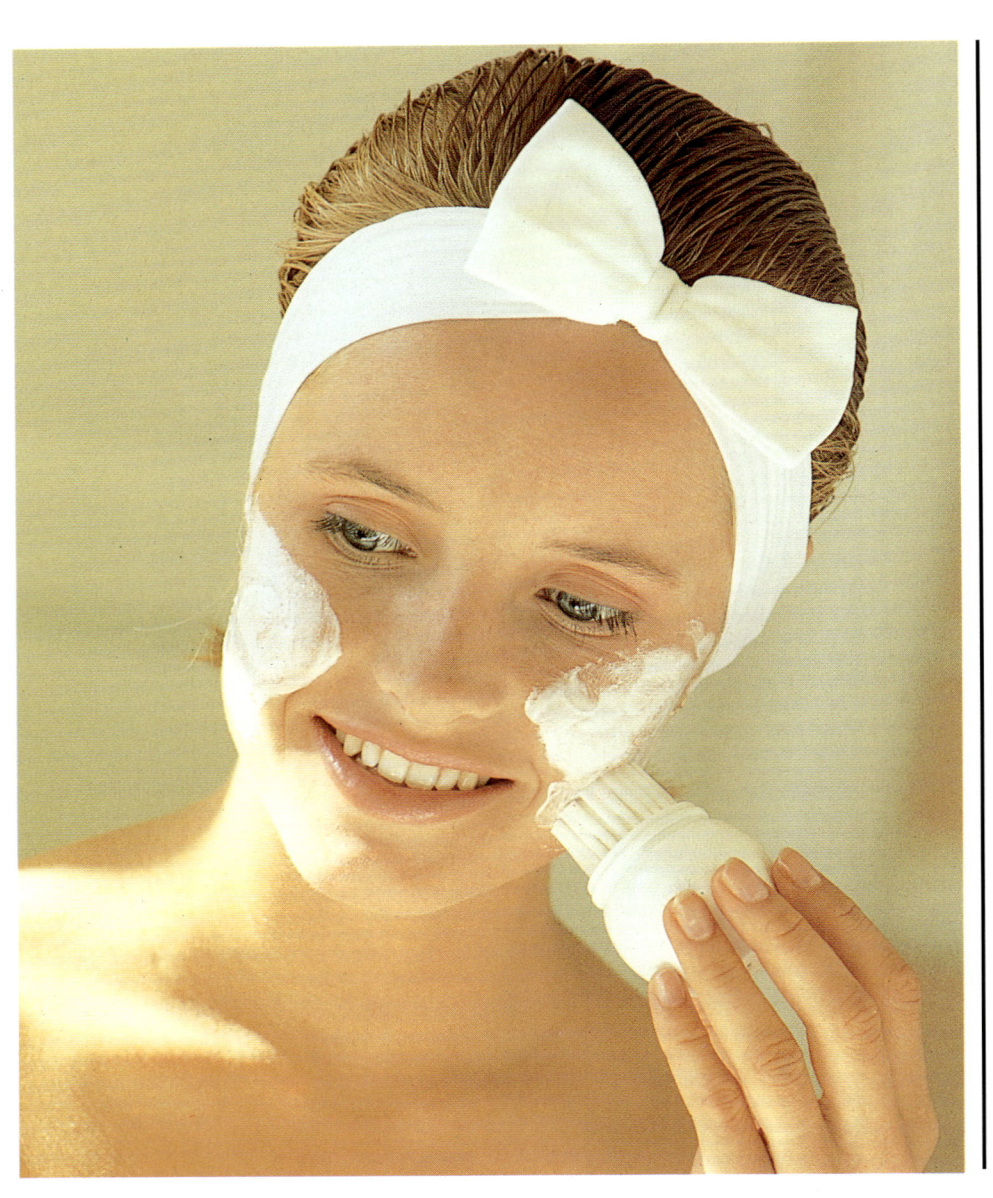

EXFOLIATION

Exfoliators, or skin sloughers, are speedy skin improvers. By removing the dead cells from the surface of the skin, face 'scrubs' make your skin smoother and brighter in seconds. They also help skin that is prone to spots stay clearer and increase the cell turnover so the skin looks younger for longer.

It is important to choose a product that is very gentle so that the grains do not scratch the skin.

Tips for using an exfoliator
- Use a facial scrub on cleansed, damp skin.
- Rest your thumb against your skin (this ensures that you don't use the full power of your arm) and use very light, circular movements.
- Never rub your skin until it changes colour and do not use exfoliators near your eyes.
- If your skin is fair, sensitive or very fine, use a gentler peel-off mask instead of a facial scrub to lift away dead cells and revitalize your complexion.
- Exfoliation is very useful for black skin, which can look ashen in colour, but a peel-off mask is better than a face scrub, as black skin is vulnerable to changes in pigmentation and face scrubs can trigger this if too abrasive.

SKINCARE

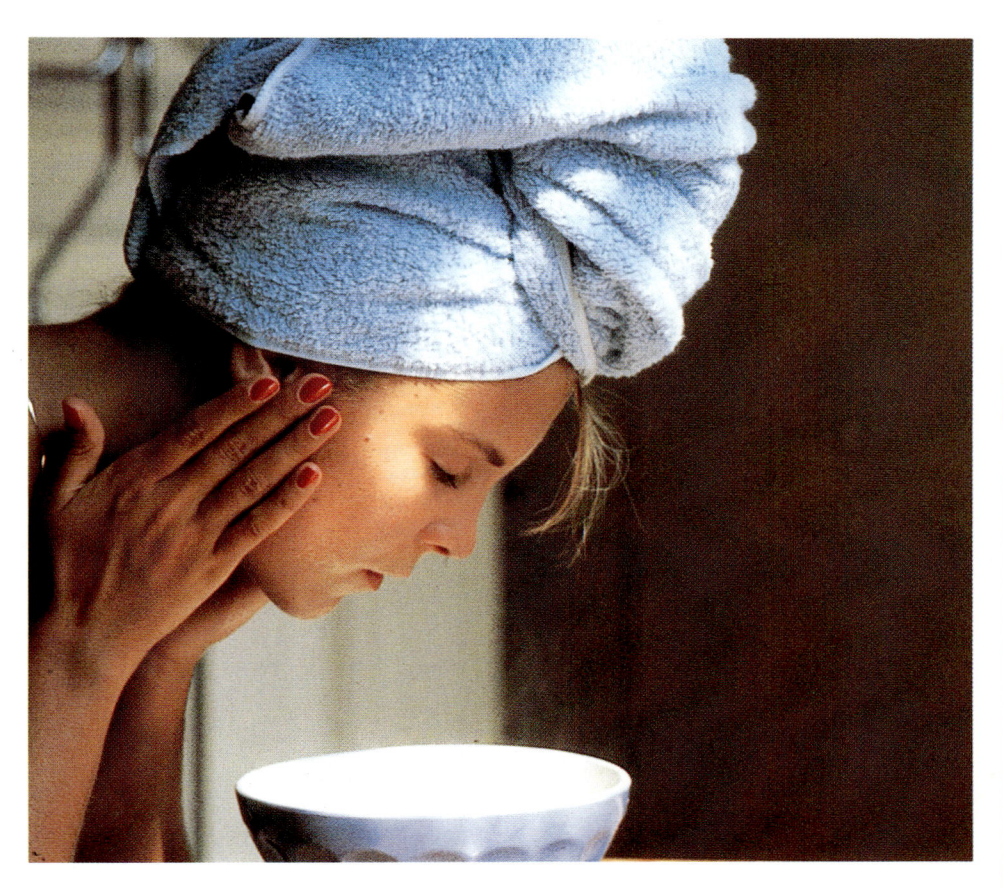

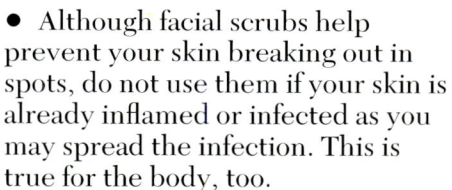

- Although facial scrubs help prevent your skin breaking out in spots, do not use them if your skin is already inflamed or infected as you may spread the infection. This is true for the body, too.

MARVELLOUS MASKS
Masks are a really good way to pep up skin in no time at all.

Cleansing masks, which often contain clay or fruit, absorb excess oils. The enzymes in fruits such as papaya have a deep-cleansing action and leave the skin glowing.

Moisturizing masks give drier skin a real boost, smoothing out fine lines and refreshing the face. Some moisturizing masks also contain toning and firming ingredients, such as seaweed, herbs and aromatherapy oils and are excellent as complexion-improvers before a party or after a late night.

STEAMING
Steaming is an effective way of cleansing the skin. You can add herbs, such as soothing camomile.

If you have sensitive skin or skin that is prone to broken capillaries, however, specialists recommend that you do not cleanse with steam.

Tips for steaming
- Cleanse your skin first.
- Pour water that is almost boiling into a bowl and lean over the steam. Draping a towel over your head and the bowl will prevent steam escaping.
- Be very careful not to get too close to the water (stay 30 cm, 12 in or so away). Do not steam for more than a few minutes.
- Apply a cleansing mask afterwards, while your skin is still warm, or cleanse your skin again and massage moisturizer into it.

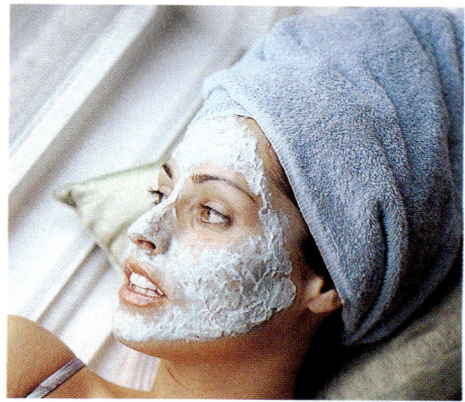

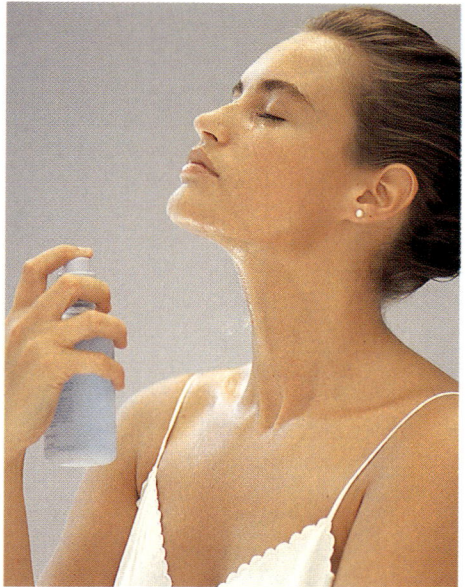

EARLY MORNING SKIN WAKE-UPS
To revive a pallid complexion try the following quick tricks:

- *Spritz your skin with cool water from a mini plant spray kept in the refrigerator. Replenish it frequently with fresh water. Pat your skin gently and moisturize while it is still slightly damp.*
- *Alternatively, cleanse your skin quickly and apply a moisturizing mask before you have breakfast or get dressed. Then remove the mask and apply a tinted moisturizer.*
- *Go out for a brisk walk in the fresh air.*

FABULOUS FACIALS

For a luxurious beauty boost, expert care and advice, try a salon facial precisely tailored to your skin's needs.

Having a facial at a beauty salon can bring immediate improvement to many skin conditions and give the complexion a fresh new look. Dryness that is due to sunbathing or the ageing process for instance, acne and blackheads, or a skin that lacks vitality, are some of the problems that can be helped.

The bonus of a salon facial is that the therapist has in-depth training and can advise you as to whether your skin is in good condition for your age, bearing in mind your lifestyle. She will choose products to treat individual areas of the face and can combine several types of treatments to tend precisely to your skin's needs. These treatments include the following:

Steaming This warms and softens the skin, making it easier to remove blackheads.

Massage Many therapists believe that this is the most important element of a facial. A beauty therapist may massage for up to 20 minutes, focusing on key acupressure points. Massaging the skin increases the skin's micro-circulation and improves lymphatic drainage. Lymph is a natural fluid produced by the lymph glands and acts as the body's waste disposal system: unlike blood, lymph does not have a 'pump' to circulate it but relies on muscle activity to move it around the body.

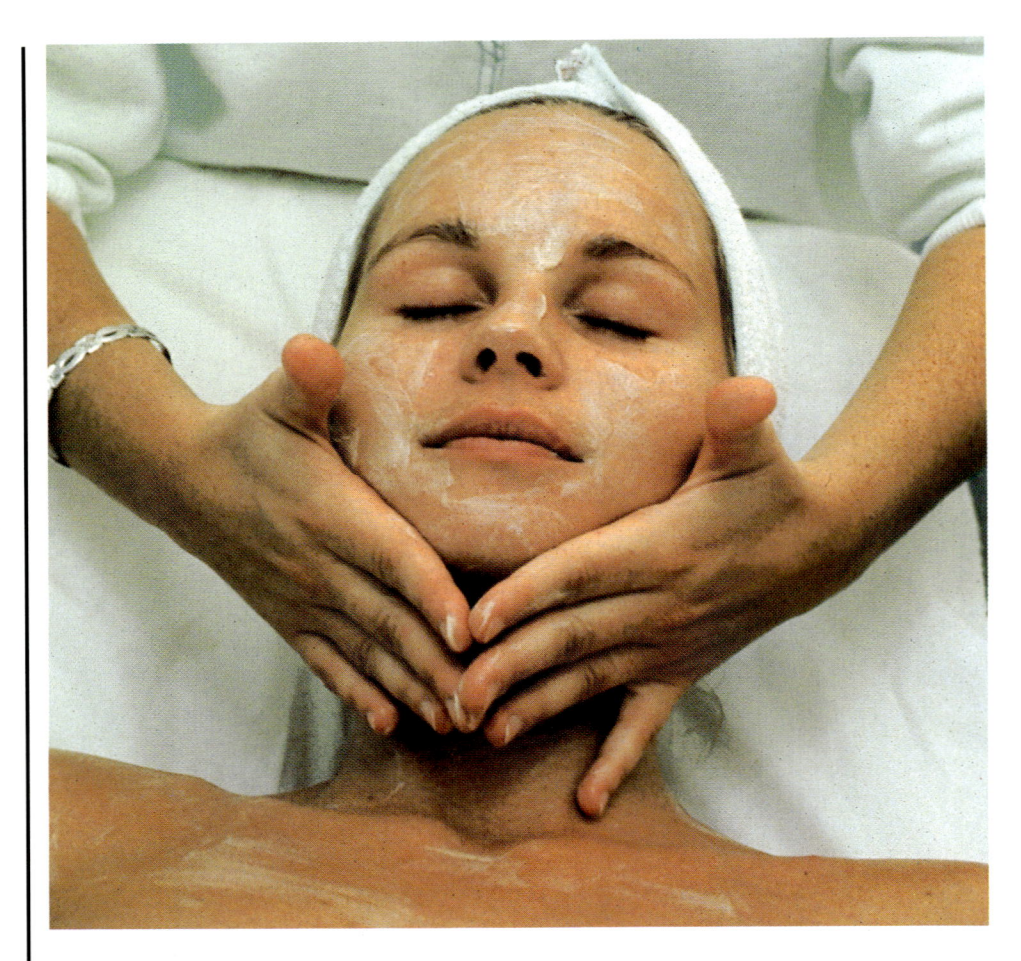

Because of the complicated bone structure in the face the lymph can become congested here, causing a tired-looking complexion that may be prone to spots.

Galvanic current Using gels chosen according to skin type, the therapist applies galvanic current via a roller. The gel is drawn into the pores and causes perspiration, thereby removing grime. The treatment is completely painless!

Ampoule treatment Very concentrated, active ingredients contained in sealed glass phials, or ampoules, are massaged into the skin. The seal ensures the ingredients remain fresh. Extracts of herbs, royal jelly, wheatgerm, vitamins and collagen are some of the elements used for their intensive and fast-acting results. Although collagen has been found to have too large a molecule to penetrate the skin, it is used for its beneficial softening and moisturizing effect.

Alternative therapies Many beauty therapists are now trained in alternative medicine and may use a technique such as auricular therapy (massage of key points on the ears) or reflexology (oriental foot and hand massage, where the therapist massages areas of the feet and hands which relate to specific areas of the face and body), both of which will improve general health and the condition of the skin.

Zone therapy, in which key acupuncture points are stimulated, is reputed to have anti-ageing benefits.

Aromatherapy facials using essential oils extracted from plants are very popular. As well as using them for massage or a mask, the therapist may add them to the steamer.

How often should you have a salon facial?
Once a month is ideal for most skins, although neglected or problem skins may require attention once a week until the skin shows improvement. If you cannot afford the time and money every month, it is a good idea to go to a salon at the change of a season so that you can check your skincare routine is on the right track.

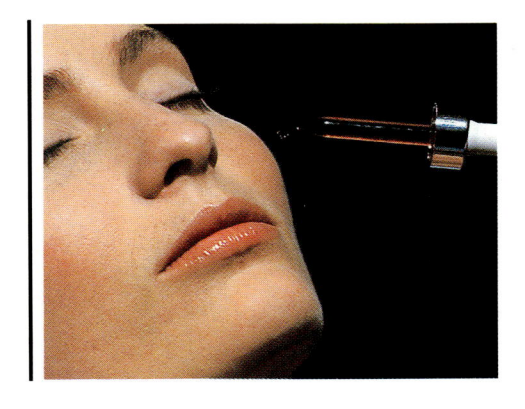

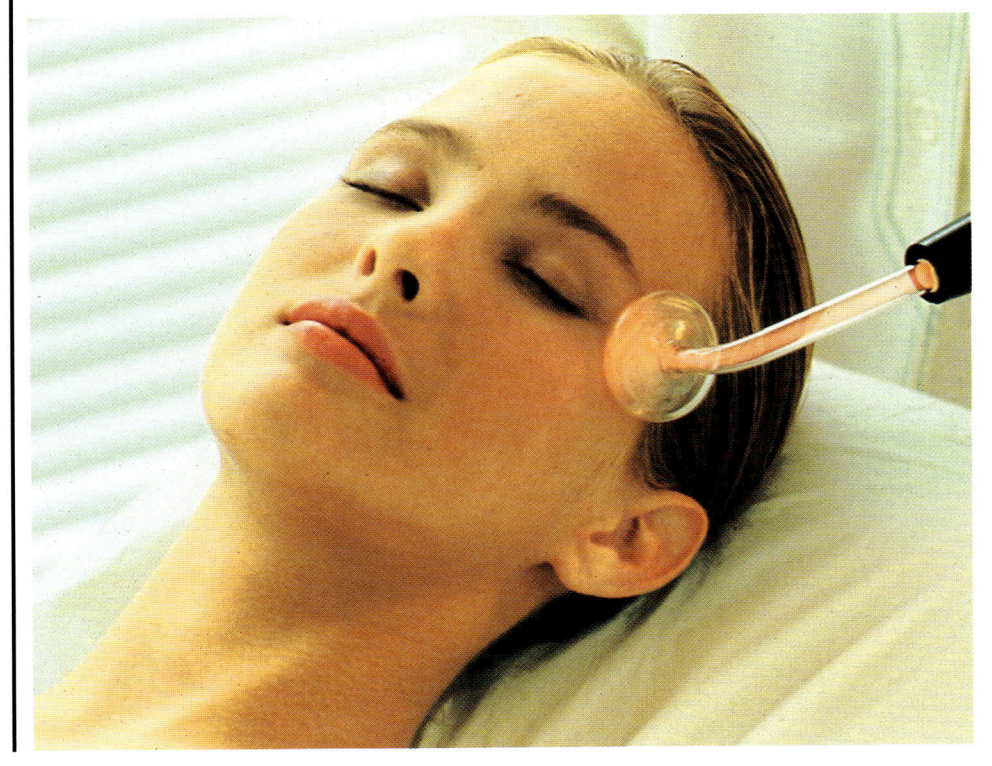

ANTI-AGEING STRATEGIES

Keep your skin looking young with simple precautions you can easily incorporate into your daily life.

Protecting and caring for your skin today will, without doubt, benefit you in years to come. While genetic factors play a crucial role in determining how well your skin will age, there are preventative measures you can take to avoid premature ageing.

The free radical theory
It is widely believed by the scientific profession that highly reactive molecules, known as free radicals, are responsible for the changes that constitute ageing. Free radicals are produced during normal body functioning when oxygen interacts with certain fats. While the body is usually able to 'mop up' these free radicals, when the body's supply of free radical 'scavengers' is reduced the molecules cause cell damage.

Anti-oxidant vitamins, especially the vitamins A, C and E, have been found to neutralise the destructive effects of free radicals in the body.

Protection from the sun
Most of the changes that come with the decades are sun-related and therefore avoidable (see pages 64–9). These changes include: fine lines at the corners of the mouth and eyes which show during your twenties and thirties; colour loss by the late thirties to forties; 'crows' feet', frown and forehead lines, and shrinkage of the upper lip that become more visible in the fifties; and in the sixties, jowls, age spots and broken blood vessels.

Some dermatologists say that, when adequately protected, the skin can repair accumulated damage by as much as 30 per cent. As ultraviolet light surrounds us constantly, it is recommended that we wear moisturizers that contain ultraviolet filters every day.

As exposure to sunlight produces free radicals, a new trend in sun protection products is to include vitamins E and/or C. Ultraviolet light, smoking and other forms of pollution produce an inflammatory reaction in the cells. New skincare products which contain anti-inflammatory ingredients help prevent damage.

Stop smoking!
As well as damaging your lungs, the ageing effects on the skin are dramatic. Smoking damages the skin's collagen, etches lines around the mouth and eyes, and causes drier, rougher skin.

Beauty from within
As well as combating skin-ageing free radicals, the A, C and E vitamins have other essential roles in maintaining your skin.

Vitamin A, found in foods such as broccoli, carrots and spinach, is essential for the growth and repair of skin tissues. Vitamin C is needed for collagen production and for maintaining a healthy immune system, while vitamin E is a vital anti-oxidant that aids normal growth and development.

It is important to eat fish oils and unrefined vegetable oils and to avoid the 'bad', saturated fats.

Sleep
The body diverts blood away from the skin to the 'essential' organs as a result of lack of sleep, giving your complexion that fatigued look and slack muscle tone. Adequate sleep is one of the best beauty treatments available!

Collagen treatment
Lines and wrinkles can be injected with collagen (which is extracted from animal sources), an anti-ageing strategy that must be done by a professional. Top-up treatments are needed every 3–12 months.

AHA skin peels
Alpha hydroxy acids, or AHAs, are extracted from sources such as apples, grapes, lemons and passion fruit (in the form of fruit acids), milk (as lactic acid) and sugar cane (as glycolic acid). Applied to the skin,

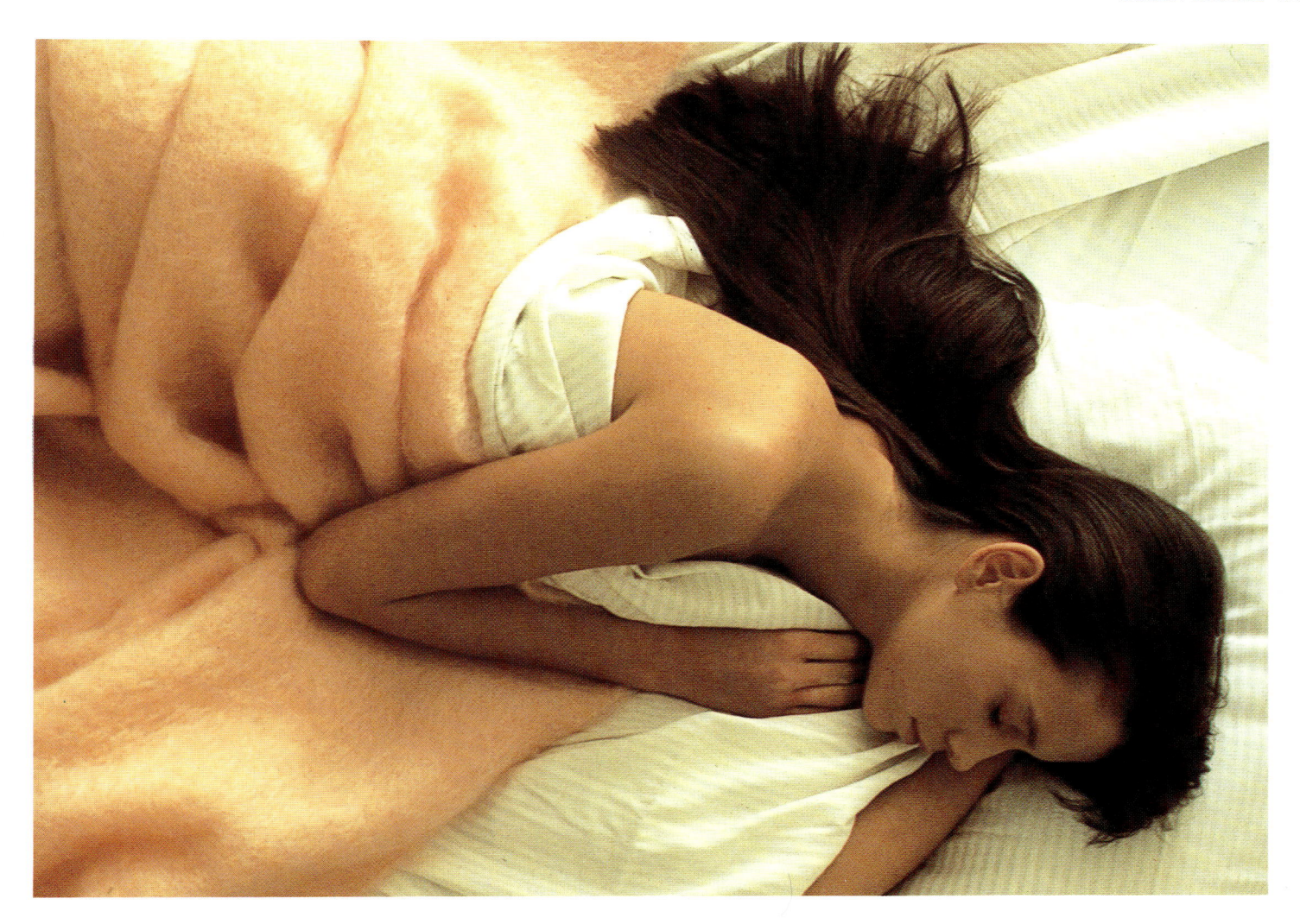

they act as a skin peel, increasing exfoliation and stimulating the turnover of new cells. While dermatologists can use a stronger solution for immediate effect, products bought over the counter need 4–8 weeks to take effect.

Retin-A
Also known as tretinoic acid, Retin-A is an acne treatment that has been found to stimulate the growth of new collagen and to reduce wrinkles and fine lines. It has yet to receive government approval for use as an anti-ageing product and cannot be used by women of child-bearing age.

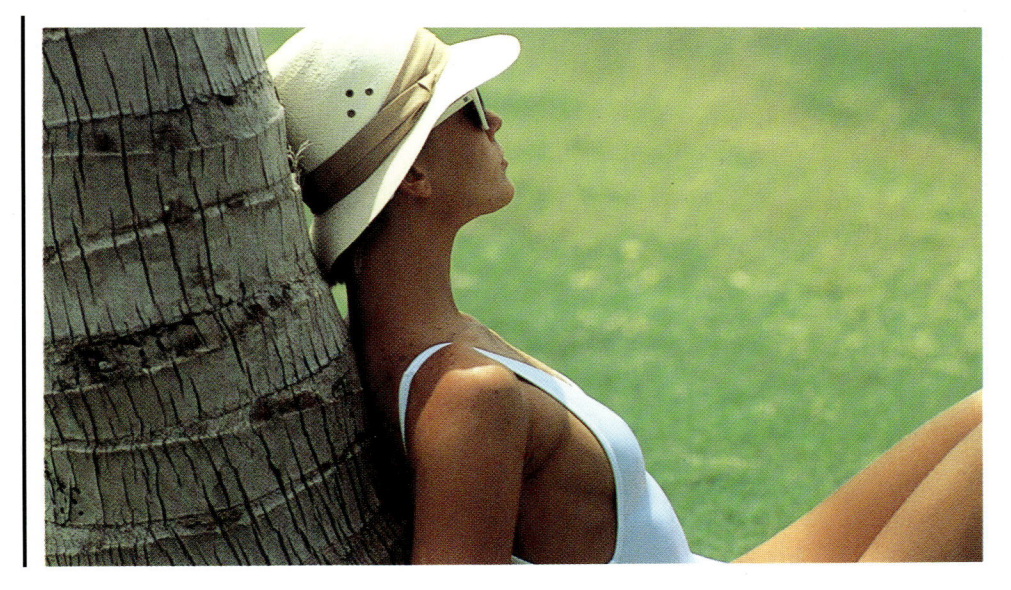

ENVIRONMENT

Protect your skin against adverse external conditions with action plans for every environmental situation.

In addition to changing with age, your skin can also change from day to day. The environment and the climatic conditions in which you live are major influences on the condition of your skin. Long-distance travel is a specially stressful situation for the skin. However, if you make simple adaptations to your skincare routine, you can stop problems *before* they start, avoiding the need for rescue operations that require time and effort.

DRY, HEATED ATMOSPHERES

Air-conditioning and central heating make life difficult for your skin. The humidity in some offices is lower than the Sahara Desert! As a result, the atmosphere robs your skin of precious moisture, leading to general dryness and flaking, and chapped – even cracked – lips.

Normal, dry and sensitive skins
These skin types suffer especially in dry atmospheres. The skin on your face may feel tight and you will be able to see fine lines on its surface. If this happens, use a richer, more high-powered moisturizer.

Oily and combination skins
If your skin tends to be oily and you get spots, you may find that a hot indoor environment stimulates the sebaceous glands and makes the situation worse.

Use an oil-free moisturizer, blot any oil coming to the surface of the skin with a tissue and be sure to cleanse thoroughly night and morning.

Action plan for overcoming the effects of a dry, hot atmosphere
- Place bowls of water near radiators. The drier the room the faster the water will evaporate. Alternatively you could invest in a humidifier.
- Keep a check on the temperature indoors and, if possible, turn the thermostat down.
- Drink water throughout the day rather than tea or coffee. Remember that they are diuretics and cause water *loss*.
- Don't sleep in an over-heated room. This can cause fluid retention in the face, leaving you with a puffy complexion and bags under your eyes the next morning.

THE DEEP FREEZE

Cold, harsh weather conditions are the worst environmental challenge your skin will face.

Chilly temperatures restrict the blood circulation to the skin, so it looks pale and devitalized. They also make the texture of your skin rough to the touch and it often looks dull. The protective acid mantle is reduced too, as the glands are less active in cold weather. In addition, cold winds and dry atmospheres take moisture from your skin. After the age of thirty your skin's moisture levels naturally decrease, so it is even more vulnerable to adverse environmental conditions.

The effects cold weather have on your skin are as much as fourteen times worse when the air is also dry and can be ten times worse in high winds.

If you are skiing, your face is in for an even tougher time. At high altitudes, the lack of oxygen increases the skin's sensitivity to cold and the sun's ultraviolet rays dehydrate and age the skin.

Action plan for overcoming the effects of cold weather
- If you wash your face, do so at least half an hour before you go outdoors. This gives your skin a chance to dry thoroughly. If your face is slightly damp, the wind has an extra-drying effect.
- Wear a richer moisturizer.
- Wear night cream to replenish moisture lost from the skin during the day.
- If your skin is flaking, avoid *abrasive* scrubs. Use a very gentle complexion exfoliator.

SKINCARE

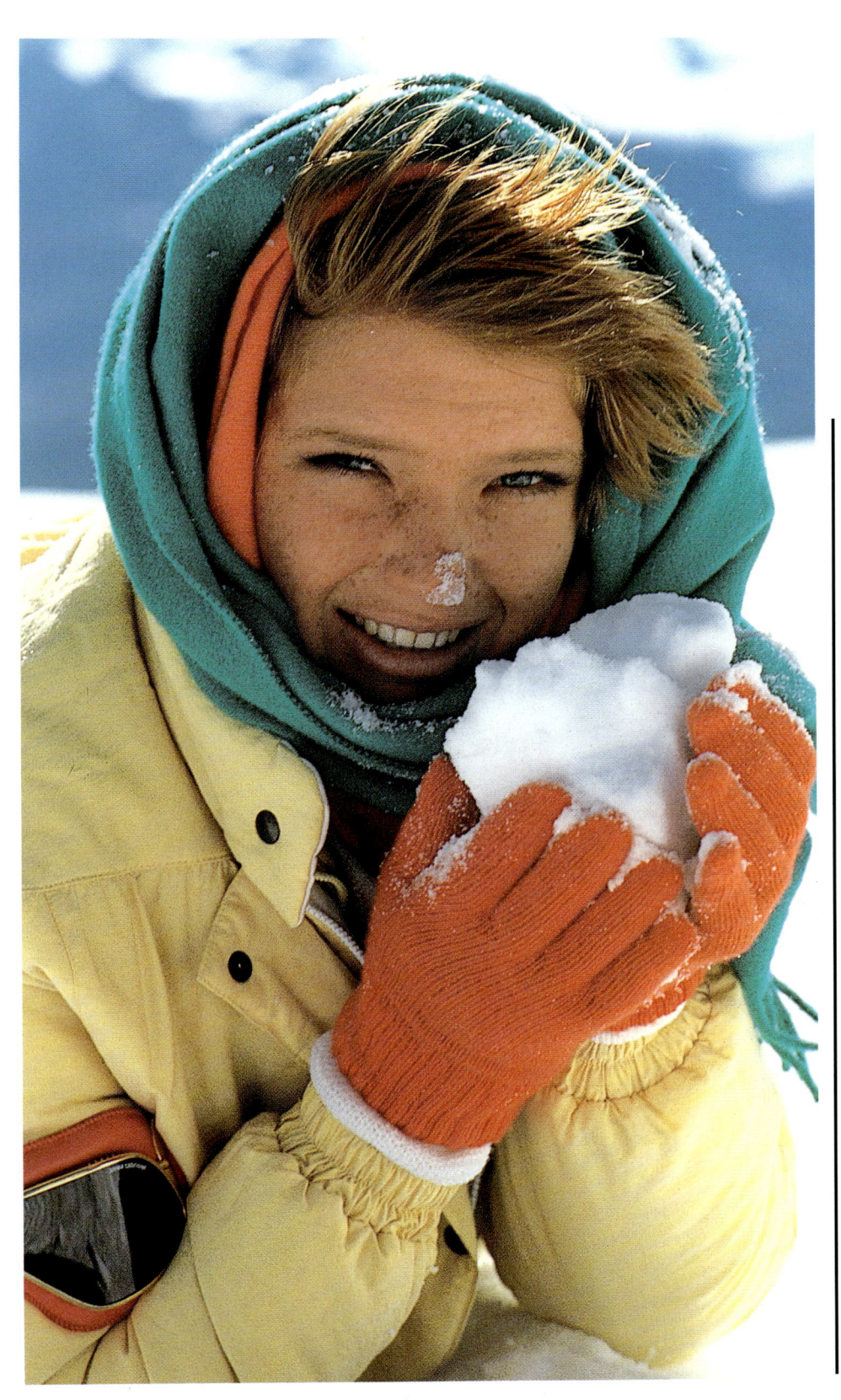

- Remember to care for your hands and nails, too, as the skin here can also suffer in cold weather.
- Always apply waxy lip salves or balms to your lips which are especially vulnerable to dehydration.
- Add oils and moisturizing gels to your bath and apply body lotions every day.
- Never come in from icy cold weather and immediately roast yourself in front of a hot fire, as you will dry your skin excessively; the rapid contrast in temperature can also break capillaries, leading to red thread veins.
- If you are skiing or are outside in sunny, but cold weather, apply protective lotions on any exposed skin. In cold weather you will not be warned by the heat of the sun on your face that it may be burning. If there is snow it will reflect the sun, increasing its damaging effect. You will need special sun protection products if you are going to be out in sub-zero temperatures. Other products contain a higher percentage of water and may freeze on the skin, breaking the tiny capillaries. Use products specifically formulated to protect the skin in cold and windy conditions and use sunblocks on your lips. Reapply sun protection products frequently during the day.

HUMID HEAT

In humid, hot climates, cleansing is a top priority in order to remove oil and dirt, especially if you have oily or problem skin.

Action plan for overcoming the effects of humid heat
- Keep a mini skincare kit with you. Pack in it small or travel-sized bottles of wipe-off cleanser and toner and, if you need to, cleanse quickly at midday as well as morning and night, using tissues.
- Just use moisturizer where you need it and choose light or oil-free types rather than heavier creams.
- Wear a water-based foundation, especially if your skin is oily. If you prefer not to wear foundation during hot weather, just sweep on a little translucent or bronze powder to control any shine.
- Look out for oil-blotting lotions that can be worn under foundation to keep your skin matte and shine-free. Apply only over the T-zone.
- If you are working in a city, consider having facials more regularly to cleanse your skin of pollution residues. Your pores open up in hot weather and so absorb these residues more readily than when it is cooler.

HOT DRY WEATHER

Warm climates are not necessarily humid. When the weather is hot and dry, it is important to ensure that you protect your skin against moisture loss by wearing a moisturizer.

Apply a light, oil-free moisturizer where your skin tends to dry out easily and reapply it during the day if necessary.

POLLUTION

Air pollutants such as exhaust and industrial fumes, and indoor pollutants such as dust and cigarette smoke, are absorbed by the skin's hydrolipidic (water and oil) film.

Over time, exposure to pollutants means that instead of performing its role of protecting the skin, this film starts to act as a skin irritant and this can result in weakened, compromised skin function and a complexion that becomes noticeably more sensitive.

Pollution also increases the production of free radicals, which accelerate skin ageing. Cell inflammation also leads to damage. Some dermatologists believe that passive smoking is more damaging than the sun over long periods of time.

In one test, carbon monoxide reduced cellular functioning by 24 per cent, exhaust fumes reduced functioning by 65 per cent and cigarette smoke affected it by 70 per cent.

Moisturizers and make-up that include 'anti-pollution complexes' with skin shielding, soothing and anti-inflammatory ingredients are increasingly available.

These complexes include plant extracts such as horse chestnut, ginseng, linden flowers, seaweed and some vitamins, especially A, C, E and B5.

Check that your diet contains good quantities of vegetables and fruits that are high in the A, C and E vitamins too, to protect your skin cells from the inside out.

Impairing the hydrolipic film can also leave the skin vulnerable to dehydration. Moisturizers which restore suppleness and which provide a protective barrier (known as filmogenic) to cut down moisture loss are particularly important in a polluted environment. These moisturizers should also contain ultraviolet filters.

You should remember to cleanse your face thoroughly but gently every evening. De-sensitizing facials that also deep-clean the skin are available in beauty salons.

Air purifiers are sold in department stores, chemists and health food stores. You can also surround yourself at home and in the office with plants which will absorb some of the pollutants.

TRAVELLING LIGHT

The air in planes is notoriously dry, leaving you feeling dehydrated and lethargic and your skin drained of energy and moisture. The tissues beneath the skin can become congested, too, and puff up, making you feel even more uncomfortable.

Action plan for overcoming the effects of flying
- As part of your final preparations before leaving, apply body lotion after you've showered or bathed. If you are travelling to a hot country and use self-tanning moisturizer, this will give your skin a colour boost for when you arrive.
- Carry a skincare kit in your hand luggage. As soon as you can, remove your make-up, freshen your skin with toner and spritz it with a mineral-water spray. Apply moisturizer and eye gel to ease any tendency to puffiness. If you are on a long-haul flight, repeat this routine when your skin feels dry, or use a moisturizer with extended moisturizing power – some moisturize the skin for up to twenty-four hours.
- Drink plenty of water and fruit juice to prevent dehydration.
- Avoid alcohol, tea, coffee and cola drinks as these actually have a diuretic effect.
- Move around as much as you can to stimulate your circulation.

SKINCARE 63

SPORTING CHANCE
You should cleanse your skin before and after you exercise and make sure that your sports kit and hair are as clean – and bacteria-free – as possible since they come into contact with your skin. Loose-fitting sports clothes in natural fibres are also kind to your skin. Do not wear a heavy moisturizer when exercising.

If you are going to be exercising outside, protect your skin by wearing a sunscreen. You can buy oil-free screens – gels for instance – which are terrific for oily skins. Apply sunblocks to vulnerable areas, such as lips, particularly if you are going sailing or windsurfing. Wearing sunglasses designed for your sport is also a good idea as they will protect your eyes and the skin around them from ultraviolet light and glare.

Always take a shower immediately after you've been swimming, so that the salt or chlorine in the water cannot dry on your skin and irritate it. When you are playing an active game, such as tennis or volleyball, pat perspiration from your face and body with a clean towel between sets and drink a refreshing glass of chilled water.

If you use the sauna or steam room at a health club, try not to stay in too long. Steaming in moderate amounts is good for your skin, but if you stay in too long the skin becomes dehydrated. Leave the steam room if your skin starts to turn red. Two to three minutes is usually plenty. Do not stay in more than about ten minutes, whatever your skin type.

Do not use a sauna or steam room if you are pregnant, if you feel unwell or have sensitive skin.

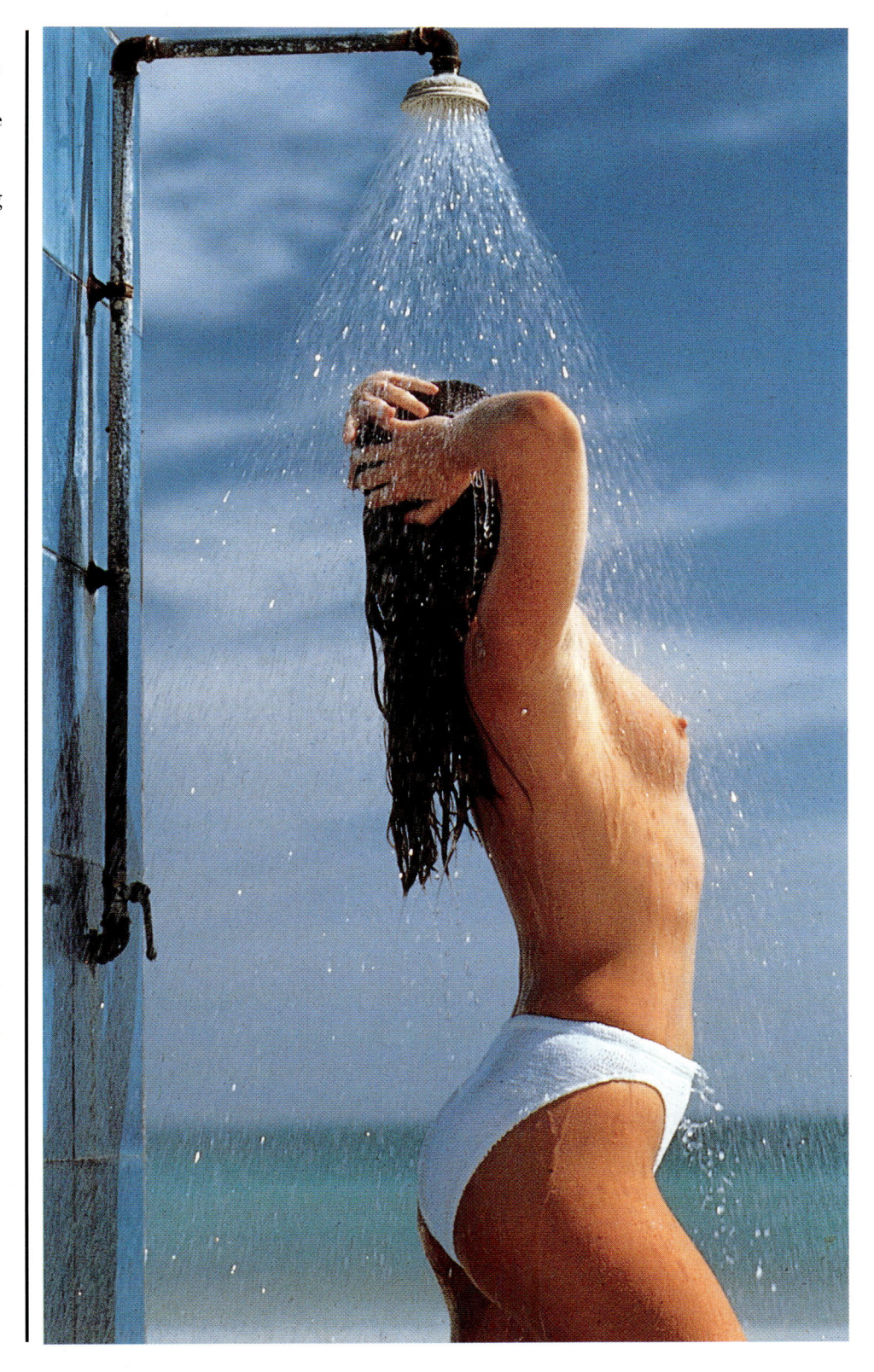

64 SHORT CUTS

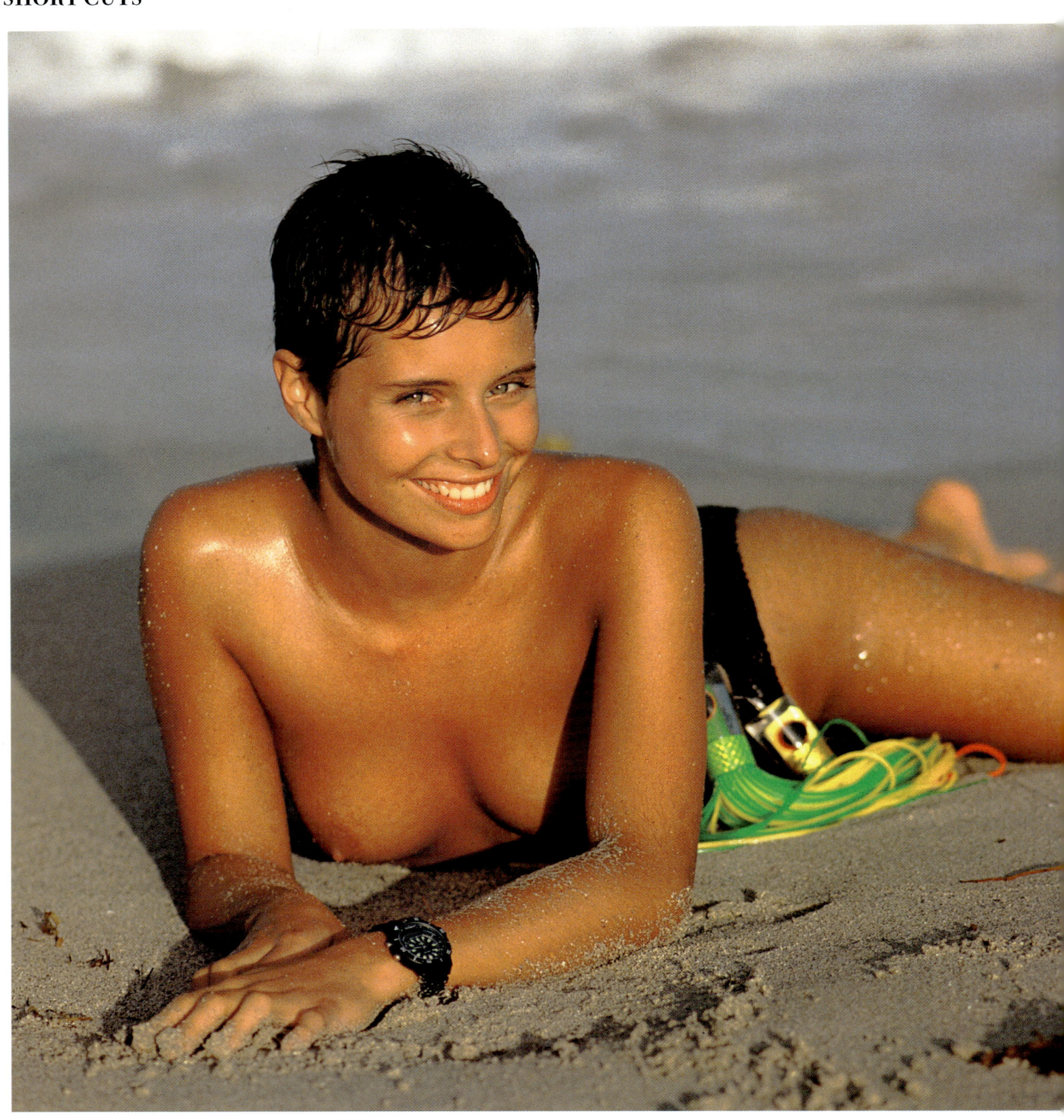

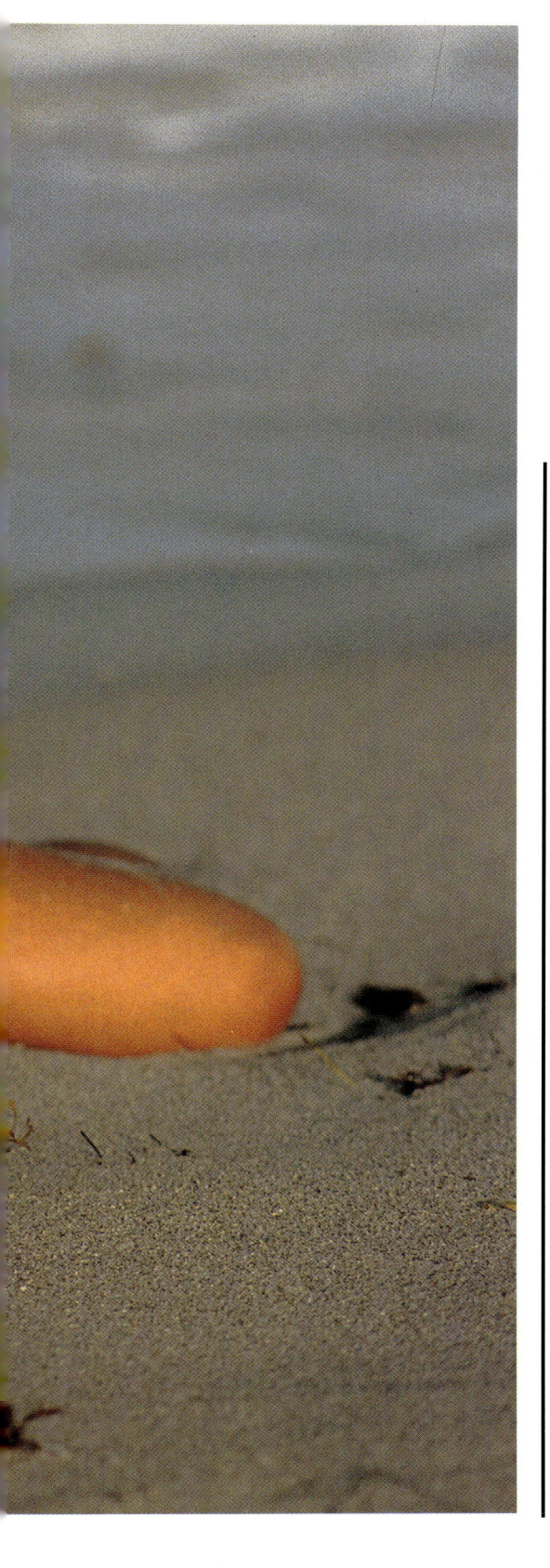

SUN AND TANNING

The key to the safest tanning is high protection with gradual exposure.

A tan makes us feel and look good. While dermatologists warn us of the dangers of sunbathing, there is a bright side to the sun. The sun's rays enhance our feelings of well-being – we feel relaxed and revitalized. They help our bodies to synthesize vitamin D which improves the absorption of minerals. There is also evidence that the full-spectrum light we receive from the sun reaches the brain via the eyes, stimulating the production of hormones, making us feel more energetic and improving our mood. We now know, though, that if we are not careful we can pay a heavy price for a golden tan.

UVB and UVA are bands of ultraviolet light from the sun, which sun products can filter or screen. UVB causes the skin to go red, and, if unprotected for long enough, to burn. It also stimulates the skin's pigment-forming cells, a natural protective measure. UVB is the main cause of skin cancers (which themselves are linked to a history of burning, especially in childhood) and premature ageing of the skin. In Northern Europe, UVB is at its strongest during the summer months, while in hotter climes it's more constant throughout the year.

UVA is less damaging than UVB, but it is thought to increase UVB's burning effect. It penetrates the skin more deeply than UVB and plays a larger role in ageing the skin, i.e. loss of tone and wrinkles. UVA is also more likely to cause sun-sensitive reactions. It is present at virtually the same strength all year round, even in Britain, which is why many dermatologists are now recommending wearing a moisturizer with built-in sunscreen on a daily basis.

In Australia, which has one of the highest rates of skin cancer in the world, sun protection is taken very seriously. Life guards can throw you off the beach if you're not properly protected. School children too are sent home or kept in if not adequately lotioned up. Draconian may be, sensible certainly. Incidences of skin cancer are expected to fall.

BE AWARE!

Skin cancer is the third most common cancer occurring in women in the 15–34 year-old age group. If you notice any changes in the size or shape of moles on your skin, itching or bleeding, you should see a specialist as quickly as possible. A common site for skin cancer in women in on the legs. With men, it is often found on the back.

With early detection, skin cancer is curable. Be aware and take preventative measures, too – avoid burning and always cover up with a high protection sunscreen. Sunscreen worn on a daily basis is the single fastest way to protect the health and appearance of your skin, both now and for the future.

PROTECTION: THE SHORT CUT TO STAYING YOUNG
The good news is that protecting your skin from the sun and tanning *gradually* will cut the cost of sunbathing. You will develop fewer lines and greatly reduce the chances of suffering skin disease.

The key to safer tanning is to know your skin type and to use adequate protection.

Time your exposure to the sun
Your skin has built-in natural protection against the sun. The skin's pigment – melanin – will prevent your skin from burning for a short time if you are not wearing protection. This protection time ranges from ten minutes for very fair skins, which have very little melanin, to many hours for black skins, which contain a lot of melanin. If you multiply this natural protection time by the factor number of your sunscreen cream, you can work out how long you can sunbathe before you start to burn when wearing the sunscreen. The sunscreens recommended below should be used for at least the first two to three days while the skin steps up its production of melanin and you tan.

After this time, you can use a sunscreen with a lower factor, for example from SPF15 to SPF12, if your skin is not red or tender.

Sun protection tips if you are red-haired and freckled with pale eyes
This skin type always burns extremely easily and never tans. Your skin's natural protection time is just ten minutes, so the recommended sunscreen for you is an SPF15 or higher.

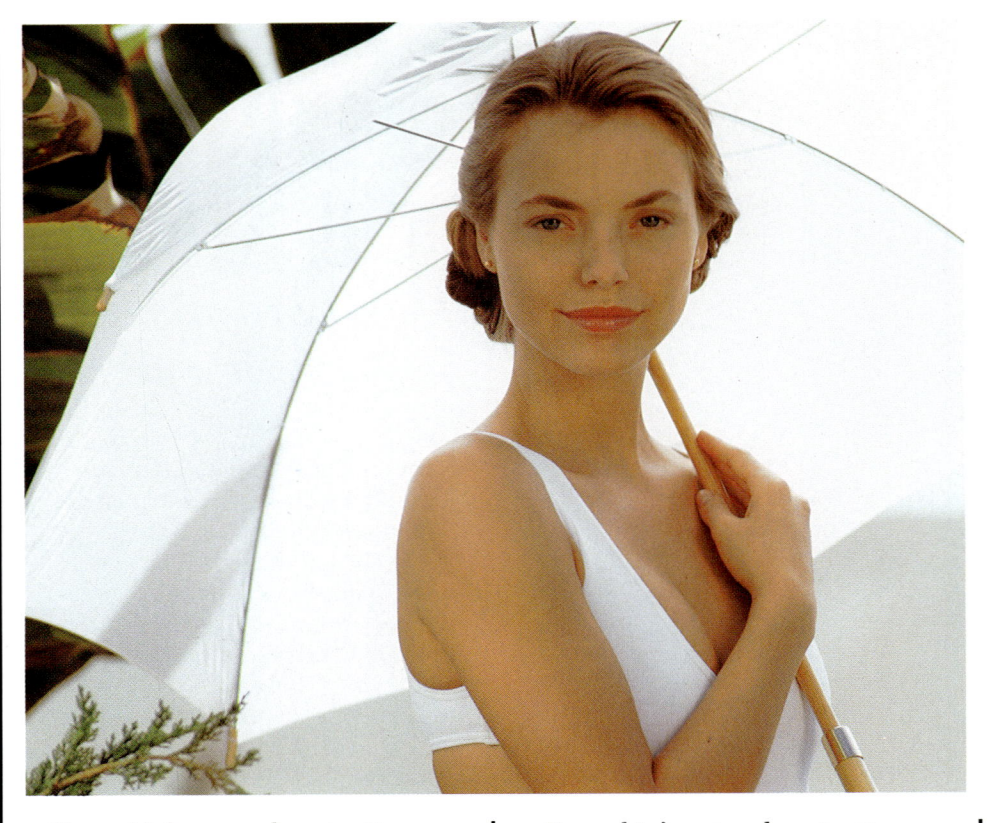

Fair skinned and blue-eyed
This skin type burns easily and tans minimally.
Your skin's natural protection time is ten to fifteen minutes. The recommended sunscreen for your skin is an SPF15 or higher.

Dark hair and eyes and pale skin
This skin type can burn and tans gradually.
Your skin's natural protection time is twenty minutes. A sunscreen of SPF10 or higher is recommended for you.

Olive skin and dark eyes
This skin type hardly burns at all and always tans, but still needs to be protected.
Your skin's natural protection time is between twenty and thirty minutes. The recommended sunscreen for your skin is an SPF6 to SPF8 or higher.

Dark olive skin
This skin type rarely burns and generally tans well.
Your skin's natural protection time is many hours. A sunscreen of SPF4 or higher is recommended.

Black skin
This skin type rarely burns and is deeply pigmented.
Your skin's natural protection time is many hours. A sunscreen of SPF2 or higher is recommended.

TAKE EXTRA CARE
In addition to taking into account your skin's natural protection time when you sunbathe, you should also consider the following factors:

Time of day The sun's ultraviolet rays are most intense between 11 am and 3 pm.
Temperature We gauge the strength of the sun by the warmth we feel, but the *infra-red* rays, which raise the temperature on the thermometer, are not a guide to the damaging potential of the *ultraviolet* radiation. Even on a cloudy day the ultraviolet rays are still quite powerful. Beware as well, when it is windy – the wind makes it seem cooler and we are lulled into a false sense of security.
Surroundings Sea, sand, snow and white buildings reflect light and can dramatically increase the effect of ultraviolet rays.

Latitude The sun is always overhead at the equator, giving your skin more concentrated doses of ultraviolet rays because they pass through less of the atmosphere before they reach you.
Altitude If you are on holiday in the mountains you're closer to the sun and the atmosphere is thinner, increasing the risk of sunburn.

All-round protection

It is important to screen out both UVB and UVA rays, so choose a sun product that has a high ratio of both.
Extended protection Many sun preparations now offer waterproof or water-resistant protection – great if you're playing sport in the sunshine or in and out of the water. Even this type of product needs reapplying though, so check the label carefully and follow the reapplication instructions to ensure you're properly protected.
Lips and eyes These need extra care, so use specialized products whenever possible. Wear sunglasses, too, to prevent you from squinting and to protect from glare.

Sunscreens and skin repair

There is an added advantage to using sunscreens. Studies have shown that, if the skin is protected in this way, it can actually repair the damage done during previous periods of exposure to the sun. New collagen is formed and laid down on top of the damaged, cross-linked connective tissue.

After-sun skincare

- Shower off salt or chlorinated water before it dries on your skin, which may cause irritation.
- Use shower gels after sunbathing rather than soap, which will further dry sun-damaged skin.
- Lavish after-sun lotion on your face and body. It will contain skin-soothing and cooling ingredients, such as aloe vera. You could also try aftersuns with fake tan to enhance your natural colour without damaging your skin. Fake tans for face and body can, of course, be used any time to create the illusion of a golden tan. The latest formulations are technologically more advanced so you won't be left with those tell-tale orange streaks that characterized early self-tanners.

Sunbeds

Dermatologists strongly advise against using them. The risks of damaging your skin are high and one-third of the people who use them don't get a tan at all.

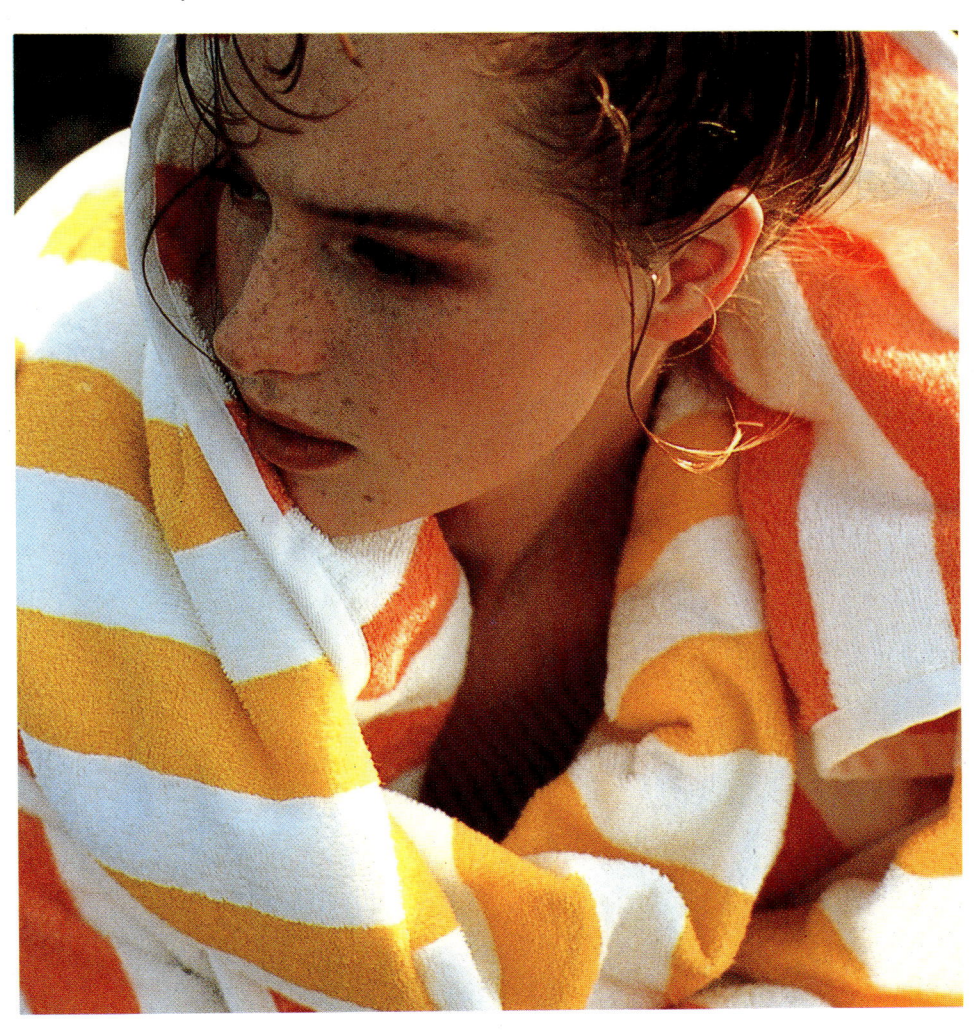

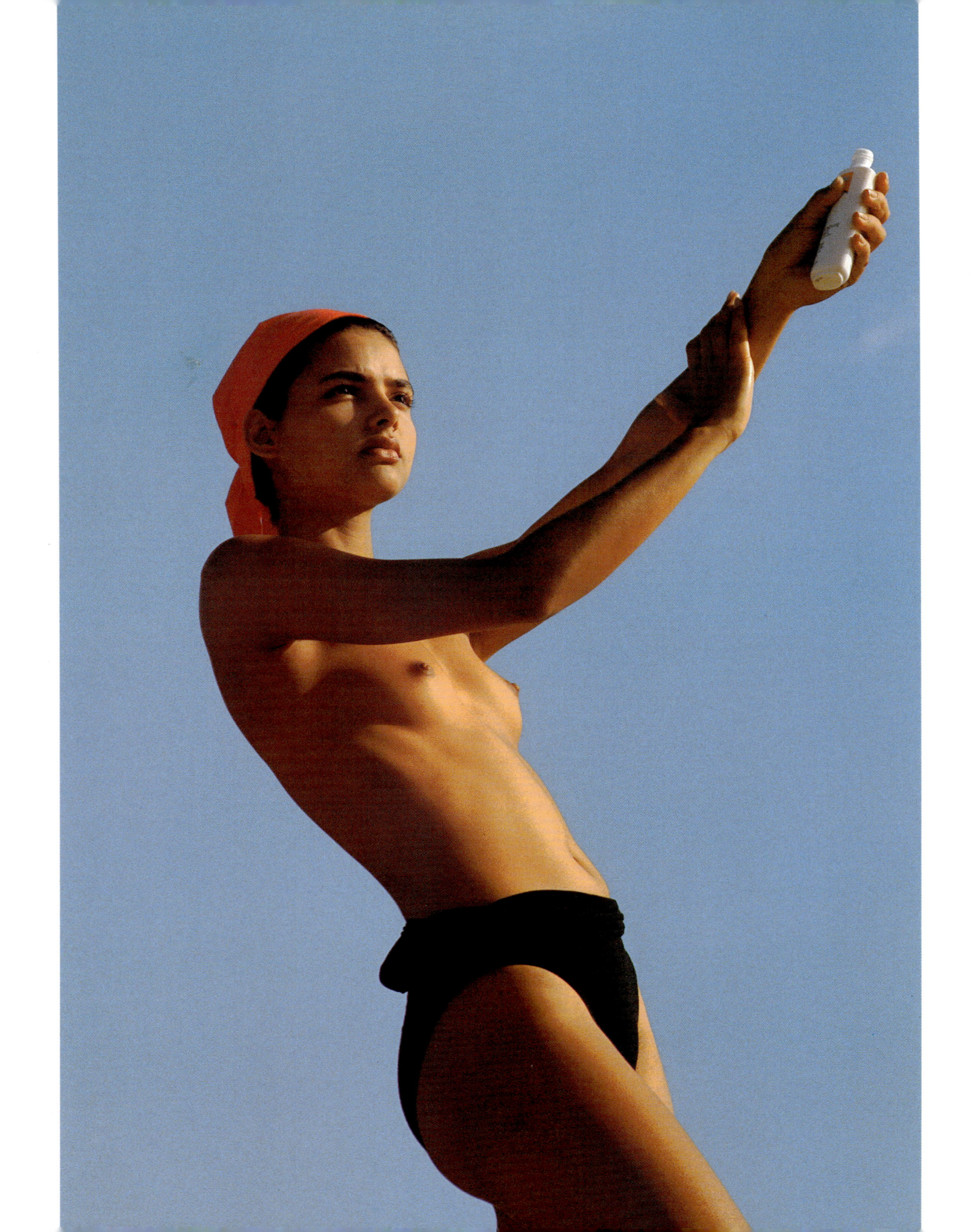

SHORT CUTS TO SOLVING SUN PROBLEMS

Sunburn

Sunburn has long-term detrimental effects on the skin and should be avoided. Contrary to popular myth you do not have to burn to get a tan. And, just in case you're still wondering, you can still get a tan using high protection factors. If you do burn, however, keep your skin cool and clean and soothe it with calamine lotion or natural yoghurt. Aloe vera is another good sunburn calmer, as is the essential oil from the bark of the tea tree. Simply add 2–3 drops of it to 10ml of a carrier oil such as wheatgerm or avocado, available in most health food stores and chemists.

If you burn badly over most of your body, you may need to rest in bed and drink plenty of fluids. You definitely should not sunbathe the following day, or until the redness has gone. Seek medical advice for severe burns.

Prickly heat

This spotty rash occurs as a result of blocked sweat glands, mostly appearing on the chest, back and arms, and you can take steps to prevent it.

Avoid strong sunlight, especially between eleven in the morning and three in the afternoon when the sun is at its strongest. Wear high-factor sunscreens that screen out both UVA and UVB rays. Take cool showers or bathe frequently, patting the skin dry afterwards. Also avoid activities that make you sweat a lot.

If you do develop prickly heat, stay in the cool, apply calamine lotion or talcum powder and wear loose clothing. Prickly heat is often confused with polymorphic light eruption (see right).

Heat exhaustion and heat-stroke

Avoid succumbing to either heat exhaustion or heat-stroke by resisting the temptation to lie in the hot sun for hours on end. Keep your body cool by going for a swim at regular intervals.

Don't fall asleep in the sun. If you begin to feel woozy or headachey, retreat to the shade immediately and cool yourself down with cold compresses or a tepid bath and sip liquids. Orange juice is good because it replaces potassium lost through sweating.

Drink at least two litres (three to four pints) of water a day, and don't rely on thirst as an indicator of dehydration – you could easily be dehydrated and yet not feel thirsty. Don't drink alcohol or caffeinated drinks as these have a diuretic effect, adding to dehydration.

If, despite these precautions, you develop symptoms of heat exhaustion or heat-stroke, take the following steps immediately:

Heat exhaustion There are three types of heat exhaustion, all of which can be fatal: water deficiency, salt deficiency and anhidrotic.

The symptoms of water deficiency heat exhaustion include thirst, lack of appetite, giddiness, a dry mouth and rising temperature. Rest in cool surroundings and drink half a litre (about a pint) of water every fifteen minutes for two hours. Seek medical help if your symptoms continue.

Salt deficiency heat exhaustion occurs if you have been sweating heavily during the first few days of acclimatization to a very hot climate and have not eaten properly. Fatigue, giddiness and severe muscle cramps are symptoms of this type of heat exhaustion. If you think you may be suffering from this condition see a doctor.

Anhidrotic heat exhaustion is a rare malfunction of the sweat glands, which occurs in people who have been in a hot climate for several months.

Heat-stroke The symptoms of heat-stroke are that your body temperature rises but you do not sweat as this heat-regulating mechanism is not functioning correctly. You develop a severe headache, feel faint or disorientated, stagger or start to convulse. The skin is hot and may feel dry. 'Sunstroke' is an incorrect term – you can get heat-stroke without being in the sun.

Heat-stroke can be extremely dangerous, or even fatal, so call an ambulance or ask someone to drive you to the emergency department of a nearby hospital.

Photosensitization

The skin can react to plant and fruit extracts and juices (figs in particular), drugs or chemicals when exposed to the sun, resulting in a sore, itchy red rash or blisters.

Soothe with cold compresses, showers and calamine lotion.

If you are going to sunbathe, avoid using perfume, aftershave, anti-bacterial soaps, artificial sweeteners, medications containing diuretics or tranquillizers.

Polymorphic light eruption

This is a common condition whereby the skin is abnormally sensitive to sunlight. It usually starts in the spring when sunlight becomes stronger and lasts throughout the summer, causing itching, redness and a variety of rashes. It is thought that UVA plays a particular role in PLE and one clinical trial reported good results when sufferers used a sunscreen with very high levels of UVA protection.

YOUR SKIN PROBLEMS SOLVED

There's no need to suffer in silence. Here are the solutions to some of the most common skin problems.

Q *I have small red veins around my nose. What treatments are available?*

A Thread veins are dilated capillaries that may have ruptured. They can occur at any age and affect any skin type, not just dry and sensitive skins. They occur most frequently on the cheeks, the bridge and sides of the nose, under the eyes and on the legs.

They are caused by sun damage, alcohol, drinking very hot drinks such as tea or coffee, eating spicy foods, high blood pressure, exposure to harsh weather conditions and steroid products applied to the skin.

You can disguise the veins using a concealer stick or you can go to a beauty salon where they will remove them by using either electrolysis or sclerotherapy.

With electrolysis a fine needle, which transmits shortwave electrical current, is used to cauterize the blood vessel, blocking off the flow of blood. Two or three sessions may be needed, depending on how many veins need to be removed. The skin swells for a couple of days and scabs may form at the point where the needle was inserted.

Sclerotherapy is used to treat more severe broken veins, particularly leg veins (but not varicose veins). A chemical is injected into the vein that makes it collapse and close up, the blood drying out and fading away.

Q *Can I avoid getting spots and what are the quickest ways to heal them?*

A The precise cause of acne is not known, although hormones play a key role in the appearance of spots. Acne often starts in teenage years because of this, and can last into the thirties, or longer. It can also flare up in women of thirty or even forty plus who have never previously suffered, because of a change in hormonal activity.

There are circumstances that can aggravate inflammation of the skin in some people:
- a very humid atmosphere
- certain medicines
- insufficient sleep
- pre-menstrual hormone fluctuation
- stress and emotional upsets
- the contraceptive pill
- the link with diet has not been proven, although an unbalanced diet and zinc deficiency may contribute
- certain ingredients in cosmetics may be a factor.

If you develop blackheads or acne, follow these precautions:
- Don't use harsh cleansing products or abrasive scrubs as this may increase the skin's oil production and will also dry the surface of the skin.
- Never pick at or squeeze spots – this pushes inflammation deeper into the skin and causes permanent damage.
- Salon facials and professional removal of blackheads are beneficial.
- Using clay masks at home absorbs excess oil.
- Contact your doctor if the problem is severe. One form of acne can pit and scar the skin. This can be avoided with specialist treatment. But if you just have the odd spot, the best advice is to leave well alone and don't worry!

Q *How can I avoid stretch marks and are there any ways to remove them?*

A Stretch marks are caused by rapid fluctuations in weight, through dieting or as a result of weight gain during pregnancy, for example.

There is almost nothing you can do to avoid them in pregnancy as much depends on your hormones, although controlling your weight gain will help. Keeping your skin firm and elastic with body lotions can also be helpful. In addition, vitamins and minerals in your diet have been shown to maintain strong connective tissue.

Unfortunately, once the stretch marks have formed, no treatment or cosmetic will remove the scars. However, they will fade, even if they do not disappear completely, with time.

Q *How can I prevent cold sores occurring?*

A Cold sores are the result of a virus known as the herpes simplex virus 1. Once you have the virus it stays with you for life, although some people never have more than one outbreak. It can be activated by strong sunlight, colds and menstruation. Wear a high protection sunscreen to help prevent cold sores. Apply medication as soon as you feel the tell-tale tingling sensation. Cold sores are extremely contagious and you must keep them clean and dry. Do not touch them or pass them to others through contact such as kissing.

Q *How can I conceal dark circles under my eyes?*

A Dark circles are a very common complaint and can worsen with time as the surface skin thins. Try to get adequate sleep and on waking, tap the skin lightly with the fingertips, using a refreshing gel – this will improve circulation. Use a fine film of concealer, blending carefully.

Q *Could the flaking, red patches that have developed on my skin be psoriasis?*

A It sounds very likely. Psoriasis, unlike eczema, does not itch. It affects most commonly the scalp, elbows, shoulders, lower back and knees. The rough, red patches flare up at random and it may be triggered by shock, fatigue, depression and certain drugs and aggravated by stress. The complaint sometimes occurs two or three weeks after a throat infection. Studies are being carried out to determine the precise cause of psoriasis, which occurs when the skin cells turn over too quickly. The condition is often hereditary.

Your doctor can prescribe tar products or treatment by a form of ultraviolet, depending on the extent of the problem. Some doctors may suggest corticosteriod products. Alternative therapies such as acupuncture, using herb and plant oils and homeopathy can sometimes prove useful, as can bathing in mineral salts.

Eczema can also be helped by acupuncture and homeopathy. There are several forms of eczema, some of which are triggered by allergic reactions to particular chemicals. Your doctor can arrange tests to identify the cause.

Q *Is eczema the same condition as dermatitis and what are the best treatments?*

A Eczema and dermatitis are now used as interchangeable descriptions, and there are many types with different causes. It is important to consult your doctor or specialist for a precise diagnosis. This inflammation of the skin causes dryness, flaking and sometimes blisters.

In its mildest form, eczema is simply a tendency to dry skin but in severe cases it can affect the whole body, causing itching, inflammation and discomfort.

Eczema causes the skin to become itchy and hot and areas of hardened skin may develop from continual scratching. Infection may result.

The most common type of eczema is atopic eczema, which usually first appears in infancy and is strongly linked with asthma and hayfever.

You should use pure cotton bedding and clothing, as wool and some synthetic fibres can aggravate the condition. Washing powders that contain enzymes can cause skin problems. Allergies to nickel, rubber, dyes, medications, plants and the house dust mite can trigger eczema and stress can aggravate it.

Treatments include the application of special emulsifying oils to your bathwater and emollient creams after bathing when the skin is still damp.

Topical steroids may be prescribed by your doctor. Antihistamines can also be prescribed to relieve itching and antibiotics to treat an infection.

Treatment with Chinese herbs has proved successful for patients whose eczema did not respond to topical steroids. It is advisable to seek the advice of your doctor and an eczema association before embarking on this treatment.

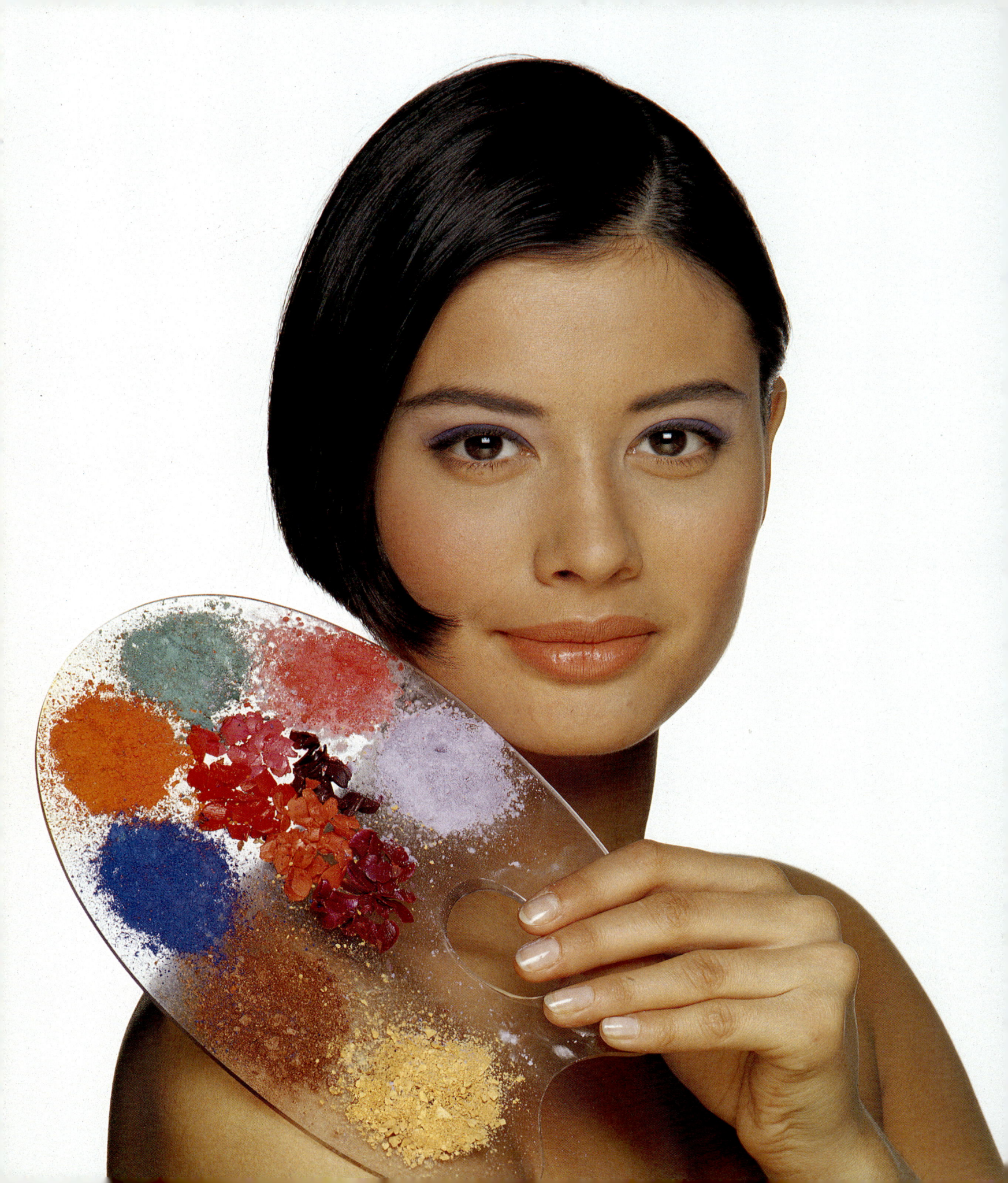

MASTERING MAKE-UP

Make-up is an art, but easy to master once you know the basics. In the following pages you will discover tips and tricks to help you maximize your looks fast, as well as plenty of inspirational ideas for creating looks for different occasions.

COMPLEXION PERFECTION 74

EYES RIGHT 78

LIP SERVICE 82

5-MINUTE MAKE-UP 84

THE NATURAL LOOK 86

THE CLASSIC FACE 88

MODERN GLAMOUR 90

WORKING GIRL 92

COSMOPOLITAN COLOURS 94

PARTY TIME 96

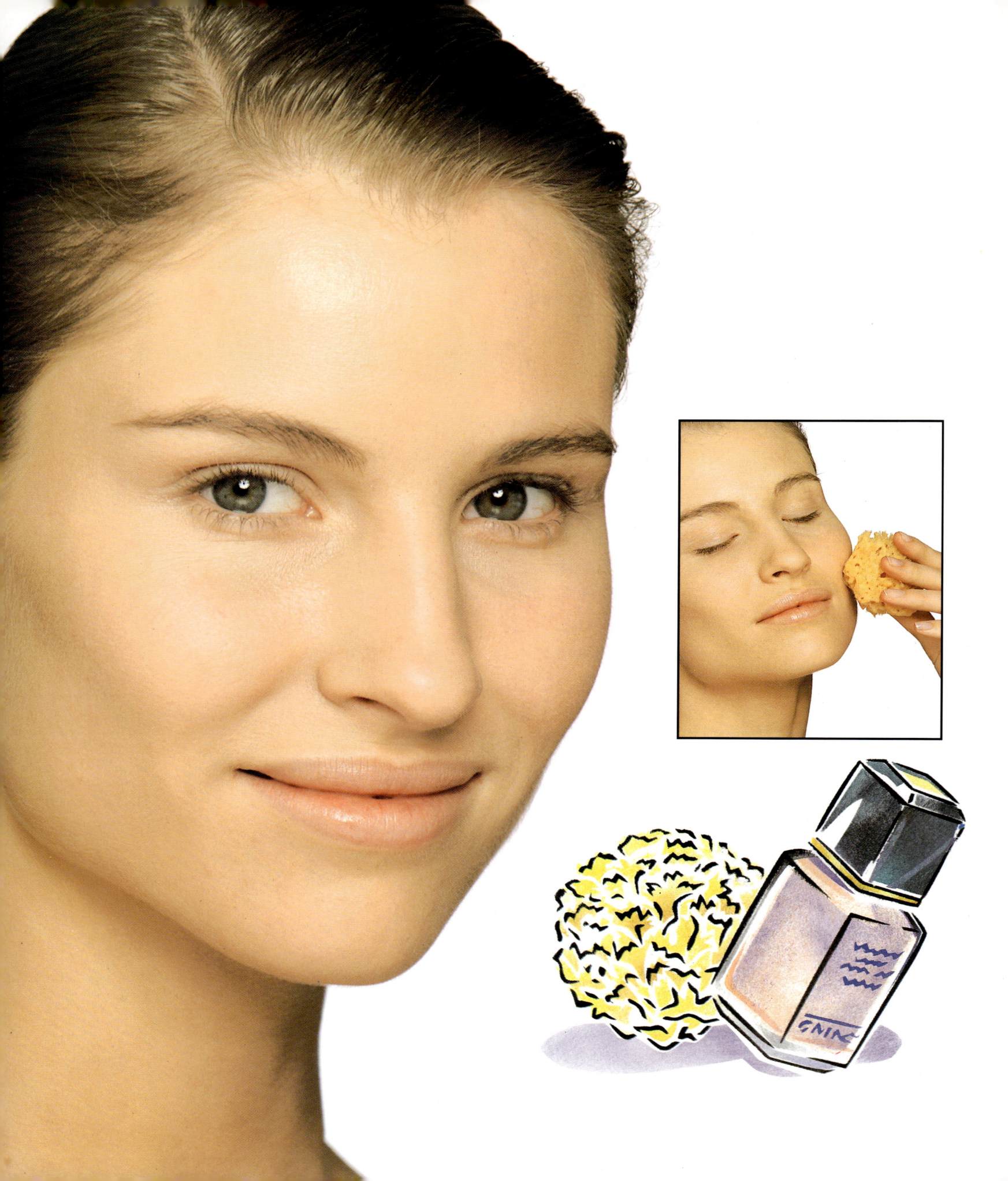

COMPLEXION PERFECTION

Carefully chosen products combined with professional techniques give you a flawless finish fast.

The key to successful make-up is getting the base right. This means choosing the right products for your skin type, learning colour and application techniques and having a knowledge of quick complexion enhancers for long-lasting polished perfection.

FOUNDATION
This has several beauty benefits: it evens out skin tones, smoothes the skin's texture, provides a base for other make-up, and keeps colours true.

Choose a colour that is close to your own skin tone – going a few shades lighter or darker will look unnatural and mask-like. Not all skins need foundation.

Colour check
Apply a little on your jaw-line (don't use the back of your hand, as the skin here is darker and coarser than on your face). With a good match, the foundation will almost disappear. It is important to check this in daylight. If you can't find an exact match buy a couple of foundations – one slightly darker, one slightly lighter than your skin tone – and blend them to your own ideal shade.

Modern mixes
Foundation and powder in one handy ready-mixed compact are the short cut to a natural-looking complexion. They are smoothed on with a sponge and suit most skin types, except very dry skins.

Tailoring foundation to your skin
Bear in mind your skin type and needs when buying your foundation. It shouldn't look obvious or feel uncomfortable. If it does, it is likely that you have chosen a product incompatible with your skin.

Remember the following when choosing foundation:
- If you have dry skin, look for a creamy, moisturizing formula.
- For oily or combination skin, an oil-free or water-based make-up is best as it minimizes shine (the high powder content in water-based foundations gives a matte finish).
- Tinted moisturizer does exactly what it says – leaves a tint on the skin and moisturizes. It is terrific for summer on tanned skin or for skin that is naturally clear and even toned, as it gives virtually no coverage; it doesn't work on open-pored or oily skin.
- Some cosmetic companies offer a personalised foundation and powder service, where the products are made on the spot to match your skin tone and type exactly.

Many foundations now also incorporate sunscreens to protect your skin from harmful ultraviolet light, which is an added benefit.

Application tips
For foundation to look like a second skin, you need to apply it correctly.

Always begin your make-up routine by cleansing and moisturizing your face. You should apply your make-up in the light in which your complexion will be seen, checking there are no shadows. It may seem obvious, but if you make up in inadequate or unbalanced lighting, this will cost you precious time later as you try to retouch mistakes.

Dampen a make-up sponge and then squeeze it well in a towel so it is just slightly damp. A triangular wedge shape or a natural sponge is best for applying foundation – they cover more efficiently and blend better than fingers.

Using the back of your hand as a palette to mix from, dab dots of foundation on your forehead, cheeks, nose and chin. Work the sponge in quick, downward and outward movements, remembering to blend to just under the jaw-line to avoid any 'tide-marks', but don't take foundation down on to your neck. Fade the foundation out towards your hair-line.

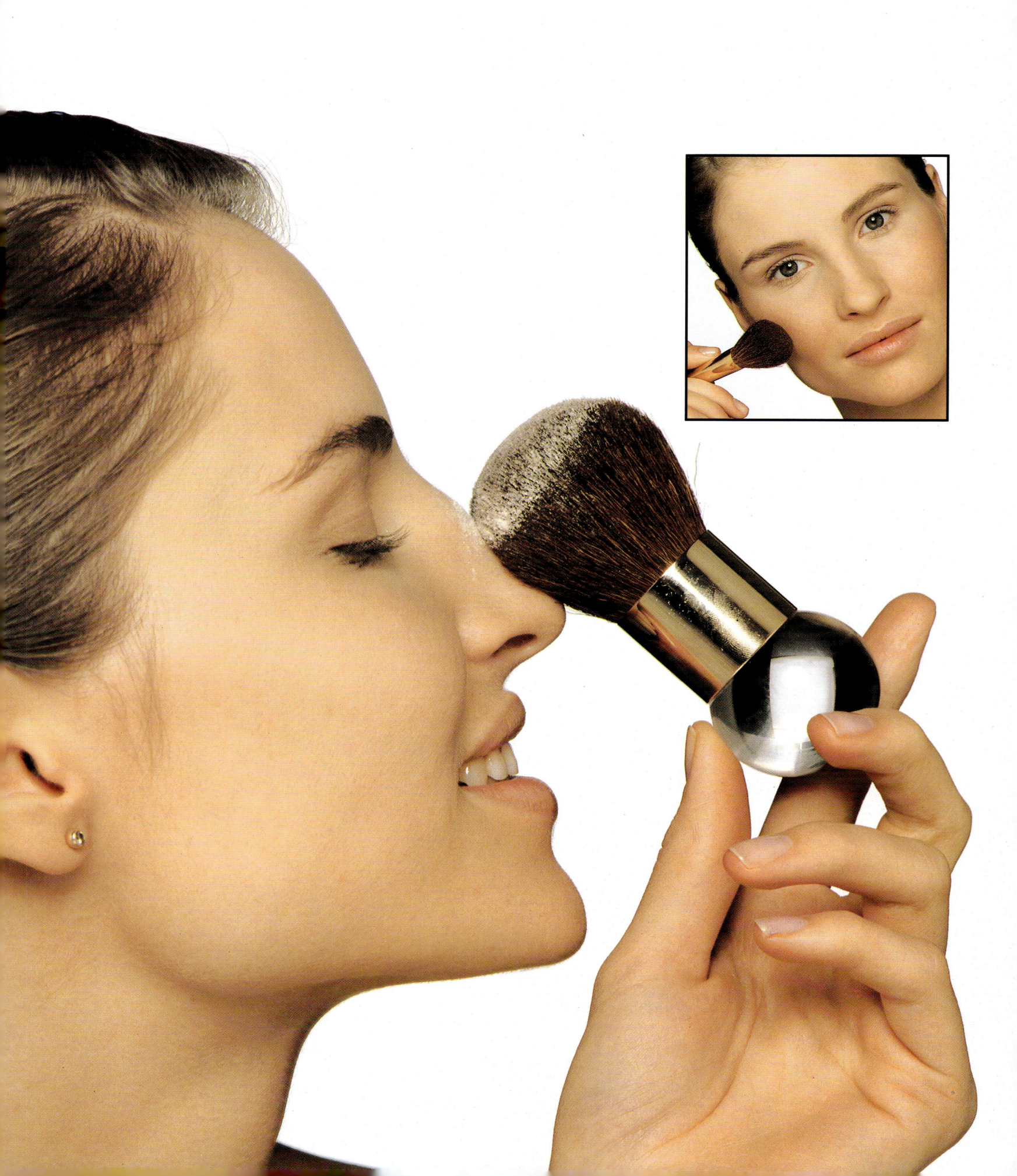

MASTERING MAKE-UP

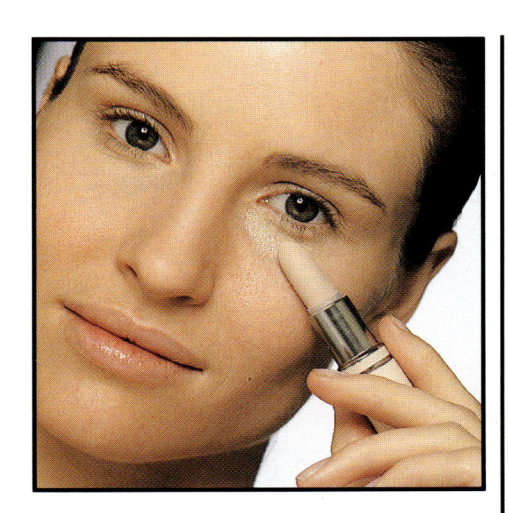

CLEVER CONCEALER
Concealers are fast, effective tools for disguising blemishes, shadows, scars and red veins.

Application tips
Pick a shade slightly lighter than your foundation and apply it *over* foundation. Sweep on lightly from the tube or dab some on your fingertip and press it on, using the barest minimum, then tidy up the edges with a flat, slim brush.

POWDER
Face powder, which went through a period of not being fashionable, is back as an indispensable beauty tool. Its traditional function is to 'set' make-up, giving it a finished look. However, modern, fine-textured powder can be a good base in itself, worn simply over moisturizer. This is a terrific time-saver when you are in a hurry or don't want to wear foundation, but don't want to be completely barefaced either.

Application tips
Loose powder should be applied with a large, soft brush (larger than your blusher brush) or pressed on with a velour pad in order to set make-up thoroughly. Brush off any excess with your powder brush.

Pressed powder is applied with a pad and is particularly suitable for retouching make-up during the day. For the most natural finish (matte and invisible) use a translucent powder. It reflects light to give the skin a luminous, satiny quality. Heavily pigmented powders are out-dated, usually look artificial and are generally best left well alone!

Colour correction powders are brush-on instant beautifiers. They come in pressed or loose form and are simply applied over foundation in the areas they are needed. Use them individually as follows:
White adds luminosity to the complexion and is particularly good for evening.
Mauve/violet warms up a sallow complexion.
Green tones down high colour.
Pink gives a healthy glow to pale skin.
Blue tones down high colour.
Apricot gives a healthy glow to olive skin that lacks brightness.

BLUSHER
The fastest face shaper, blusher adds a gentle bloom of colour to the cheeks and shape to the face.

On the whole, powder blusher is simpler and quicker to use than cream, but whichever you prefer, remember not to overdo it. It is, after all, intended to mimic the natural glow of your cheeks.

Choose a blusher colour that will co-ordinate with your total make-up look. Try to avoid the frosted variety – they can look attractive if you have a suntan but tend to be rather ageing otherwise.

Application tips
To apply powder blusher, using a large, soft brush, start the colour on the 'apples', or fullest part of your cheeks, directly below the centre of your eyes.

Smile and dust the blusher over your cheek-bones, upwards and outwards. Fade the colour towards, but not into your hair-line.

Well applied, cream blusher can look very natural and fresh. Using the same sequence as described above, dab a couple of dots of colour on the apples of your cheeks and blend them well with either a damp sponge or fingertips, again using an upward and outward motion.

Quick blusher tips
- *If you find you have put on too much blusher, apply a light film of foundation – this will tone it down.*
- *Apply powder blusher over your foundation and powder. Apply cream blusher before your powder.*

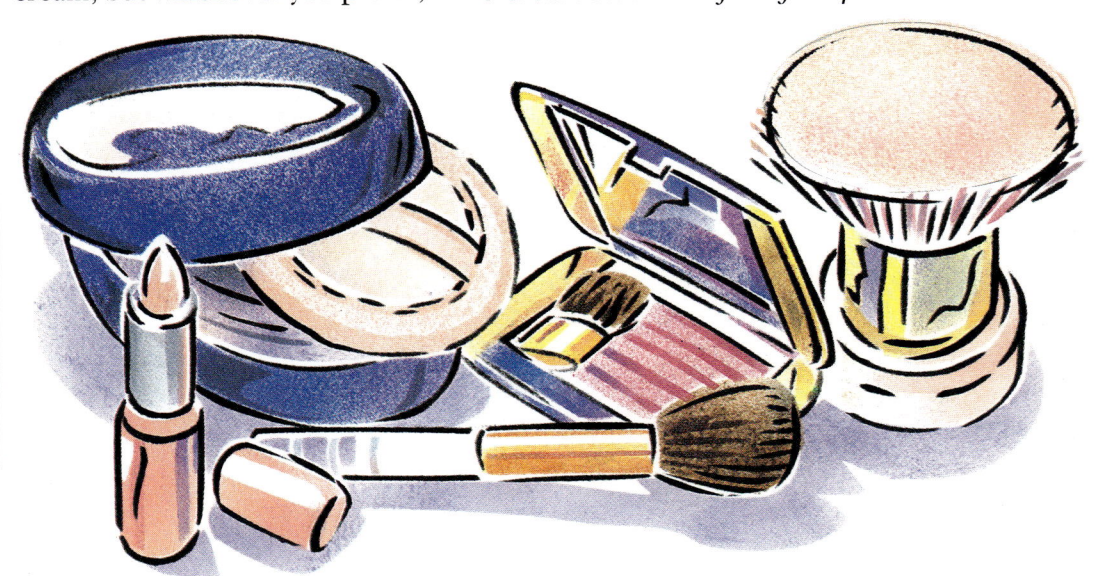

EYES RIGHT

Make the most of your eyes – choose colours that flatter and apply them so that they last.

We usually notice the eyes first when we look at someone. Whatever the colour and shape of your eyes, there are myriad ways to enhance their natural appeal.

COLOUR TRICKS

Whilst some people suggest choosing eyeshadow according to the colour of your eyes, many top make-up artists go by hair colour instead. The following are safe colour choices:
- for blondes: golden browns, taupe, lavender, apricot, light coral, black or charcoal grey (if smudged)
- for brunettes: plum browns, burgundy, black, aubergine, burnt red, deep brick, chocolate brown
- for redheads: corals, greens, blues, black or charcoal grey (if smudged), browns

Depending on where you put your eyeshadow, you can enhance and even slightly change the shape of your eyes. If your eyes are widely spaced, for example, use darker tones on the inner lid closest to your nose, and keep the colour light towards the outer corner of your eyes. You could also draw on a little colour from a pencil inside the lower lid at the inner corners. If your eyes are close together, simply reverse all this!

For bigger looking eyes, apply your shadow in a rounded shape, with the curved arc at the centre of your lids. Plenty of mascara on both top and bottom lashes completes the wide-eyed look. Should you wish to make very large eyes appear a little smaller, draw a dark brown pencil line inside your lashline, blink and reapply.

Unless you are absolutely smitten with an eyeshadow duo or trio, it's often best to buy eyeshadow singly, to avoid making an expensive mistake. Another tip: matte textures tend to be more classic choices, while shimmery, frosted shades go in and out of fashion.

Choose the right eyeshadow for the effect you want:
Pressed powder eyeshadows give excellent coverage and are useful for building up colour intensity; the colours also keep true during wear.
Loose eyeshadow powders tend to be pearly and slightly finer textured than pressed and are best used as highlighters or for a soft sheen.
Cream eyeshadow is by far the most difficult to use and it tends to sink into the crease of the socket-line after a few hours.

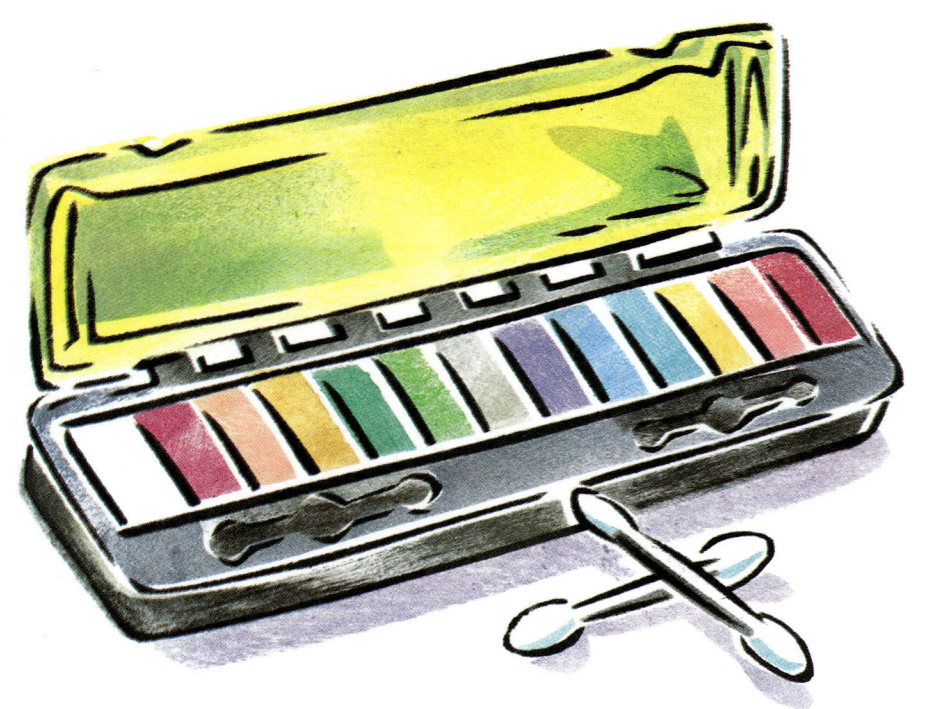

MASTERING MAKE-UP 79

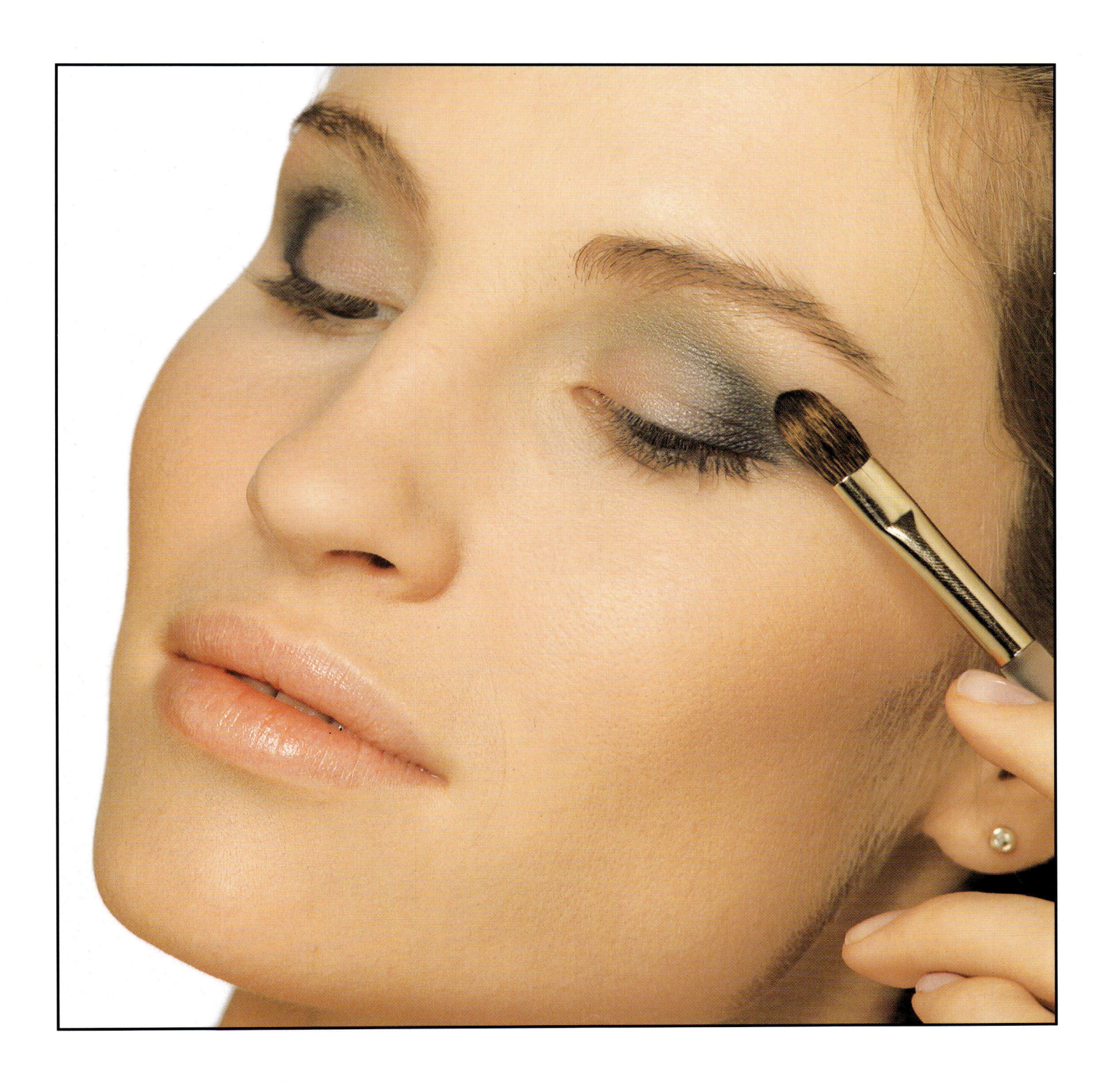

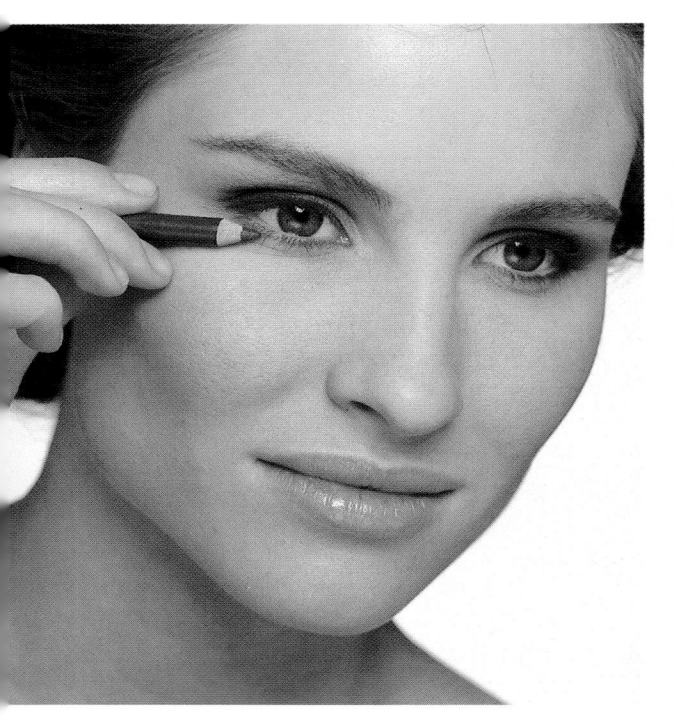

EYE-PENCIL

An eye-pencil gives instant emphasis to the eyes. It has most effect when you use it to draw a line close to your lashes (upper and/or lower) and then smudge the line with a soft brush. Beware of applying pencil or colour under the lower lashes if you look tired – it will only emphasise the fact.

Grey and brown are good for daytime, and, like eyeshadows, the more dramatic colours look great for evenings or sunny holidays.

EYELINER

Most eyeliners are fluid and you apply them with the brush provided in the cap. Well applied, liquid eyeliner gives a precise and very positive shape to the eye.

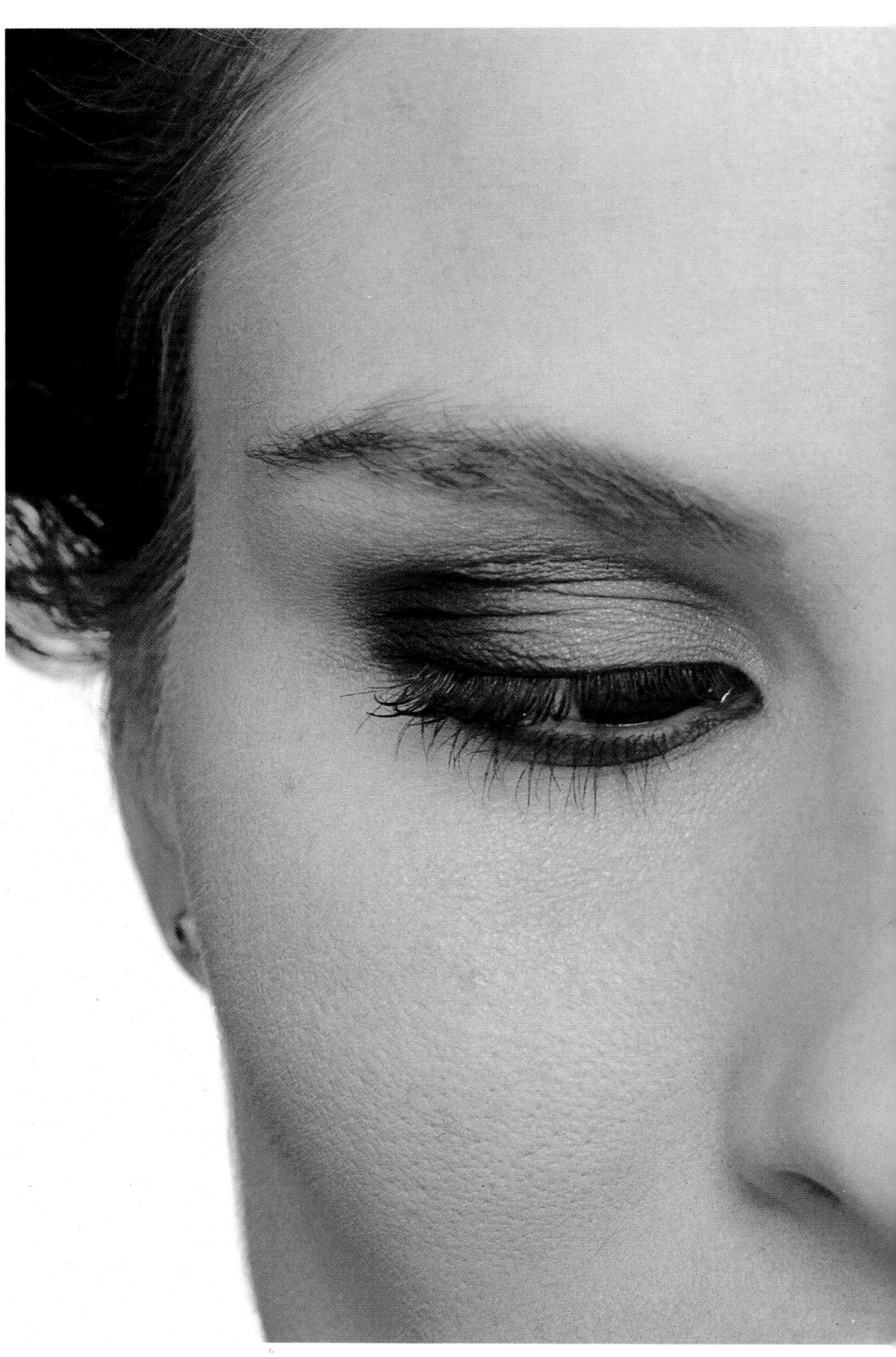

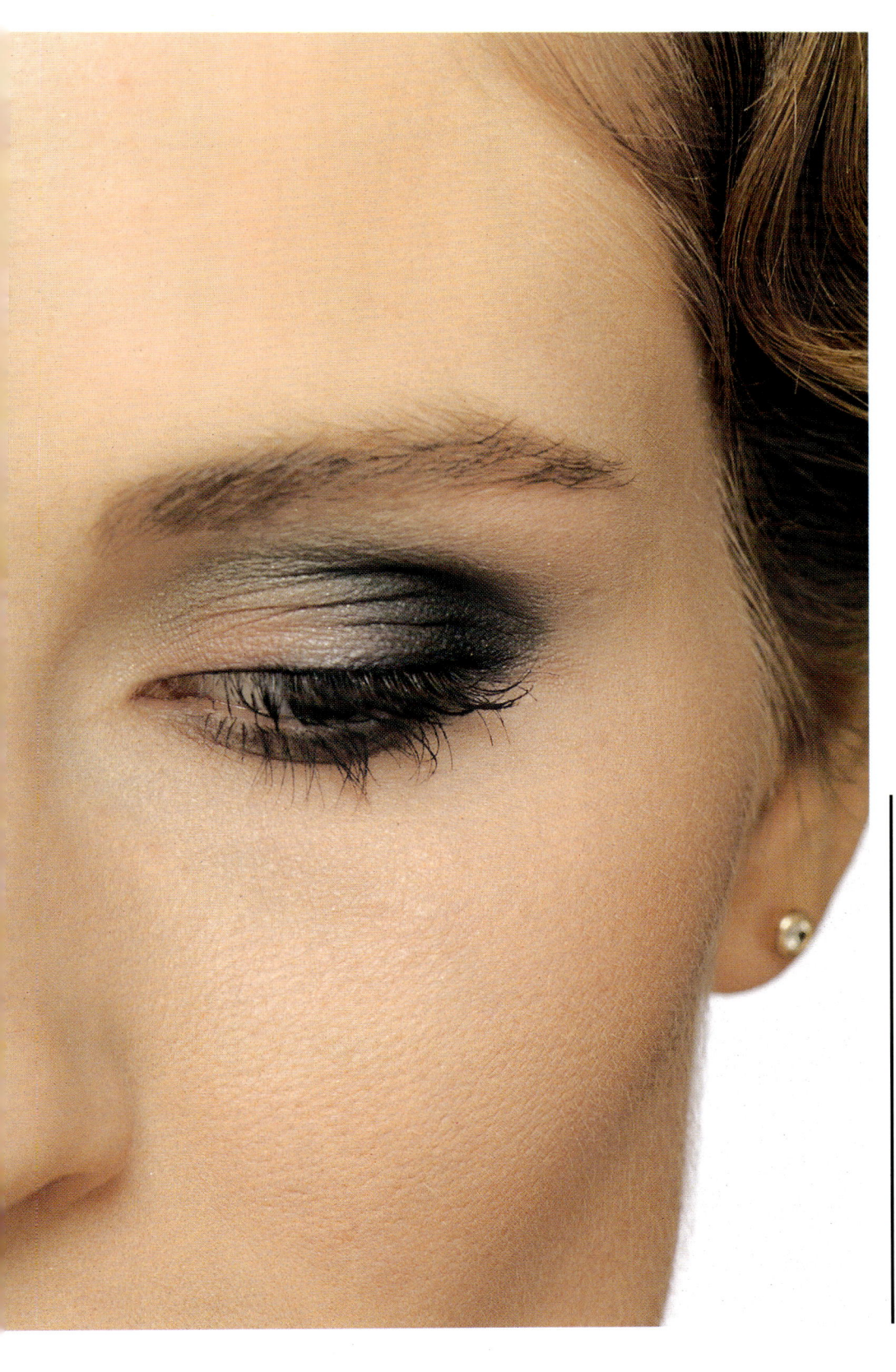

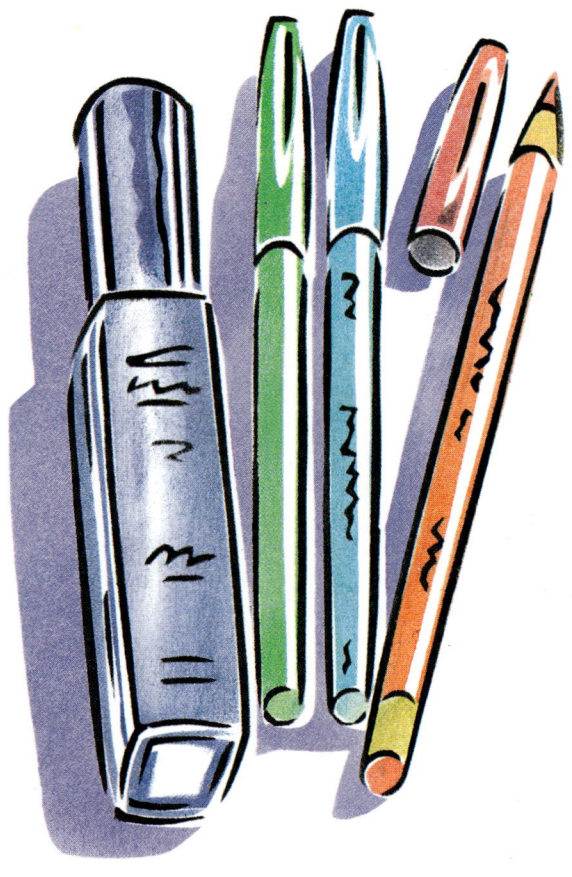

MASCARA

Normally two or three coats of mascara are ample. Comb through your lashes after the final coat so that they don't clump together.

Consider, too, having your eyelashes dyed at a salon. This looks very natural and, particularly for women with very fair lashes, saves time in your make-up routine.

Quick mascara tips
- *If your mascara is drying out, place it – sealed – on a radiator or into a beaker of warm water for a minute and you will get a couple of extra applications out of it.*
- *If you are in a rush, apply one coat of mascara to your upper lashes only. This will have the effect of instantly 'opening' your eyes.*

82 SHORT CUTS

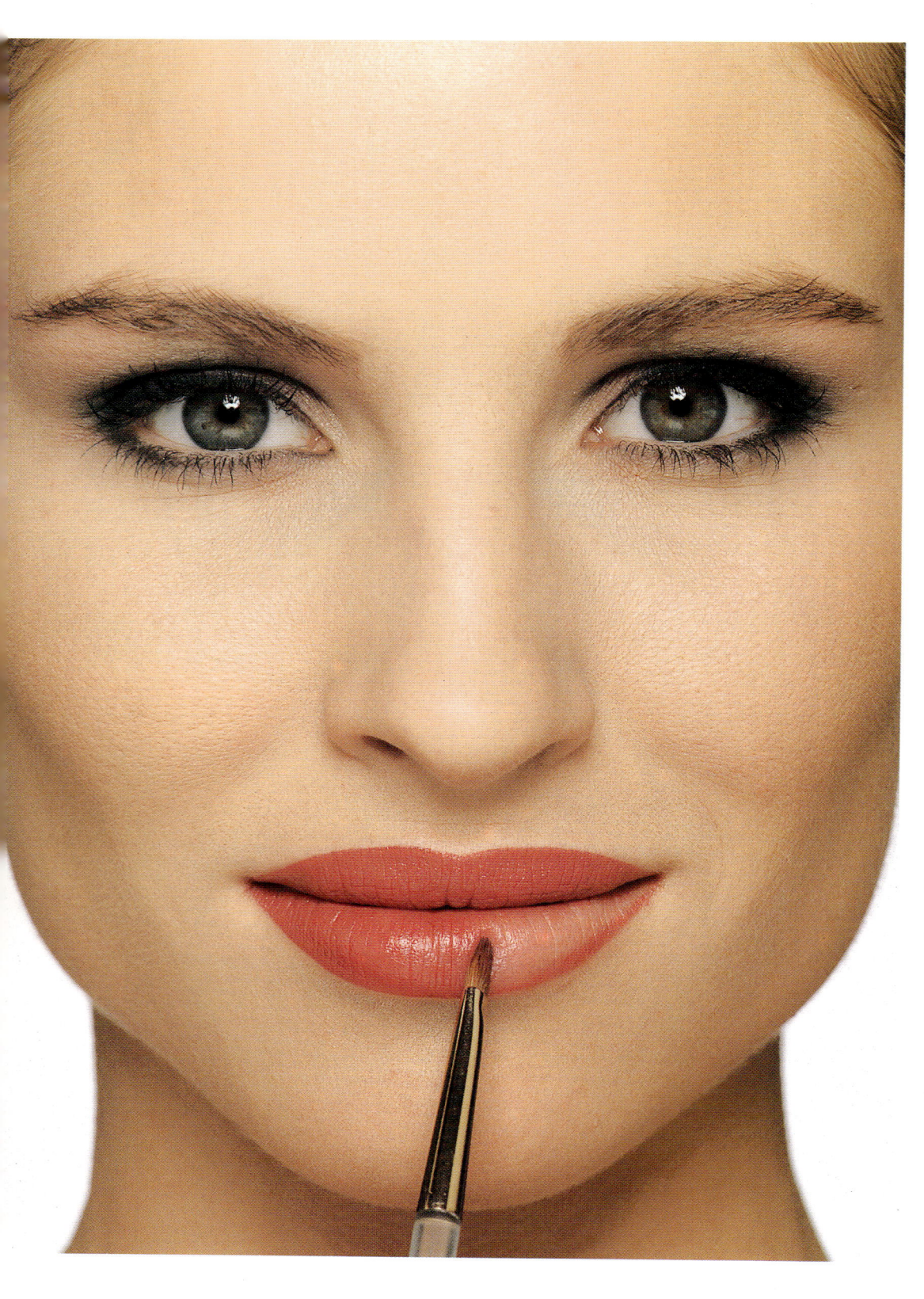

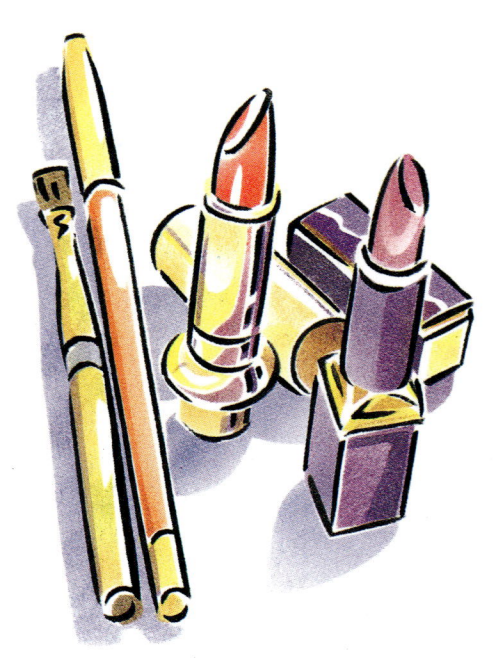

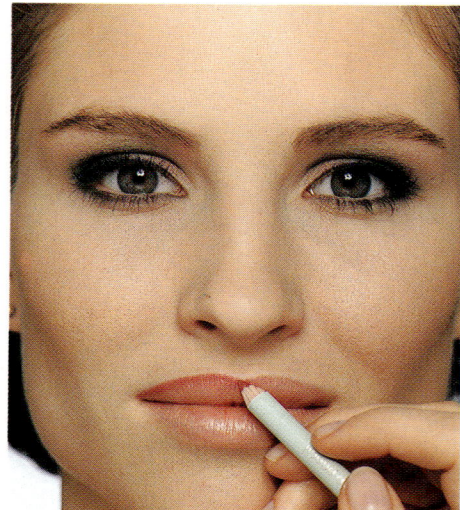

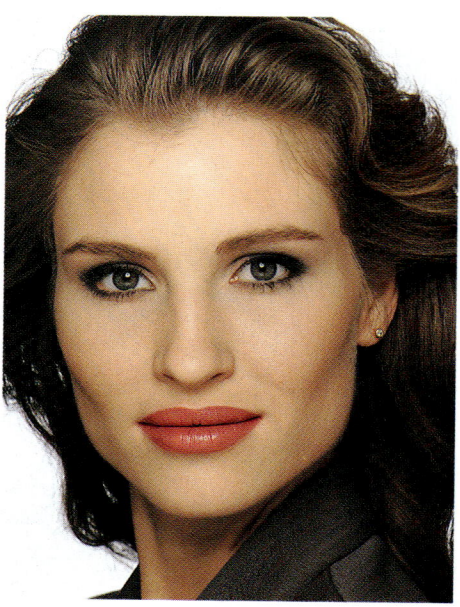

LIP SERVICE

Whether you choose palest pink or striking scarlet, here are the quickest lip tips for a perfect finish every time.

Research suggests that we choose a lip colour to reflect our moods – vibrant colours when we feel confident and want to be noticed, and paler shades when we feel introverted or even low.

Whether this is true or not, there is a cornucopia of products to colour and protect your lips – lipsticks, glosses, lip powders – many enhanced with moisturizers and ultraviolet filters. Whichever colour you choose, for whatever reason, remember these five tips:

- Before applying lip colour, prepare your lips with moisturizer or a specially designed lip primer, so that the colour goes on evenly and lasts longer without feathering.
- A lip brush gives a professional finish to your lips.
- It is not essential to use lip pencil (you can get a good finish with a primer and brush alone) but if you do want to use lip pencil, for instance with a very vibrant lipstick that needs a precise outline, it should be the same colour as the lipstick. With more neutral shades, opt for a lipliner close to your natural lip colour.
- Avoid frosted lipsticks as they rarely enhance your teeth or the shape of your mouth.
- Choose a lip colour to pull a look together, but, remember, as a general rule, blue-toned (rather than orange-toned) reds and pinks and browns will make your teeth appear whiter.

Before going out in the evening or for a special highly polished finish it is worth taking time over applying your lipstick.

Application tips

Begin by priming your lips with moisturizer and/or lip primer. If you are using a lip pencil, draw in your lip outline very carefully. The pencil shouldn't drag at your mouth, so warm it up slightly in the palm of your hand first to soften it. Try resting your little finger on your chin for balance.

Load your lip brush with colour and brush inwards from the corners of your mouth. To give your lips the Cupid's bow shape, lay the brush flat to paint a 'V' shape or curve.

Blot your lips with a tissue, dab on a little face powder and repeat with a second layer of colour.

If time is very tight, choose lipsticks that give a fairly sheer layer of colour. They are quick to apply straight from the lipstick bullet and do not need outlining or blotting.

TERRIFIC TEETH

A beautiful smile depends on healthy teeth. To achieve this, regular care is essential and this

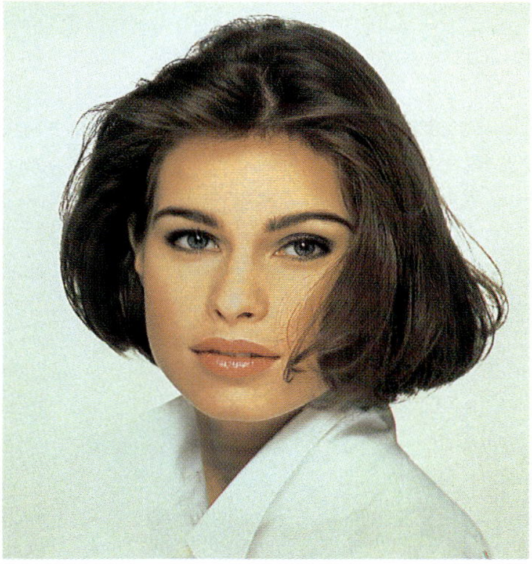

means choosing a good toothbrush. A toothbrush that has a small head is best because it will reach all your teeth and gum margins. Check too, that your brush has medium bristles with rounded ends.

Use dental floss every day to clean between your teeth, but be gentle and careful so as not to damage your gums.

Cosmetic dentistry has made a great deal possible:

- New materials mean that laminate veneers bonded to individual teeth don't pick up stains or plaque and last many years.
- White fillings are now much more widely available, replacing the silver-coloured ones.

5-MINUTE MAKE-UP

Neutral colours and simple techniques are the key to a super-quick make-up.

Here are the make-up tricks for the times when you have just a few minutes to put on a great face before you are due out of the door!

- First, plan your make-up colours to complement your clothes – lipstick, blusher and eyeshadow should all be in similar sheer tones.
- Short cut: you can buy 2-in-1 products that will work for cheeks and lips, or cheeks and eyes, to make life even simpler.
- If you wear foundation, use the sheerest base you have. Apply it using your fingertips or a slightly damp make-up sponge to clean and moisturized skin.
- Next, outline eyes with a soft brown pencil and blend the line with an eyeshadow applicator.
- One coat of mascara is sufficient. You can apply it to the top lashes only if you like.
- Defining your eyebrows immediately gives your face more impact. Use powder applied with a brush or a sharp brow pencil.
- Just a touch of powder blush is all you need for a 5-minute make-up. The secret is to sweep it on using a big blusher brush.
- Take a little loose, translucent powder onto a velour puff and dab it onto the back of your hand to remove any excess. Now press over the whole of your face to set your make-up and to prevent shine.
- Translucent lipsticks that allow the texture and colour of your own lips to show through look the most natural and are the fastest to apply. Lip-coloured shades also require less precision and so need less time to apply. No liplining pencil is required. Voila!

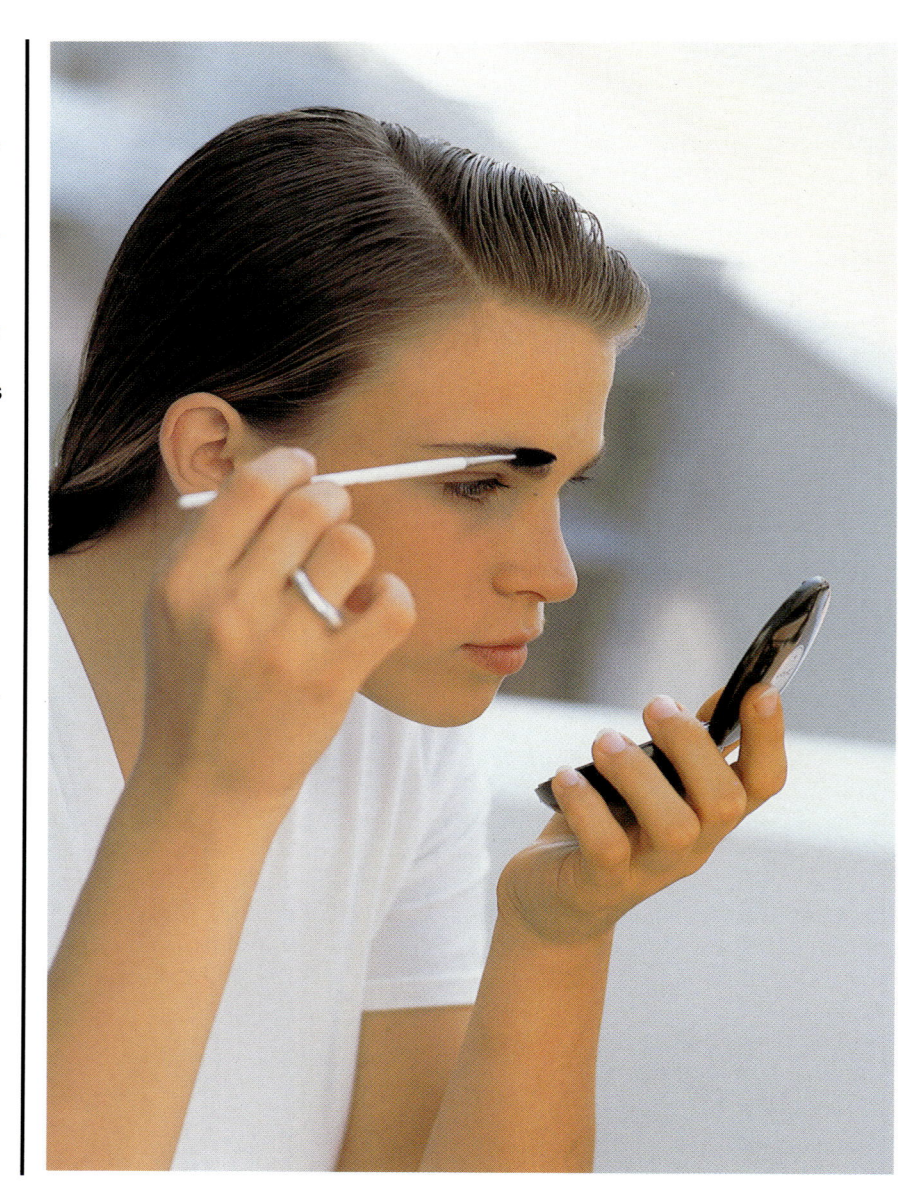

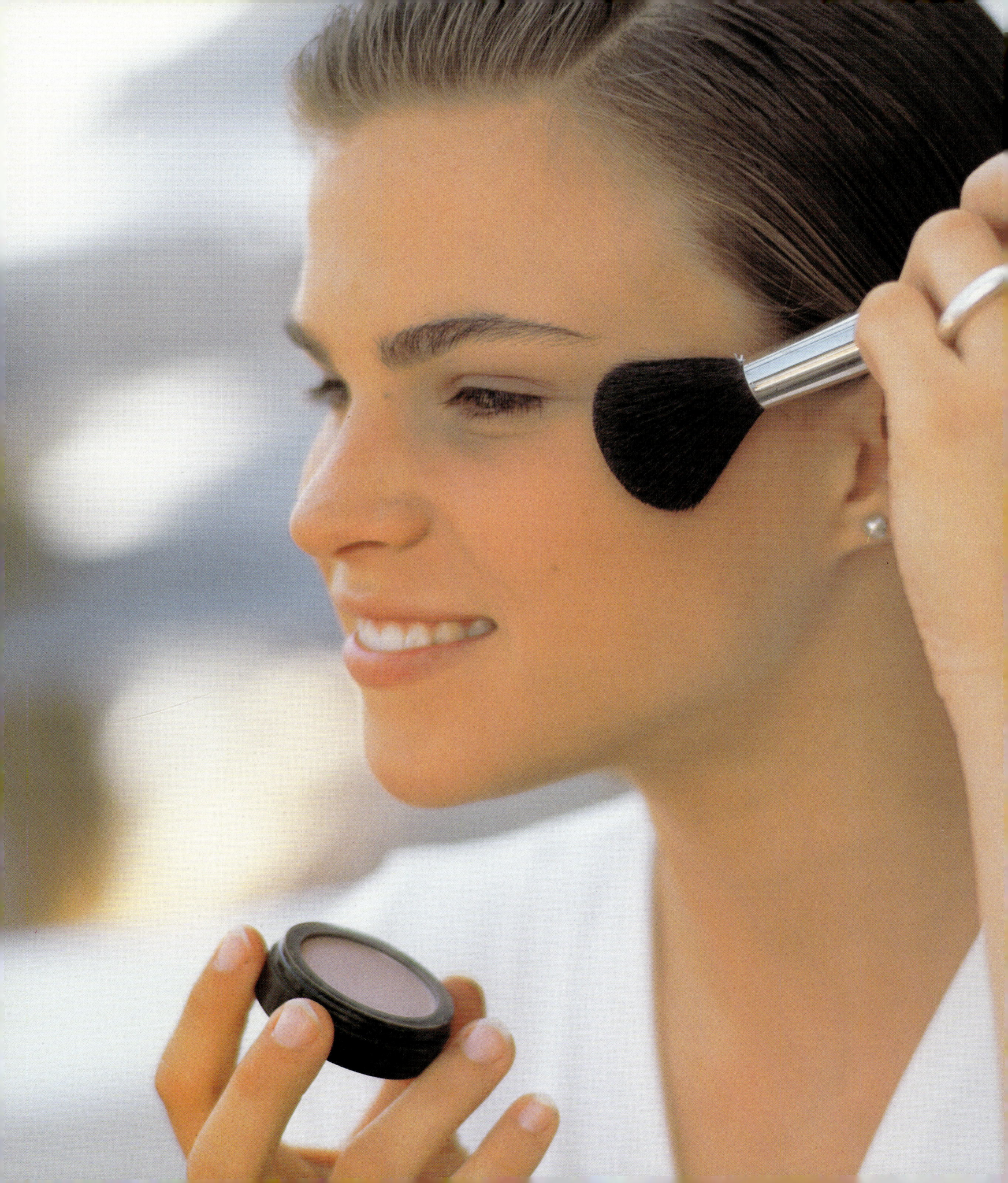

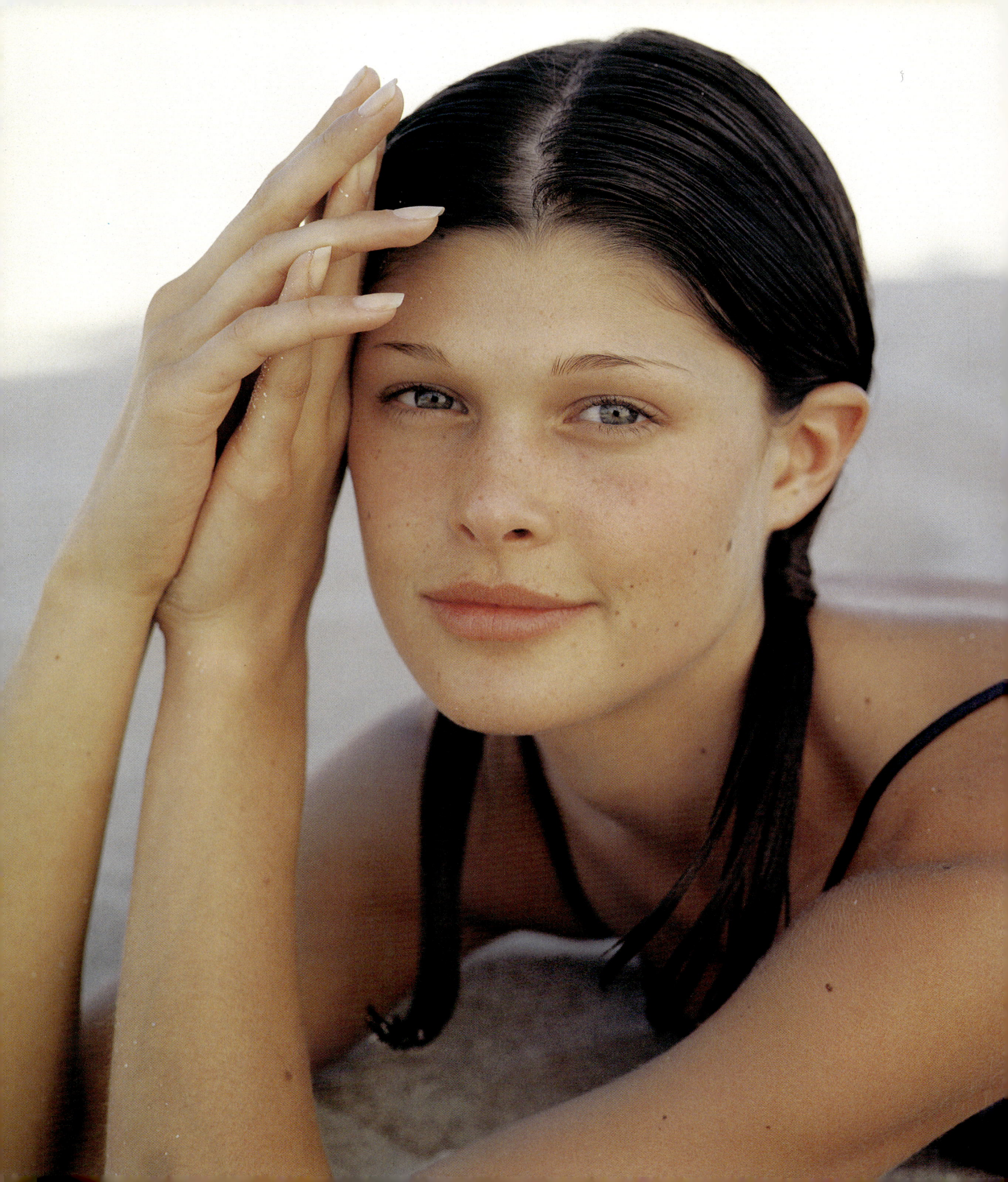

THE NATURAL LOOK

If you're looking for the fresh glow that looks right in the open air, here's a step-by-step guide to the perfect shades.

When you are on the beach, out in the country or up in the mountains, make-up can look too obvious, particularly in bright daylight. Enter the look that says 'this is bare-faced chic', the no make-up make-up that gives your complexion a very subtle glow.

It is important to use a moisturizer that contains UVA and UVB filters, ideally one with an SPF of 15.

Tinted moisturizer or a tinted gel is the ideal base (provided your skin doesn't have open pores or blemishes). Bronzing powders can work, too, if they are matte. Both tinted moisturizers and bronzers are now widely available in a range of colours, from pale beige to deep tan.

Cream or gel blusher is an essential part of the barely-there style unless you already have a natural flush to your cheeks. You should apply it very sparingly to the apples of the cheeks (instead of to the cheekbones) in a soft circle and then gently blend it out with the fingertips.

Keep mascara to the minimum and choose brown rather than black unless you have naturally dark lashes. A clear mascara, which thickens the lashes and gives them a gloss, is a good alternative and can also be used to define the eyebrows.

A touch of soft brown or taupe shadow can shape the eyes, although you may prefer to keep your lids bare.

It is important that lipsticks only enhance what is already there. Pick a supersheer shade and blot it well, after applying it direct from the tube or by dabbing the colour on with your fingertips, to stain the lips subtly with colour.

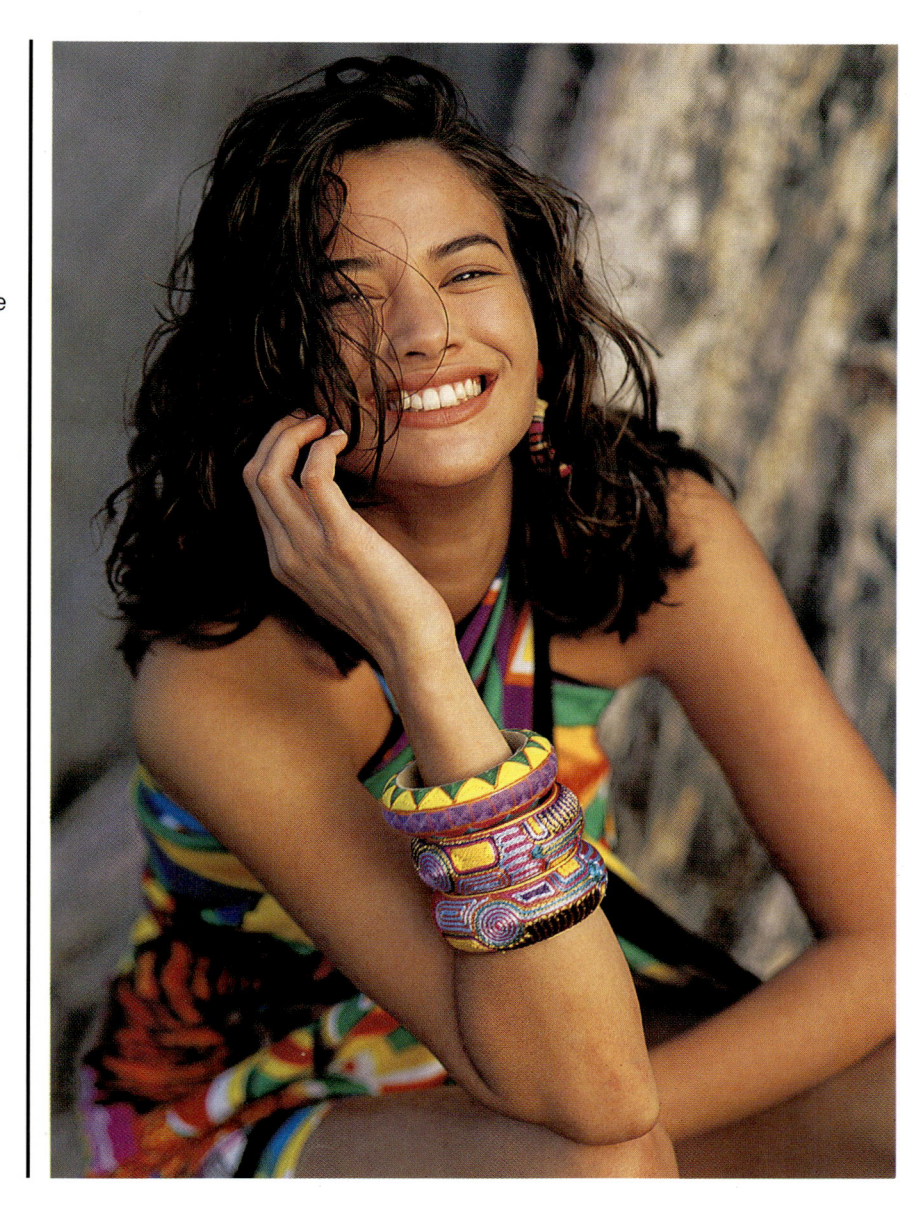

THE CLASSIC FACE

Soft and beautifully balanced, the classic make-up uses face-flattering colours to give a timeless look.

The perfect beauty of a classic make-up takes a little more time to achieve. You need to follow a few ground rules.

The essence of this timeless style is a smooth and perfect-as-porcelain skin.

Using a foundation that gives a little more coverage, apply it with a very slightly damp make-up sponge (first squeezed out well in a towel). Remember to apply it over your eye lids and lips and to take it just under your chin (blending away towards your neck).

Now apply a little concealer around your nose and under your eyes, pressing it well into your skin and blending it in.

Sweep on blusher, high on your cheekbones, in an upwards direction towards (but not into) your hairline.

A velvety finish to the skin is important. Press on plenty of soft, fine, loose powder all over the face and then dust off any excess using a big powder brush.

Use two shades of semi-matte or matte eyeshadow (semi-matte is easier to apply) to give shape to the eyes. You can try using a paler shade on the lid and a deeper colour in the socket line.

The classic look calls for plenty of mascara to lengthen the top lashes particularly.

Don't forget to treat your eyebrows to the full works. Emphasise them first with brow pencil and then blend the strokes using a foam smudger at the other end of an eyeshadow applicator.

Now outline your lips with a lip pencil that matches your lipstick, choosing a classic hue such as rosewood or cappuccino, to complete the classic look.

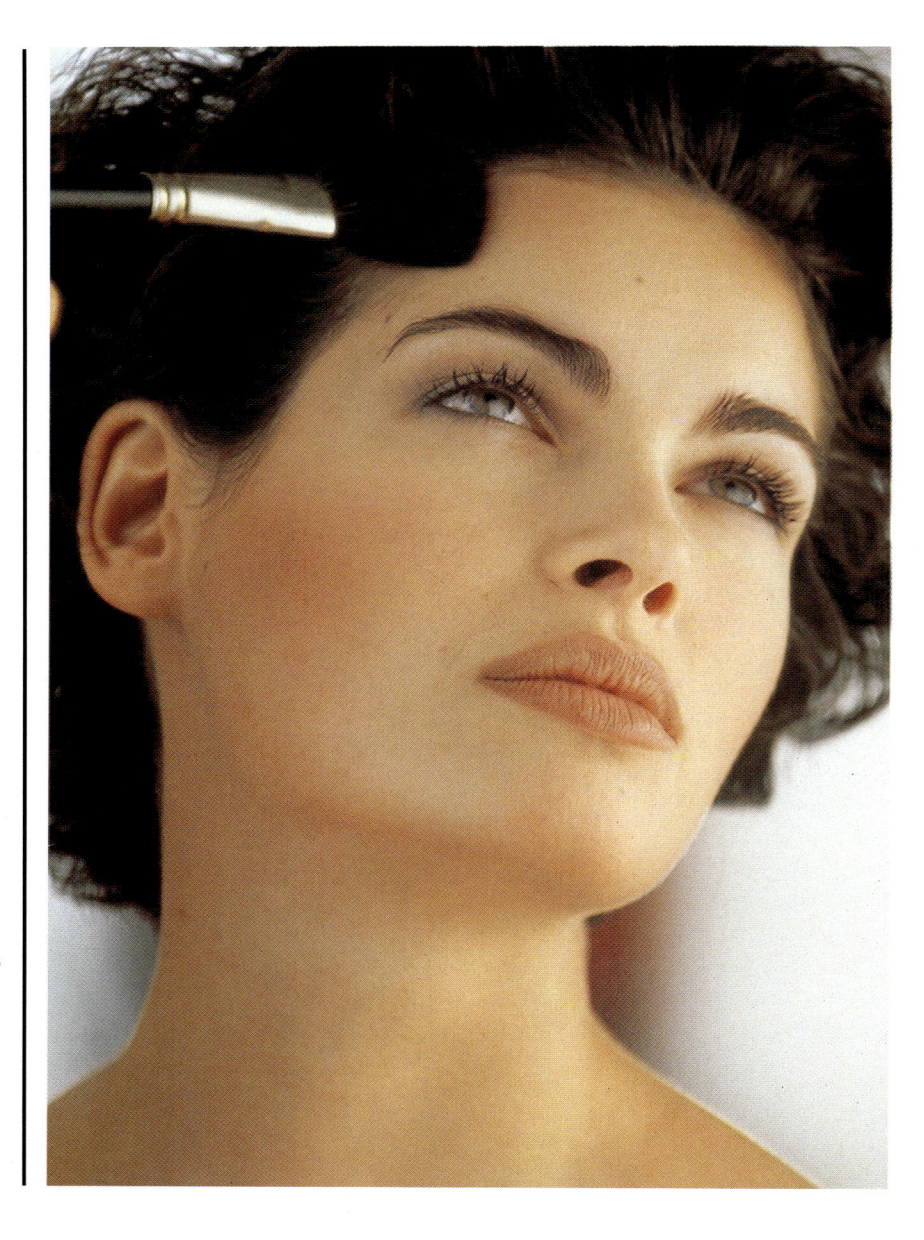

MASTERING MAKE-UP 89

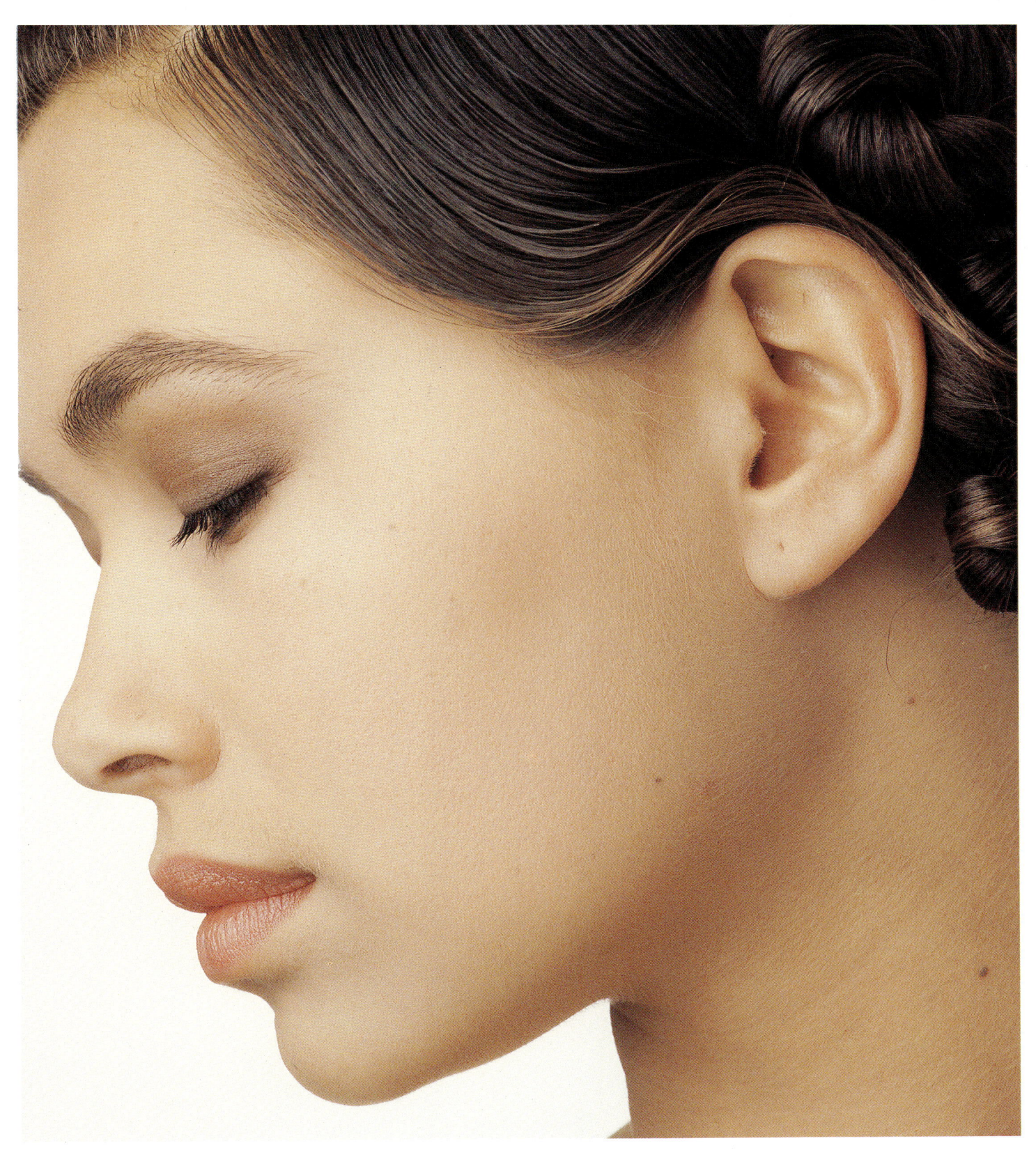

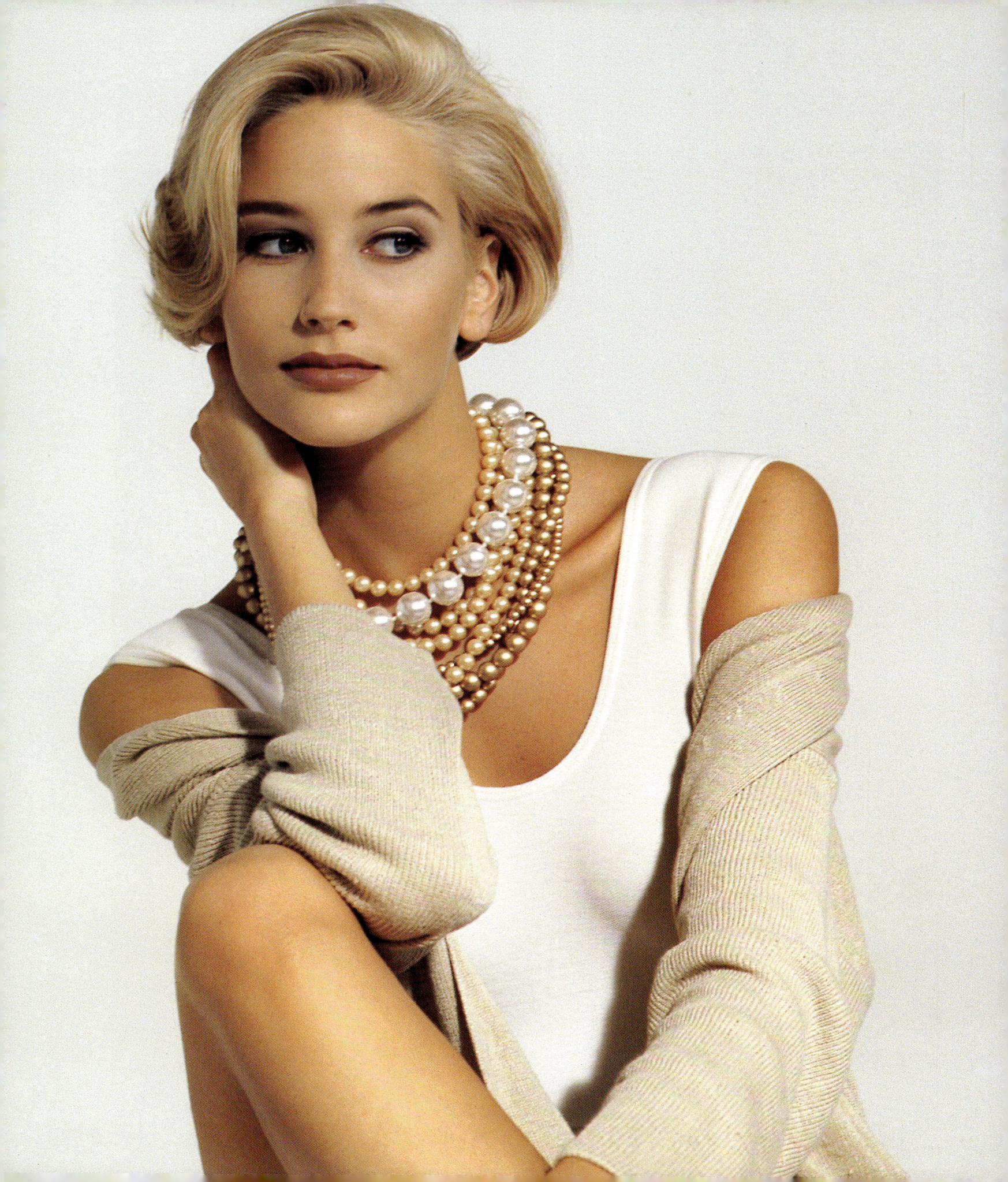

MODERN GLAMOUR

When 'natural' is too low-key, and self-assured and dynamic are your buzz-words, modern glamour is the look for you.

At first glance, yes, it's a made-up look. But look again and you'll see that this style is perfectly balanced. There's no garish technicolour, but a harmony of colour and shading. Here are the keys to achieving this contemporary finish.

The base
Begin with a clean, moisturized face that you've blotted with a tissue to lift away any excess moisturizer. Foundation, or at least tinted moisturizer, is essential to give an even-textured flawless look to your skin. A make-up artist we work with on *Cosmopolitan* suggests this trick for a sheer, cover-girl style finish: once you've applied your foundation, gently splash your face with warm water, then carefully pat dry with tissues. It sounds unusual, but it works! Next apply a loose, translucent powder with a large brush.

Eyes
Colours from the brown spectrum suit everyone. Try keeping the lids and browbone light and use darker shades in the socket line. The secret with eyeshadow is to blend with brushes, using just a little colour at first. You can add more to build up colour density. To help eyeshadow last longer, you can put foundation over the eye area. A dusting of loose powder under the eyes will catch any loose shadow particles. All you have to do is brush it away once you've applied your eyeshadow.

Use brown pencil for extra definition close to the lash lines and mascara on either top and bottom lashes or just on top. Go for black mascara if you have black or dark brown hair and brown if your hair is red, blonde or light brown.

Groomed eyebrows are vital to the modern glamour look. Aim for a classic arched curve. An eyebrow pencil can help fill in any gaps and accentuate the natural shape.

Cheeks
To add a healthy glow and shape to your face, apply blusher over the apples of your cheeks. Go for tawny, peach, apricot and browny shades. If you are using powder blusher, shake the excess off the brush before applying it. Always keep a light touch so you have a hint of colour rather than stripes! To finish, dust your blusher brush down each side of your nose, under your chin and over your temples. This will add an extra glow.

Lips
A strong lipstick is glamorous and attention-grabbing. It's also a sign of confidence. A perfect red looks great. It's high maintenance though and needs regular checking for feathering. Pinky brown, brownish red and orange shades suit most women.

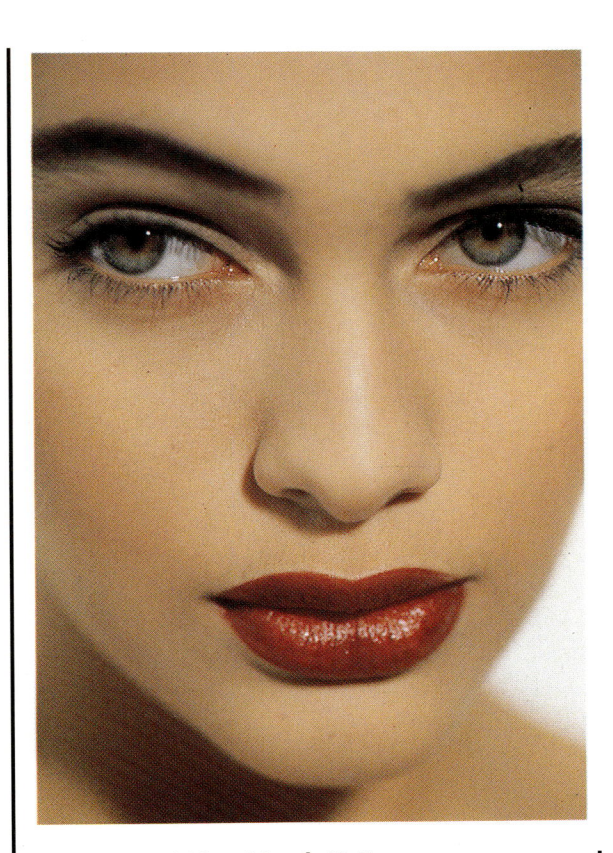

Nails
To complete the groomed, glamorous look, check your nails. Short, well-maintained nails always look good. If you don't like the idea of coloured varnish, just paint them with a clear polish so they shine.

WORKING GIRL

Make-up is an essential tool in creating a professional appearance. Take our short cuts to a super-successful face.

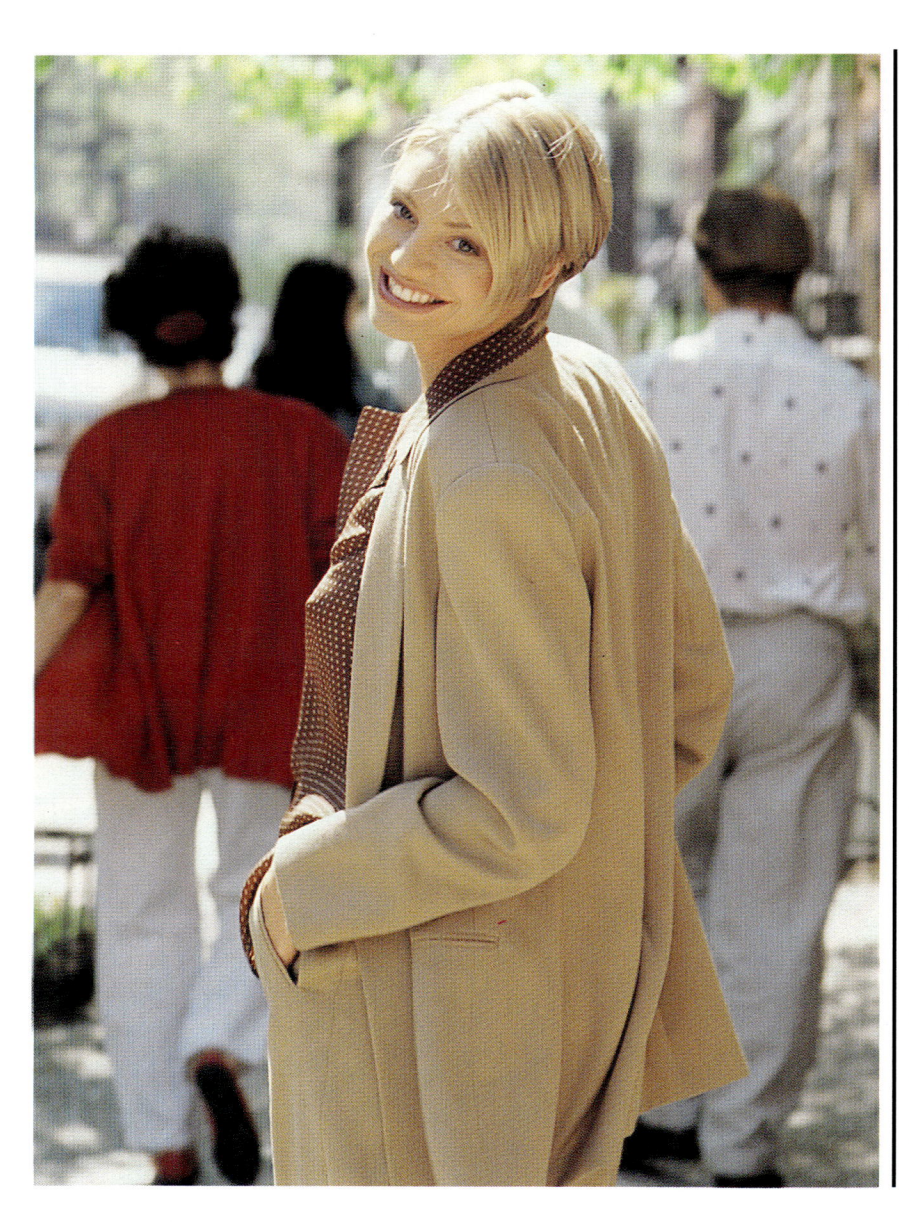

Make-up is a proven way to create both an immediate and a lasting impression in the minds of those around you.

Research has shown that people find women who wear make-up and whose hair is well-groomed and styled to be more capable, more confident and more interesting than those who do neither!

Obviously, it is important that this working image is within the framework of certain criteria, that is, not too extreme or overtly glamorous in what is a professional situation.

The key to a creating a successful image lies in striking a balance.

Work basics
Begin with a moisturizer that contains UVA and UVB filters as UVA light is skin-ageing and present constantly.

Complexion-wise, you want to avoid joining the shiny set, so if your T-zone tends to be oily, apply a blotting lotion on top of your moisturizer. These lotions are usually slightly tinted liquids that contain suspended particles of powder that act like blotting paper beneath your regular foundation or face powder. You can apply them just where you need them, rather than all over.

A natural-looking base gives a working girl the edge. Try one of the contemporary foundation-and-powder-in-one mixes which do both jobs effectively and can be quickly retouched during the day. The compacts contain a latex sponge to apply the base – the sponge doesn't need to be dampened first.

Use eyeshadows that pick up on the colours in your clothes,

playing the shades down rather than up, and keep the application techniques simple. A touch of eye pencil is long-lasting and won't need maintaining during the day. Check that your mascara is smudge-proof and that it defines the lashes without making them look thick or clogged with make-up. If your mascara tends to smudge under your eyes, try applying it to the top lashes only or consider using a waterproof type.

Keep blusher to the minimum – you may prefer to skip it altogether.

Lipsticks are often most effective when they are in strong, matte shades and so are more assertive: try true reds, burgundies, deep or rust browns. Avoid paler shades like pastel pink or peach, particularly when they are glossy or frosted.

Remember to check that your nails are manicured and also add polish. A transparent top coat is enough to give your hands that important cared-for look.

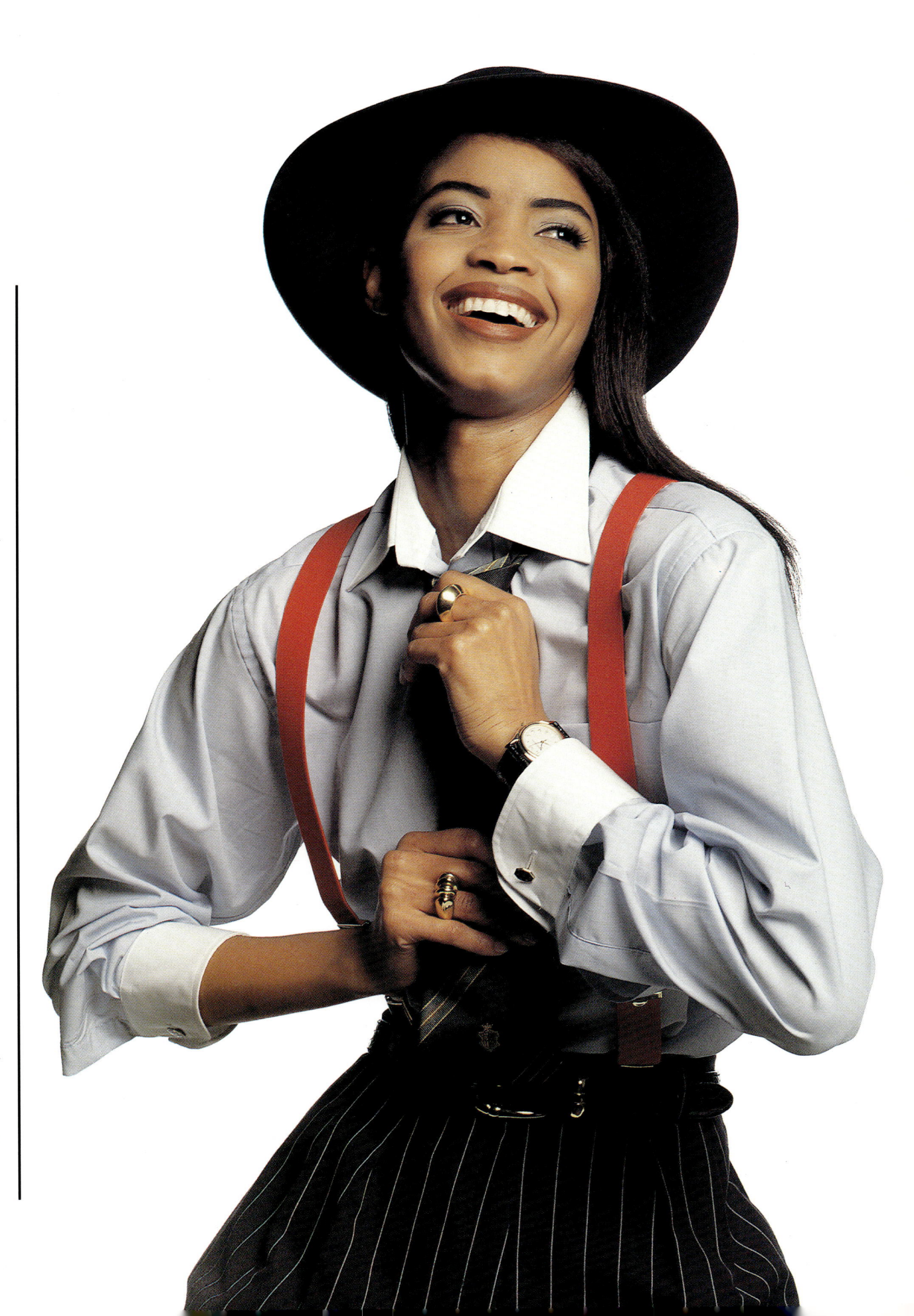

COSMOPOLITAN COLOURS

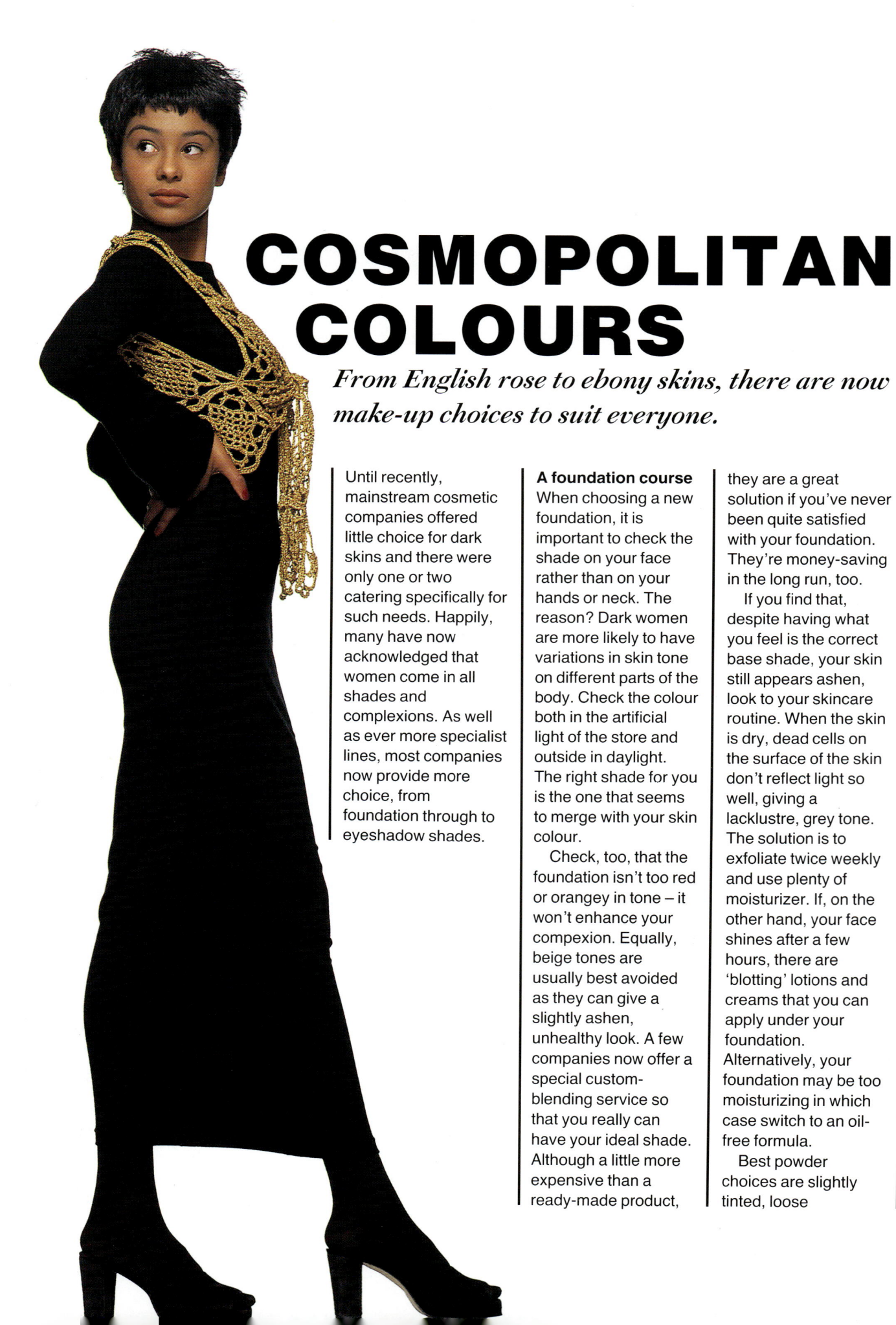

From English rose to ebony skins, there are now make-up choices to suit everyone.

Until recently, mainstream cosmetic companies offered little choice for dark skins and there were only one or two catering specifically for such needs. Happily, many have now acknowledged that women come in all shades and complexions. As well as ever more specialist lines, most companies now provide more choice, from foundation through to eyeshadow shades.

A foundation course
When choosing a new foundation, it is important to check the shade on your face rather than on your hands or neck. The reason? Dark women are more likely to have variations in skin tone on different parts of the body. Check the colour both in the artificial light of the store and outside in daylight. The right shade for you is the one that seems to merge with your skin colour.

Check, too, that the foundation isn't too red or orangey in tone – it won't enhance your compexion. Equally, beige tones are usually best avoided as they can give a slightly ashen, unhealthy look. A few companies now offer a special custom-blending service so that you really can have your ideal shade. Although a little more expensive than a ready-made product, they are a great solution if you've never been quite satisfied with your foundation. They're money-saving in the long run, too.

If you find that, despite having what you feel is the correct base shade, your skin still appears ashen, look to your skincare routine. When the skin is dry, dead cells on the surface of the skin don't reflect light so well, giving a lacklustre, grey tone. The solution is to exfoliate twice weekly and use plenty of moisturizer. If, on the other hand, your face shines after a few hours, there are 'blotting' lotions and creams that you can apply under your foundation. Alternatively, your foundation may be too moisturizing in which case switch to an oil-free formula.

Best powder choices are slightly tinted, loose

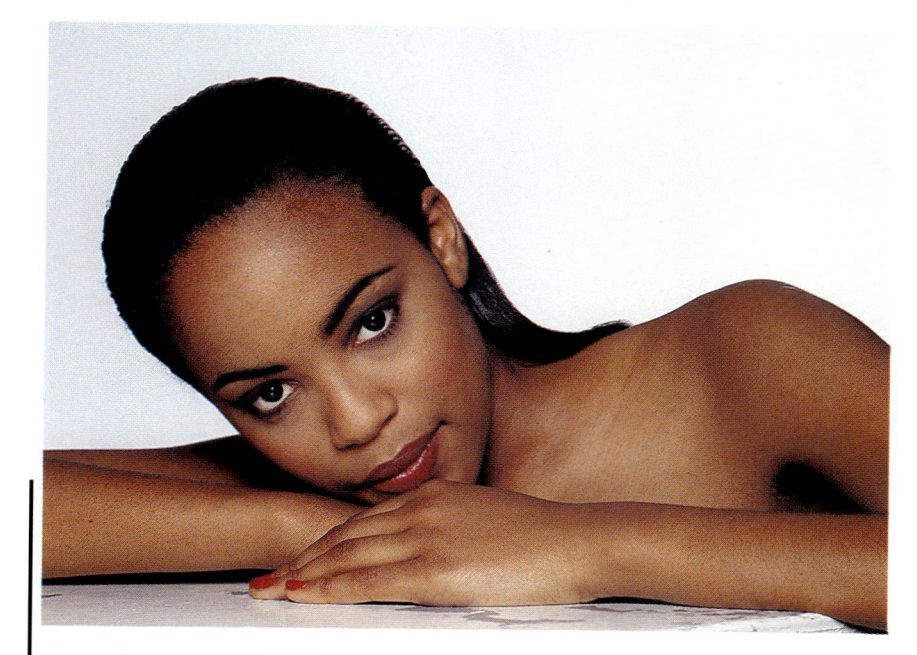

formulations which give a matte finish without appearing too 'chalky'.

Colour code

If you're dark, you can probably wear just about any eyeshadow colour. For subtle daytime make-up, browns and navy look great, with a lighter, highlighting shade on the browbones. Bright, glitzy colours are best kept for evening. Watch the balance of colour on your face. Strong lips (red or orangey) look right with neutral or dark-coloured eyes. But if your eyeshadow is bright, keep your lips less obvious, with say a pinky-brown shade, burgundy or plum. Choose black for mascara and eye liners or pencil – brown will just fade away.

Depending on your exact skin tone and total choice of make-up colours, opt for blusher with red, plum or brick tones. Keep it light, though, so your cheek-bones are enhanced rather than covered with colour. Bronzing powder works beautifully on black skin. Dust it over your cheek-bones, around your temples, down your nose and over your chin. Watch that it isn't too sparkly with silvery particles. Gold sheen from powders and shadows can look amazing, however. It picks up the yellow undertones in the skin and reflects light flatteringly off the face. Use very light gold along the cheekbones and down the bridge of the nose, plus a light touch in the centre of the chin. Teamed with browns and oranges for eyeshadow, blush and lipstick (and also mixed in with them – try a smudge of highlighting gold in the centre of your bottom lip), gold creates a warm, healthy look.

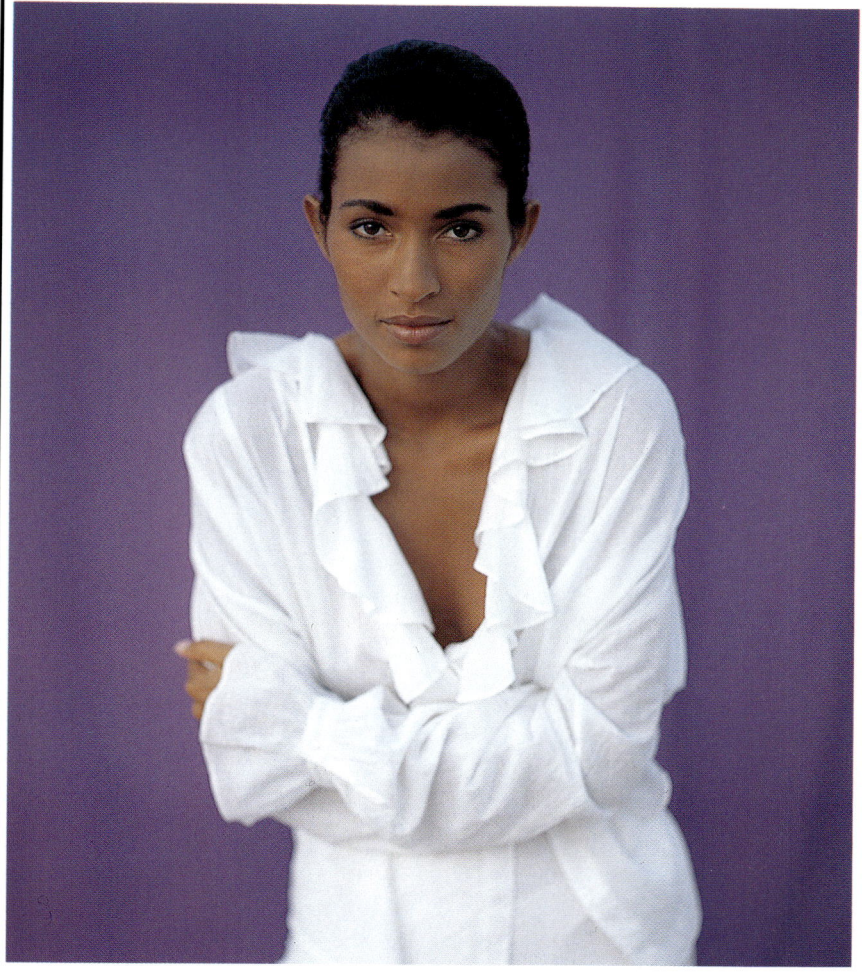

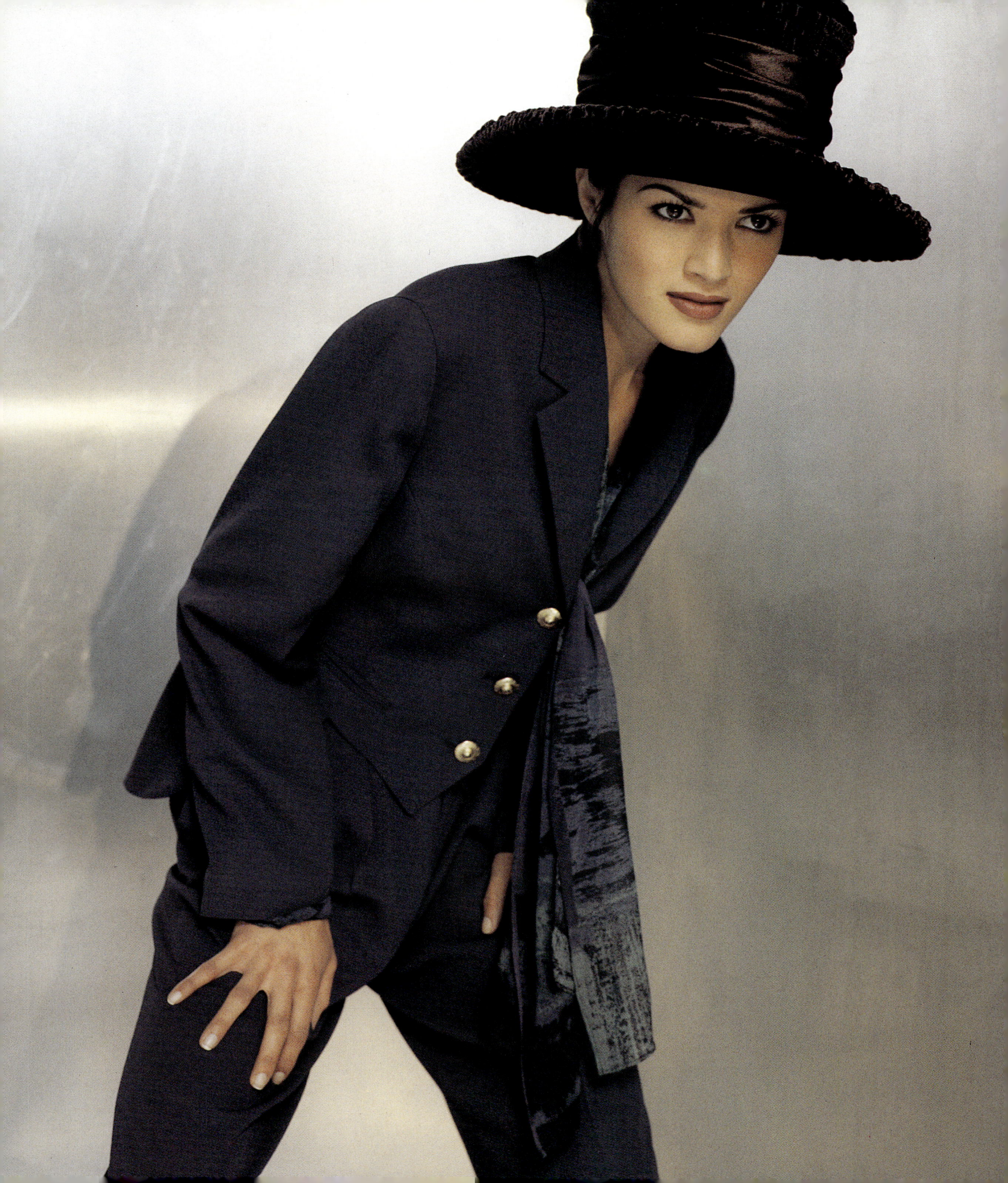

PARTY TIME

Discover how to create a glamorous evening face – it's your chance to pull out all the stops!

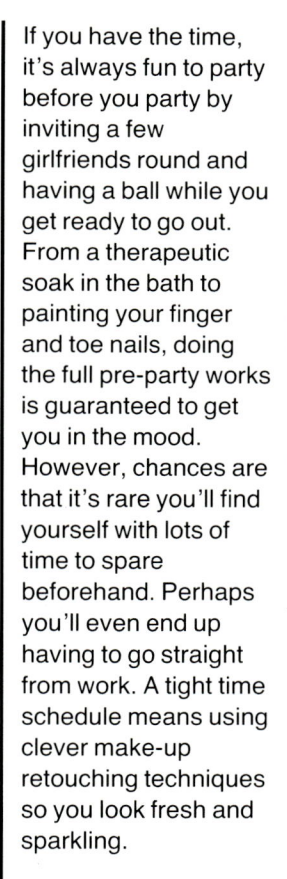

If you have the time, it's always fun to party before you party by inviting a few girlfriends round and having a ball while you get ready to go out. From a therapeutic soak in the bath to painting your finger and toe nails, doing the full pre-party works is guaranteed to get you in the mood. However, chances are that it's rare you'll find yourself with lots of time to spare beforehand. Perhaps you'll even end up having to go straight from work. A tight time schedule means using clever make-up retouching techniques so you look fresh and sparkling.

Day-into-night tips

- Start by blotting the T-zone (forehead, nose, chin and, if your skin is oily, the cheeks, too) to remove shine. You can also use a dry make-up sponge to 'lift' foundation, powder and blusher from your face. Use a cotton bud to remove eye make-up and wipe away any mascara smudges. With a tissue and a dab of Vaseline, wipe off your lip colour. If your lips are dry and flaky, use an old dampened tooth-brush to work gently over your mouth. Finally, a quick spritz of mineral water mist will refresh and hydrate your face.
- Compact foundations, of which there are many on the market, are ideal for touch-ups. You may find, however, that a light dusting of powder is all you need.
- When reapplying make-up, it's a good idea to use slightly darker shades than those you used during the day. Do blend well and use a light hand as heavy make-up can make you look less than fresh. If you are tired, do check that your eye make-up isn't too dark as it will accentuate the fact. To 'open up' the eye area, keep the shadow light and neutral, but apply a little highlighter as a small dot in the centre of your upper lids and on the browbone. Then brush your brows up and out.
- Mascara is simple to reapply. You'll probably find that just applying it to the tips of your lashes is enough. If it has become clogged, try gently pinching your lashes with your fingertips – excess fibres should then come away.
- For born-again blusher, try to think in terms of light and shade as opposed to adding colour. Evening light may make colour disappear, but sculpted cheekbones will look great. Many cosmetic companies are now offering blusher products with sculpting in mind. They usually consist of a deep matte shade and a highlighting tone. The darker shade simply goes under the cheekbones to shape, while the highlighter is stroked along the top of the cheekbones. If you still feel you want actual colour, just add a dusting of your regular blusher colour.
- Before applying lip colour, prime your lips with a little moisturizer or specialised lip-fixing product. Then blot with a tissue. A bright shade, such as red, pink or orange, gives an instant lift whether you choose a matte or glossy finish.

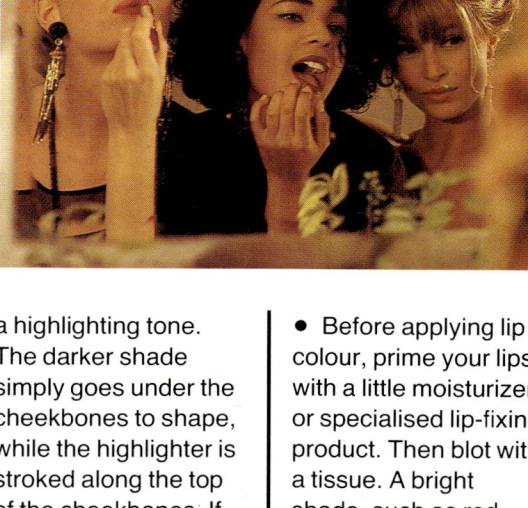

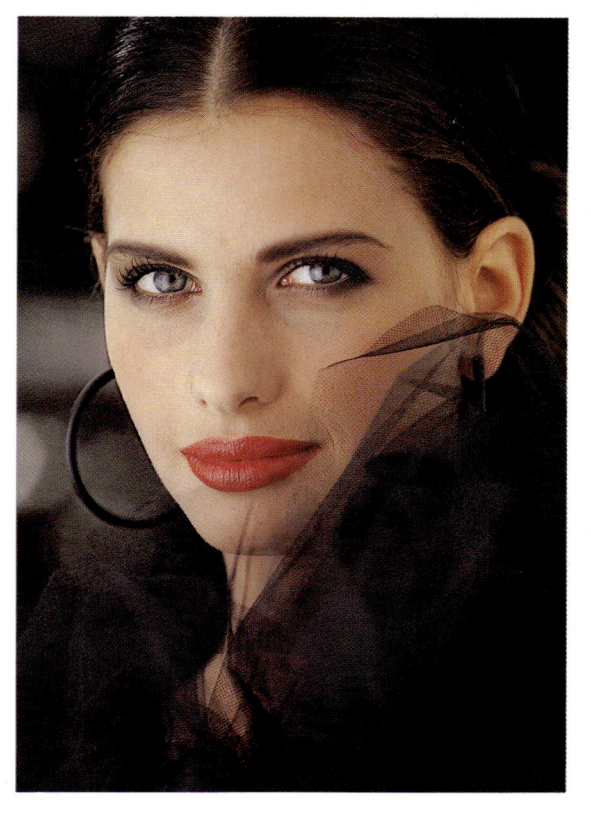

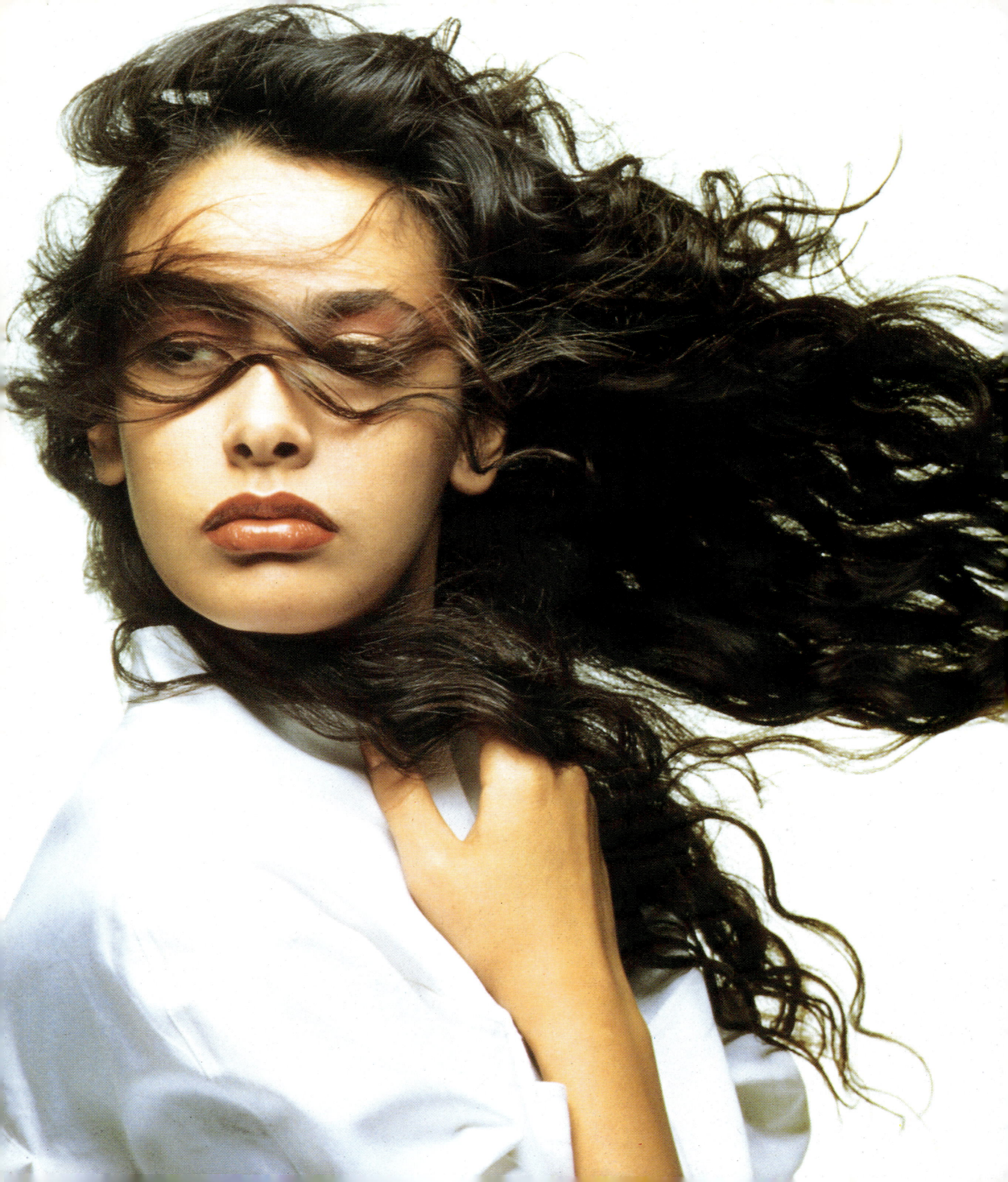

HAIRCARE

*Your hair is your most versatile beauty asset.
You can change its style, colour and shape, temporarily or
permanently, often altering your image quite dramatically.
It's important to be aware of your hair type and to look
after your crowning glory accordingly, to keep it
in peak condition. Remember that beautiful hair
is healthy hair, full of bounce and shine.*

HAIR BASICS 100
HAIR TYPING 102
HAIR PROBLEMS 104
CUTTING CLEVER 106
COLOUR SENSE 108
PERMANENT SOLUTIONS 112
SHAPE AND STYLE 114
TWISTS, PLAITS AND ROLLS 116

HAIR BASICS

Wise up on fundamental haircare – it will save you time in the long run.

There are haircare tactics and products that can noticeably improve the appearance and manageability of your hair. Follow this step-by-step guide to giving your hair the best treatment, from start to finish.

HAIR FACTS

On average hair grows about 2.5 cm (1 in) per month, with the strongest growth period for women being between the ages of 14 and 40, when you also produce the most oestrogen. But your hair never stops growing, it just slows down as you get older.

A strand of hair is made up of three layers, the medulla, cortex and cuticle.

The medulla runs the length of the hair shaft, but is often broken at intervals and sometimes people with fine hair have no medulla at all. Its exact purpose is unknown, though its presence or absence seems to make little difference to what you can do with your hair.

The cortex makes up between 75 and 90 per cent of the hair shaft, containing cells that affect the elasticity and strength of your hair and pigments giving it its colour.

The outer layer, the cuticle, is made of flat, overlapping scales that provide a protective covering for the other layers. When these scales lie flat, light bounces off them easily, making the hair look shiny.

The hairs grow out of follicles in the scalp, at the base of which lie the papillae. These absorb nutrients from the blood supply. As soon as a new hair surfaces from the follicle, through the skin, the cells die and harden (keratinize). All visible hair is then, in effect, dead.

A DIET FOR YOUR HAIR

A balanced diet benefits your hair as much as the rest of your body, but hair is one of the last in the queue for nutrients, as the vital organs of the body take precedence. Particularly important for healthy hair are the vitamins B complex, A and E, proteins, iron and iodine.

CLEANSING AND CONDITIONING TIPS

It is important to get the basics of haircare – shampooing, conditioning, drying and brushing – right, if you are to avoid problems that will take time to correct later.

Shampoo

Choosing a shampoo that works for you is often a trial-and-error process, but there are some useful guidelines:

- Pick a shampoo that is designed for your hair type as this should leave your hair feeling clean and looking shiny (shampoo should not leave any stickiness behind or dull the hair).
- Never use washing-up liquid or household detergent on your hair as they are highly alkaline and disturb your hair's pH balance.
- Avoid having a communal family shampoo – the chances are that everyone will have a different hair type – so buy a selection.
- Change your shampoo every now and then; hair seems to develop a resistance to a shampoo's ingredients after a period of time, sometimes the result of a build-up of styling products. Special shampoos to remove this residue are available.
- Don't throw away a shampoo that doesn't seem to lather. The amount of lather produced is determined by the active level of detergent used in the shampoo and does not influence its cleansing ability – it is more a cosmetic touch.

Rinse well for shiny hair

Always rinse your hair thoroughly in clean, warm water to eliminate any remaining shampoo and conditioner. If traces of these are left in the hair they make it look dull and feel sticky, and also leave particles that flake from the scalp like dandruff.

HAIRCARE

Conditioner
Conditioners cannot *mend* damaged hair but they can help prevent damage getting worse and protect the hair by leaving a film on the cuticle. They have the effect of flattening the cuticle, which makes light reflect off it so your hair looks wonderfully shiny. Conditioner also works to untangle your hair – especially useful if your hair is over-processed and so tends to be knotty.
- Use conditioner after every shampoo (on the whole of your head if your hair is dry or just the ends if it is oily) – it shouldn't leave your hair lank unless you do not rinse it properly.
- Avoid products that claim to shampoo and condition in one because the functions of *washing* and *protecting* are different and cannot really be successfully combined.
- Apply only a small amount of conditioner as your hair won't absorb any surplus and it will take longer to rinse out.

Drying without damage
Let your hair dry naturally as often as possible. With a towel, blot, don't rub the hair. When using a hairdryer point it down the hair shaft to keep the cuticle flat. Do not brush or comb wet hair more than is necessary – it is very vulnerable.

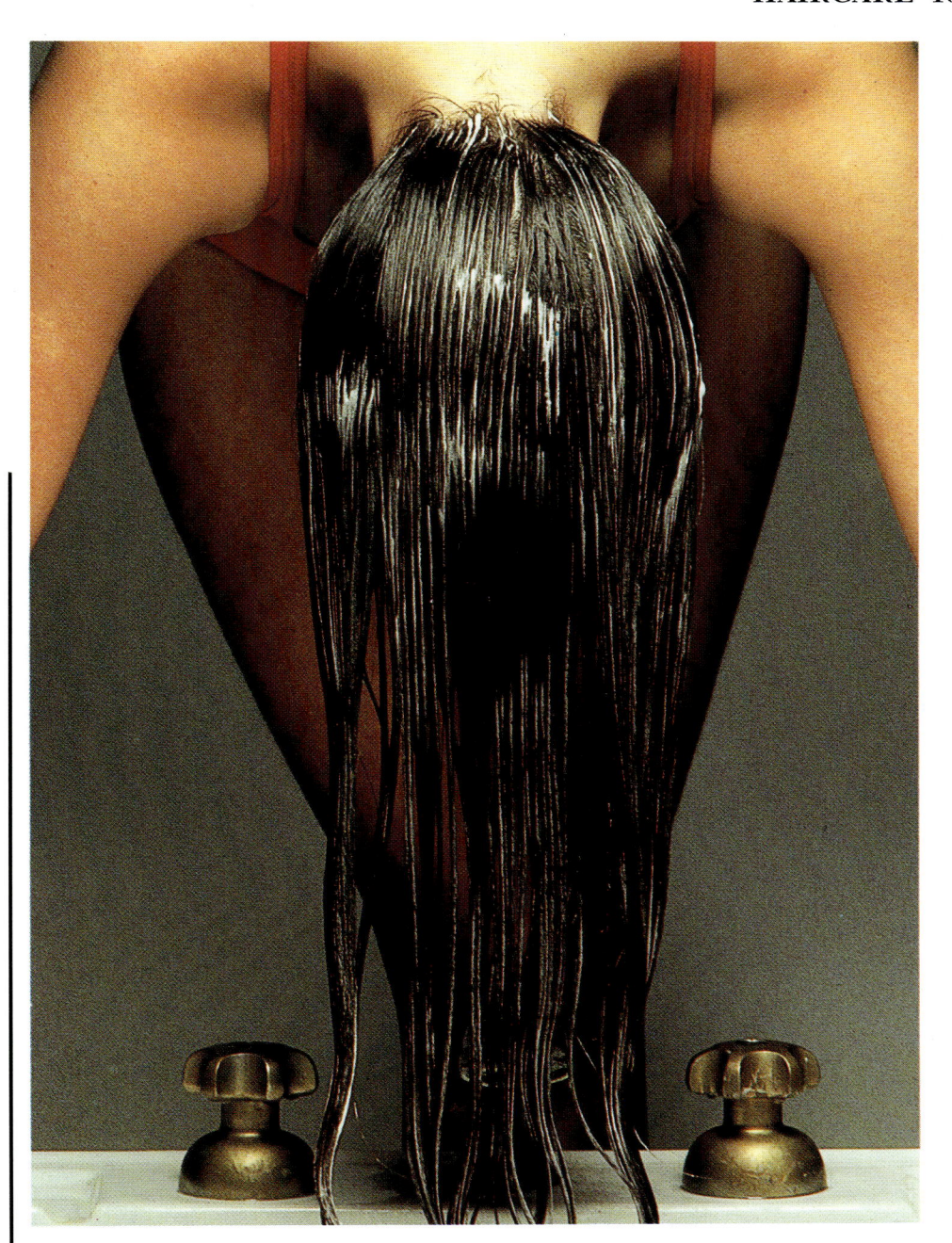

Choosing combs
When buying a comb, check that it has a smooth join down the centre. Uneven jagged plastic will damage the hair shaft. The best option is a comb that is 'sawcut' in one piece with wide, rounded teeth. Trichologists normally recommend avoiding metal combs which can cause damage.

HAIR TYPING

Knowing your hair type and caring for its particular needs is the first step to a crowning glory.

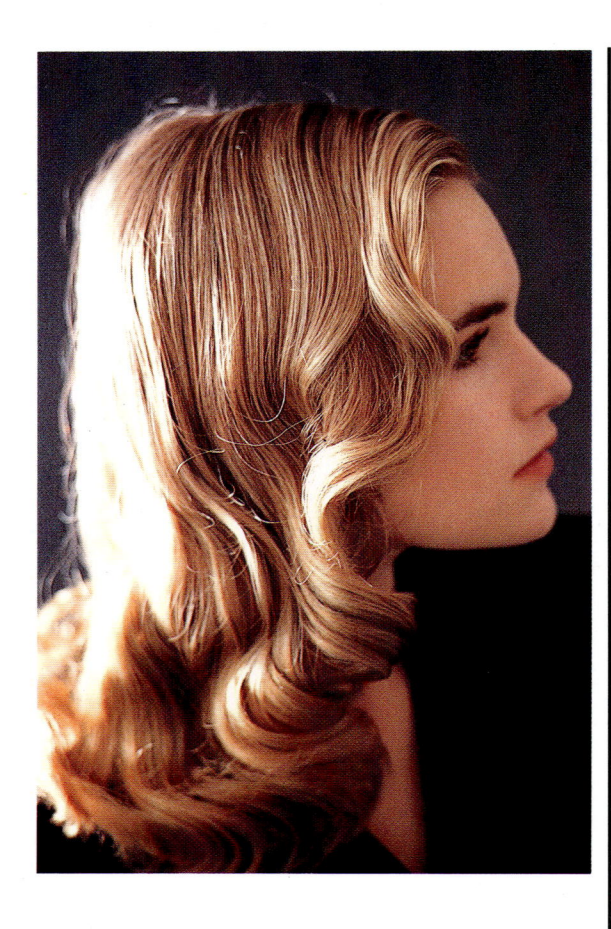

Recognizing your hair type will ensure that you give it the best possible care. There are many factors which will affect your natural hair type and alter the needs of your hair.

DRY AND/OR DAMAGED

The causes of this can be varied:
- Heredity.
- The use of too many harsh chemical treatments, such as bleaching, or incorrect use or over-use of hair dryers or heated rollers.
- Over-exposure to the sun, sea or chlorinated water.
- Not using a conditioner.

Haircare
- Shampoo and condition with moisturizing products two to three times a week, but if you prefer to wash your hair every day, use a mild shampoo and try a lighter conditioner.
- Give your hair a deep conditioning treatment once a week.
- Let your hair dry naturally as often as possible, but if you have to use a hair dryer, set it on a low speed and temperature.
- Don't use at-home perming or bleaching kits as your hair could become even more damaged – go to a salon for advice.
- Wear a bathing cap if you go swimming and a hat, scarf or special hair-protecting product in the sun.
- Foods high in protein such as fish, poultry and pulses will help combat brittle hair.
- Massage your scalp gently to improve the circulation and stimulate the sebaceous glands which produce the body's own natural conditioner for hair – sebum.

OILY

This can have several causes, including:
- Heredity.
- High hormonal activity.
- Under- or over-washing using harsh products.
- Brushing too frequently which over-stimulates the sebaceous glands in the scalp.

Haircare
- Use a comb rather than a brush and don't style or touch your hair more than is necessary, to avoid stimulating the sebaceous glands.
- Use a mild shampoo, washing your hair as often as necessary, and use a conditioner designed for oily hair, but only on the ends.
- Give your hair a final rinse with a little lemon or vinegar added to the water as this restores the pH balance of your hair.
- Avoid wearing hats

or scarves as they may make the problem worse.
- Check that your diet is healthy and balanced.

COMBINATION HAIR

This combination of greasy scalp with dry ends can be caused by:
- Chemical treatments such as perming and bleaching.
- Not having your hair trimmed frequently enough; approximately every six weeks is usually recommended.

Haircare
- As for oily hair, use a comb in preference to a brush.
- Shampoo your scalp only; when you rinse out the shampoo it will run down the hair shaft, cleaning it in the process.
- Try alternating shampoos for dry and greasy hair.
- Use conditioner only on the ends.

NORMAL

It is rare to have completely normal hair.

Normal hair is the result of sensible haircare, regular trims, few, if any, chemical treatments, and a good diet. Oh, and good genes!

Haircare
- Keep to your usual haircare routine and trims to maintain its good condition.
- Use conditioner to protect the ends and use an occasional deep-conditioning treatment.
- Try to avoid damaging your hair with too much chemical processing.

AFRO HAIR

Afro hair has curved follicles, which give it its characteristic springy curl. The hair strands are deceptively thin and are actually fewer in number per square centimetre than other hair types. As a result, Afro hair is particularly vulnerable to damage during chemical processes.

Many people with this hair type have their hair straightened, but it is a technically very complicated process and can cause terrible damage to the hair's infrastructure, leading to hair loss unless treated professionally. Do not use at-home straightening kits.

This hair type is invariably dry, as its very structure makes it difficult for sebum from the sebaceous glands to travel down the hair shaft.

Haircare
- Massaging a little specially blended hair oil into the hair after shampooing and conditioning helps to alleviate dryness.
- If you have a mixed hair type, with a greasy scalp and dry ends, avoid using too many oils as they may block the hair follicles. Instead, shampoo minimally and use conditioner only on the ends of your hair, not on the scalp.
- Braiding looks great on ethnic hair, but you should not keep your hair in this style for long periods, as the constant pulling on the scalp exerts too much pressure on the hair follicles and can lead to hair loss.

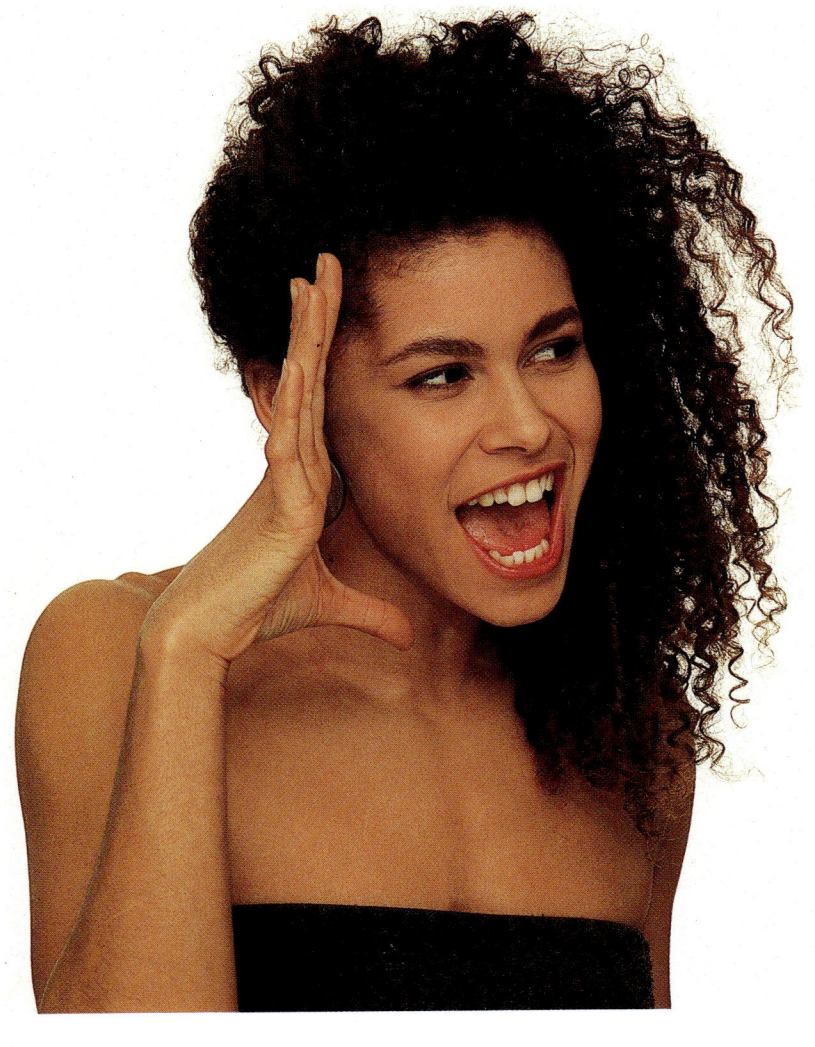

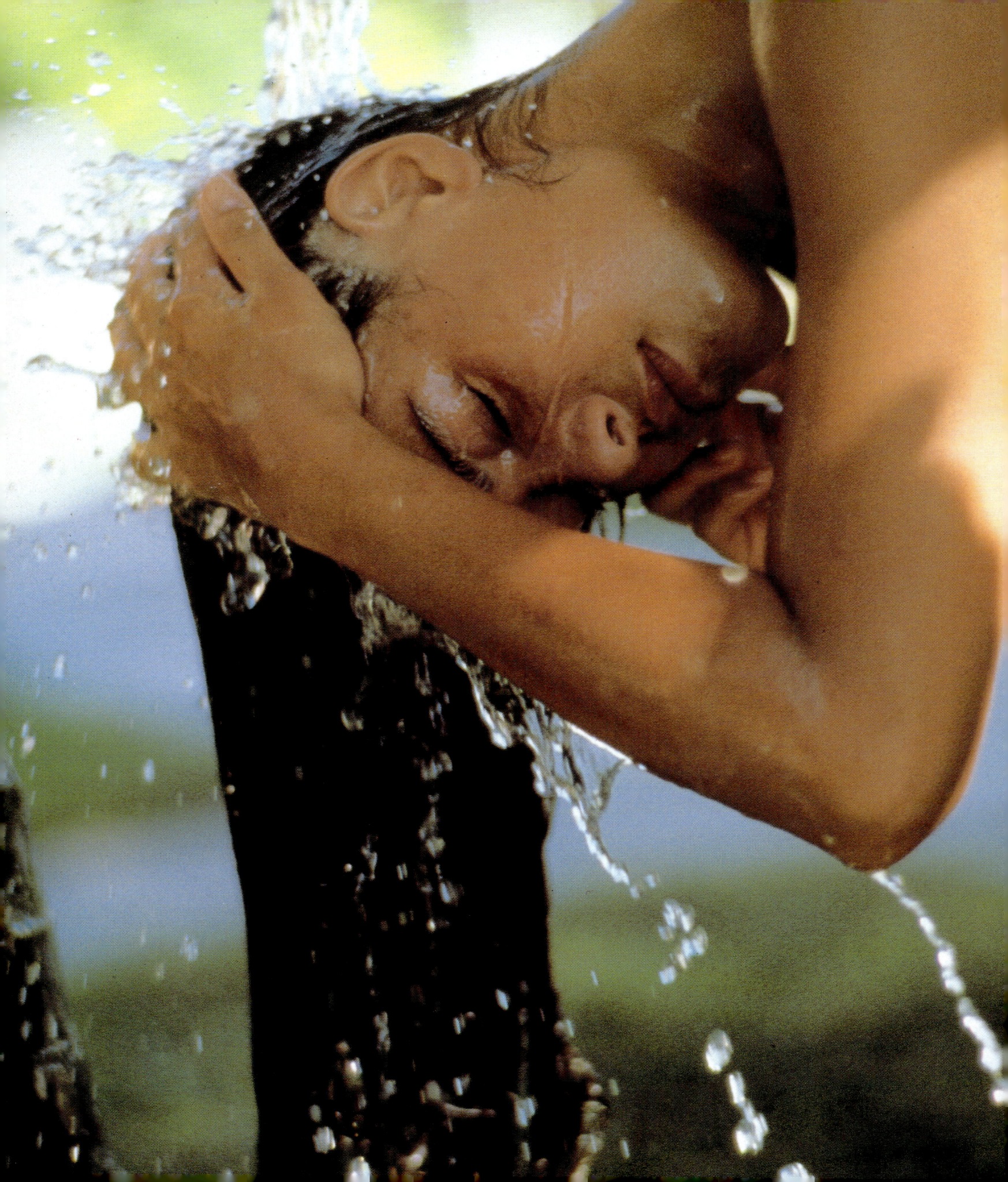

HAIR PROBLEMS

If your hair is looking less than its best, it's time for some special treatment.

Three of the most common complaints about hair are dullness, thinning and dandruff. These conditions may have any of several causes and there are a number of different treatments to try.

DULL HAIR
This may be caused by:
- stress
- not rinsing out shampoo and conditioner properly
- a build-up of the residue of styling products
- sun damage
- chemical treatments
- heated drying or styling appliances.

Treatment
- Rinse with white wine vinegar after shampooing and before conditioning.
- Dry your hair correctly (page 101).
- Silicon serums add instant shine. Just apply a few drops to dry hair.
- Use a shampoo that removes build-up.
- Avoid chemical treatments until your hair has recovered.

THINNING HAIR
Thinning hair and hair loss can be caused by:
- stress
- hormonal changes
- poor diet
- heredity
- pulling the hair while brushing or scraping it back too often into tight pony tails.

Treatment
- It is important to see a trichologist to ascertain the cause of the problem.
- Massage your scalp daily to stimulate hair growth.
- Condition your hair – it coats and thus thickens the hair shaft and has the cosmetic effect of making your hair look fuller.
- An unbalanced diet can result in thinning hair. Try to eat at regular intervals and ensure that your diet contains adequate protein, vitamins and minerals. A trichologist or nutritionist will be able to advise you.

DANDRUFF AND ITCHY SCALPS
Trichologist Philip Kingsley advises: 'Most of us at some time have a flaky or itchy scalp. The most common cause of itching is "dandruff", which describes all kinds of scalp flaking. Dandruff is produced when sweat and oil secretions change; the micro-organisms which are controlled by these secretions then multiply, causing the skin on the scalp to be shed faster. *Dandruff is rarely the result of a dry scalp.* It is usually oily because the flakes absorb oil. Dandruff and itching can get worse with stress or before menstruation, and can vary with the seasons. The foods you eat can also affect the problem. White wine and aspirin may also trigger an itchy scalp. You could be sensitive to your shampoo or conditioner – test this by a process of elimination.

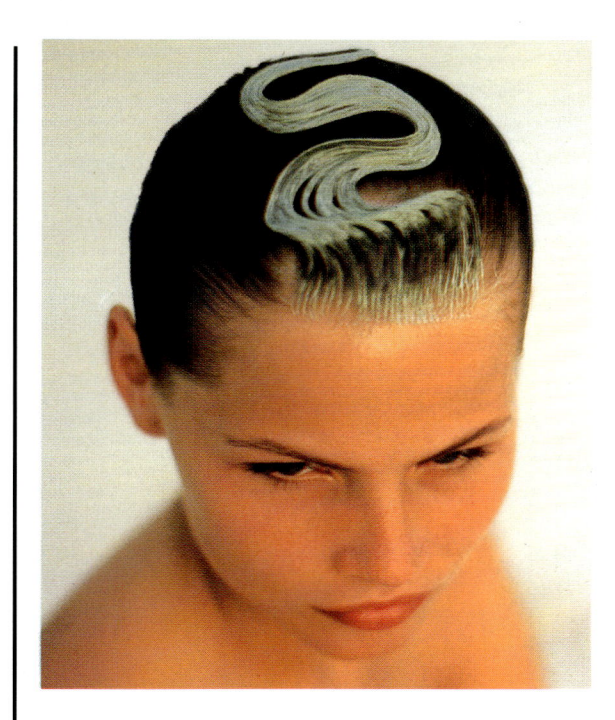

Anti-dandruff shampoos are quite effective but they can often leave the hair too oily, too dry or unmanageable. As an alternative, you can ask your chemist to make up a cream containing 1 per cent each of sulphur and salicylic acid. Rub this into your scalp for a few minutes, wash off with your favourite shampoo, then condition. Remember to keep your hair clean, washing it daily if possible.'

If self-help fails, see a trichologist.

CUTTING CLEVER

A good cut is the basis of a great hairstyle and will keep your hair in top condition.

Your hairstyle can make all the difference to whether you feel confident and happy with your appearance or dissatisfied. It is important therefore to find a hairdresser with whom you can develop a good rapport.

A stylist will adapt a cut according to your hair type and the directions of hair growth, and ensure that the style will enhance your features and flatter the shape of your face. He or she should also take your lifestyle into account and give you a cut that's easy to maintain. Do take with you photographs of styles you like, but be prepared to be flexible if the hairdresser feels they won't work on your hair type. Equally, try to be open to new ideas, as changing your hairstyle is the most effective way to inject new energy into your look.

Regular cuts
You should have your hair cut approximately every 6–8 weeks, although a very precise short style may need shaping every 4 weeks.

Changing your hairdresser
If you're thinking about changing stylists, book a free consultation or a simple service such as a trim before opting for a major new look. This will give you a chance to find out if you're on the same wavelength!

SHORT CUTS
Short hair can be cut and styled to create many different looks, from the classic short bob to the gamine urchin image. Sharp, angular styles look strong and individual; then there are soft, wavy styles that are modern classics. The added bonus with short hair is that it can look professional and smart in an instant.

Versatile bobs
The classic short bob remains modern-looking and is easy to style and wear. Blunt cut on straight hair the bob looks chic and shiny. A short bob to just below the ears looks young and fun.

Layering a bob gives the effect of movement. A layered bob can be worn full and wide, scrunch-dried and teased out with the aid of mousse, or close to the face, with the sides swept forwards. A permed bob with a straight fringe is a variation on the theme.

Your hairdresser will advise you as to whether a side parting or a fringe is best for you. Asymmetric cuts work well on the bob shape and add an element of individuality.

The urchin look
Gamine cuts that are short, layered and cut close to the head look especially chic when worn slightly tousled.

MID-LENGTH AND LONG HAIR
Whether one-length and sleek, or layered and full, longer hair can make you feel especially glamorous. It is, however, essential to keep longer hair in peak condition – keep brushing to a minimum and do it gently. Have it trimmed regularly, too, so that split ends don't have a chance to develop – they'll simply work their way up the hair shaft.

Volume with length
If you want to wear your hair long but like height on top, you could try a 'no curl' perm just on the roots. Alternatively, for temporary lift, use large velcro rollers. Roll sections of hair under, spritz with setting lotion or hairspray and then brush out.

Fringe appeal
Consider keeping interest at the front if your hair is long. A fringe can be short and straight, or longer and layered.

Pre-Raphaelite curls
Curls can be created with curling tongs or by sleeping with your hair in rags. Twist a lock of hair and wind it round your finger. Insert the end of a strip of fabric through the hole created by your finger and fasten it with a knot. Long-lasting curls can be achieved with a spiral perm.

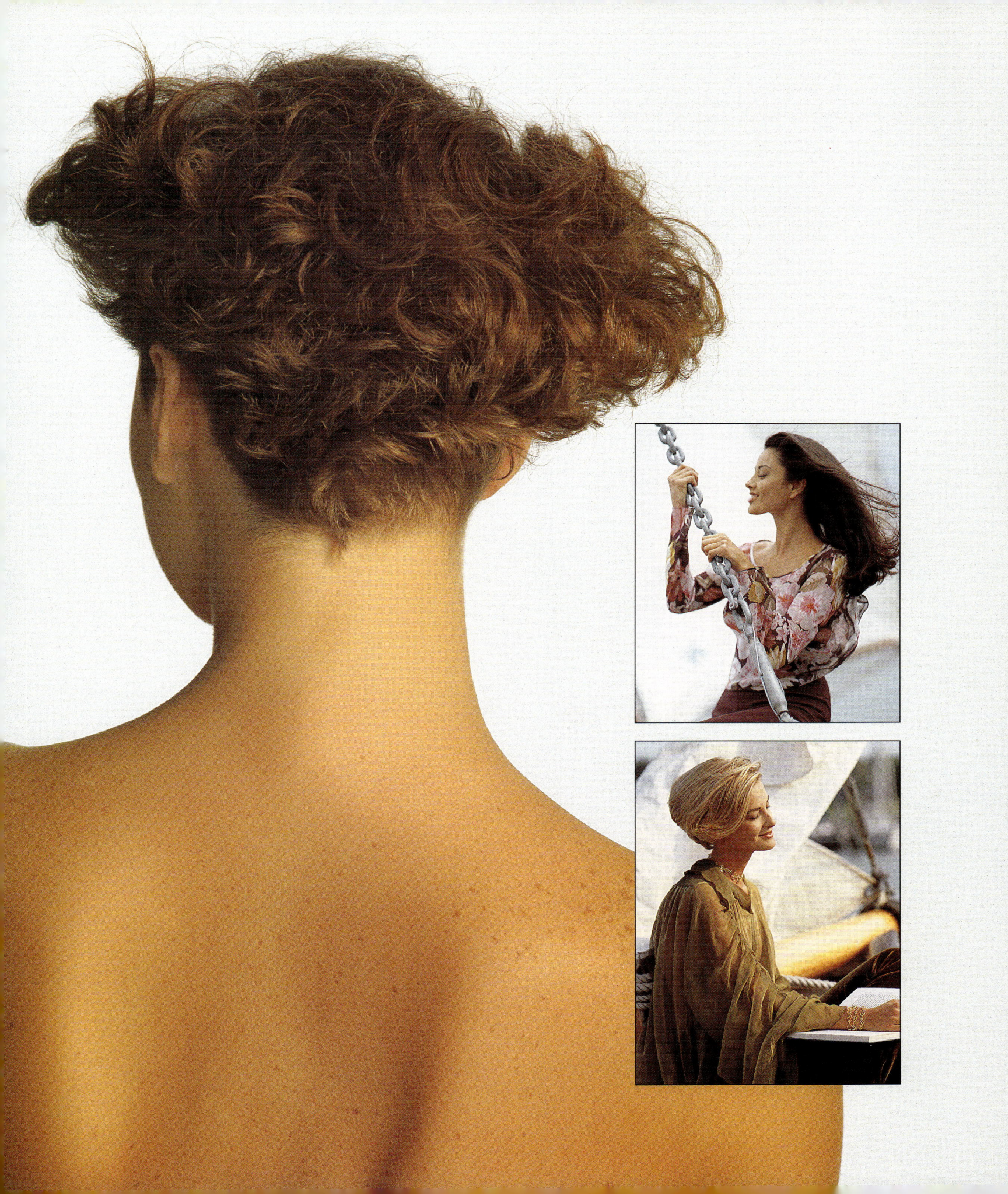

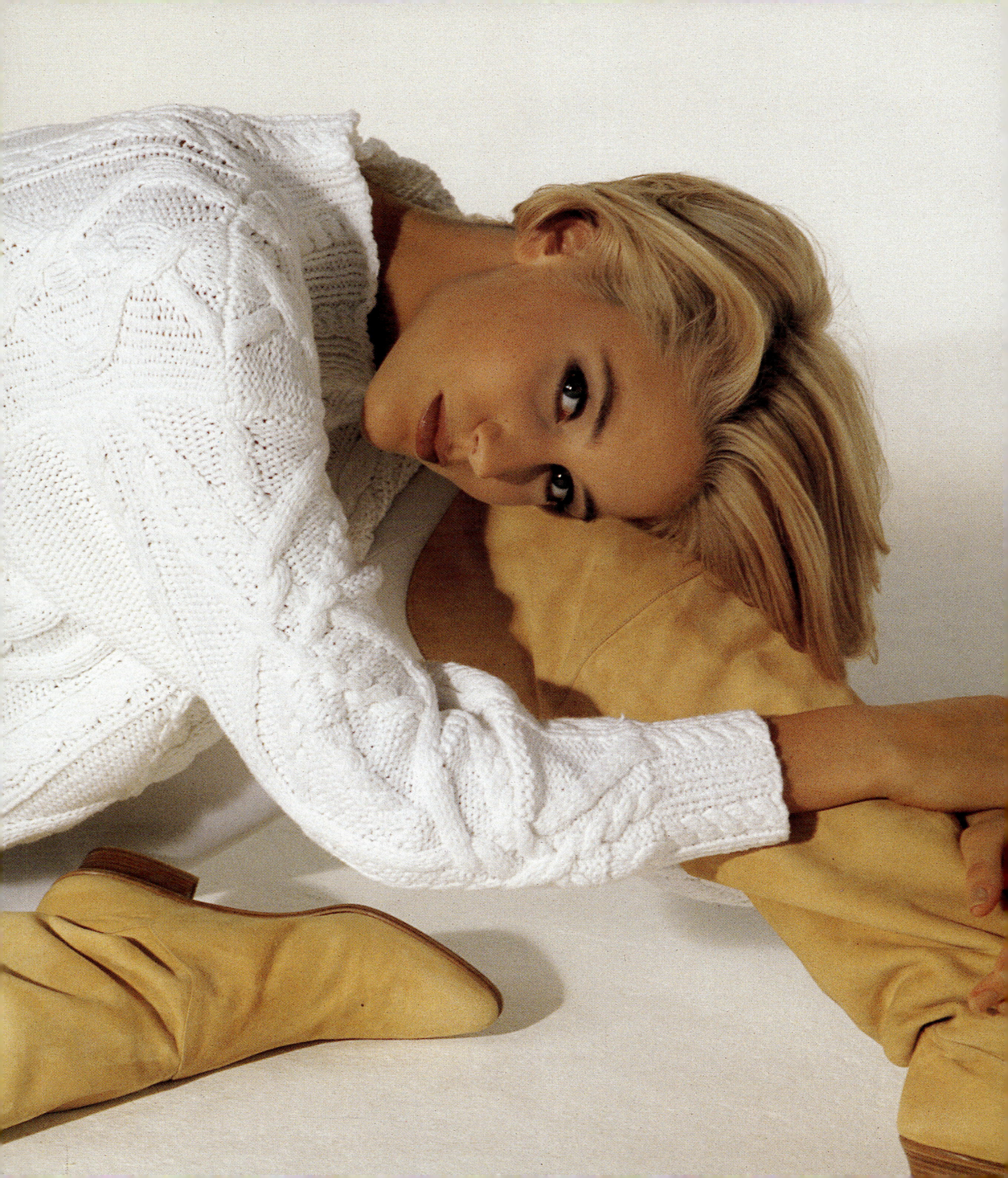

COLOUR SENSE

Colouring is one of the quickest ways to change your image. Check out all the options to find the best method for your hair.

Before you make any changes to the colour of your hair, think about your colouring, features, age and even your occupation. Remember too, that what looks great on someone else may not suit you.

It's a good idea to try on a few wigs in colours and styles that you are thinking of – particularly if you are contemplating a dramatic change. Alternatively, some salons have a specialized computer that can show you images of yourself with different tones in your hair.

If you want a more permanent colour change, rather than just a rinse, do go to a salon. An expert colourist will examine your hair and make *realistic* suggestions, taking your hair's health, porosity and natural colour into consideration, as hair colours react differently on various types and conditions of hair.

There are several different colouring techniques. Listed below are the most commonly used, what they do and how long they last. However, colouring technology is advancing so much year by year, it's worth asking your local salon what they have to offer.

Colourways
For the most natural-looking effects, just choose a shade or two lighter or darker than your natural hair colour.

PERMANENT COLOUR
This is usually a blend of a tint and hydrogen peroxide which penetrates the cortex and then is sealed in. The tint combines with your natural hair colour to produce the final shade.
- Going a few shades *lighter* seems to work better than going *darker*, which can look flat and matte.
- In a salon, tell them the history of your hair as it may affect how the tint takes; the initial treatment is always more expensive than later retouching treatments, so it is important to get it right.
- At home, don't attempt to use a tint on previously bleached hair in the hope of improving the colour – it will probably end up looking brassy.
- After tinting, be sure to condition your hair regularly.
- Tinting will normally need retouching every month or so, depending on how different it is from your natural colour.
- Permanent colour needs to grow out or be re-coloured by an expert.

BLEACHING
Bleach tends to be ammonia-based (though there are ammonia-free varieties), mixed with hydrogen peroxide. It removes the natural pigment; a blonde toner then gives it the characteristic colour.
- Bleaching damages the hair so badly that it's best to resort to it only if you can't achieve blonde with a few shades of tint.
- It is expensive and time-consuming to return to your natural colour if you find that you don't like your hair bleached blonde.
- Salon bleaching always looks better than home-bleached hair.
- Your hair will need retouching, which not only means frequent visits to the salon, but each re-application of bleach damages your hair further.

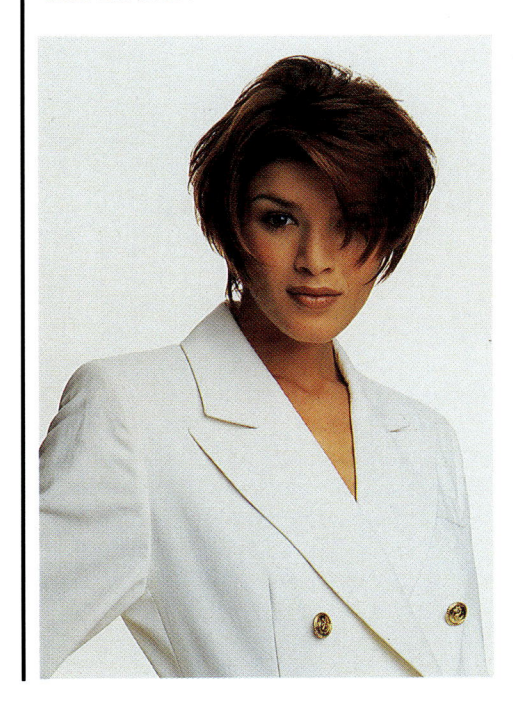

TEMPORARY COLOUR RINSES

These colour the hair by coating the cuticle and wash out quickly. They normally shampoo-in, but you can buy them in the form of setting lotions.
- Your hair colour is not dramatically changed; rinses just add depth.
- Temporary rinses usually contain built-in conditioners.
- Rinses can be used on all non-processed hair, though they work best on fair hair.
- They are cheap, quick and easy to use at home.

SEMI-PERMANENT COLOUR

These, logically, are not as permanent as a tint, but more lasting than a rinse, penetrating the cuticle only.
- Like rinses, semi-permanent colours don't produce a dramatic change unless you choose a dark shade and your natural colour is blonde, and so can be used just to brighten your own hair colour.
- There's little regrowth problem with this method as the colour fades out after about six to eight washes.
- Semi-permanent colour is reasonably cheap and it is relatively easy to achieve good results in the salon or at home.

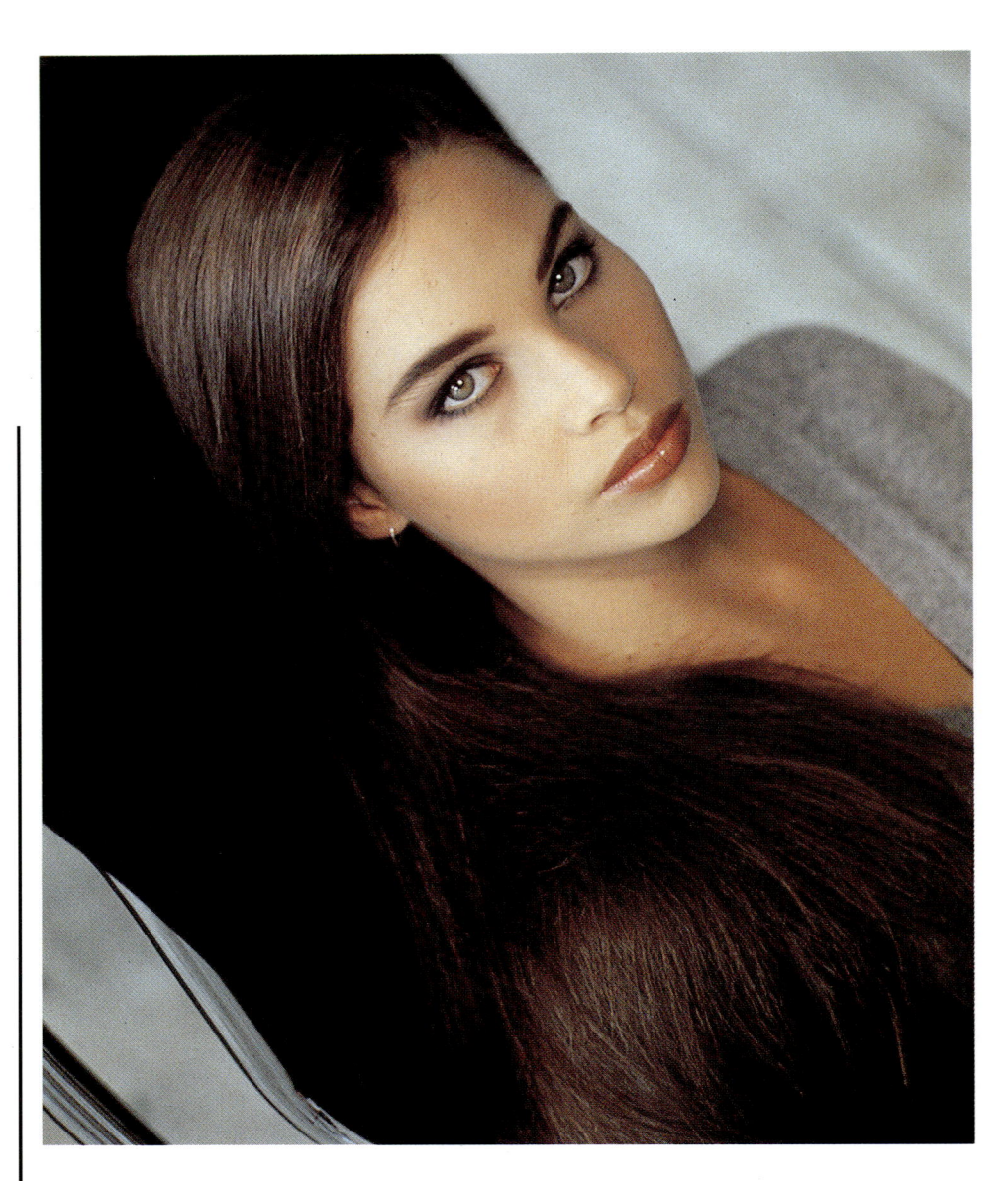

THE NEW GENERATION

There are colourants that you can use at home or have applied in a salon, which are longer lasting than semi-permanents (which last for around 6 washes) but do not require the long-term commitment of a permanent colour. They last for 6–8 weeks, but don't lighten or damage the hair. In fact, these colourants will enhance the shine factor. Available in subtle and stronger shades, they are very effective at blending in grey hair.

HIGHLIGHTING OR STREAKS

These are done by using a peroxide or tint mix that penetrates the hair cortex, applied by either the foil or cap method. Foil is usually more expensive but gives better results; pulling strands through a perforated rubber cap is a cheaper option.

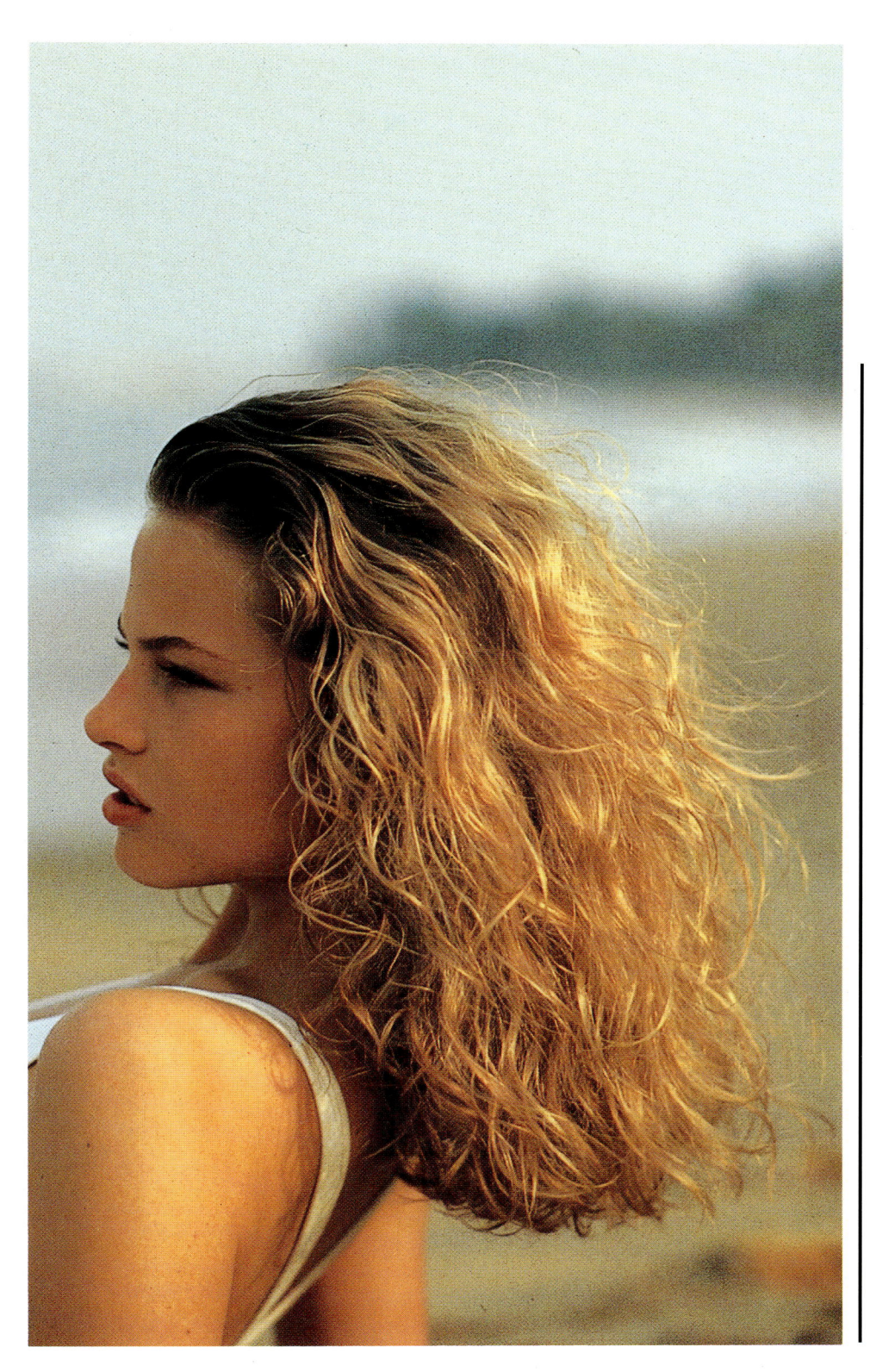

- Highlighting is kinder than total bleaching; although it still damages your hair (sometimes leading it to knot easily and become frizzy), it *can* look wonderful, like naturally sun-streaked hair, giving the of depth and movement.
- It is a technique best left to the salon, as there is too much room for mistakes with home kits.
- On average, highlights will need to be redone every three months or so, though more frequent retouching may be necessary.

VEGETABLE COLOURS

These are colourants that use natural ingredients such as camomile or henna.
- They add colour, depth and shine.
- They are fairly cheap.
- They can be used both at home and in the salon, although they tend not to work on grey hair unless they are specially designed for it, and highlighted and bleached hair may go a little orange.
- The colour fades out gradually.

Colour care
- *Don't expose coloured hair to the sun as it will probably change its shade. Wear a hat or specialized hair protector.*
- *Use shampoos produced specially for coloured hair.*

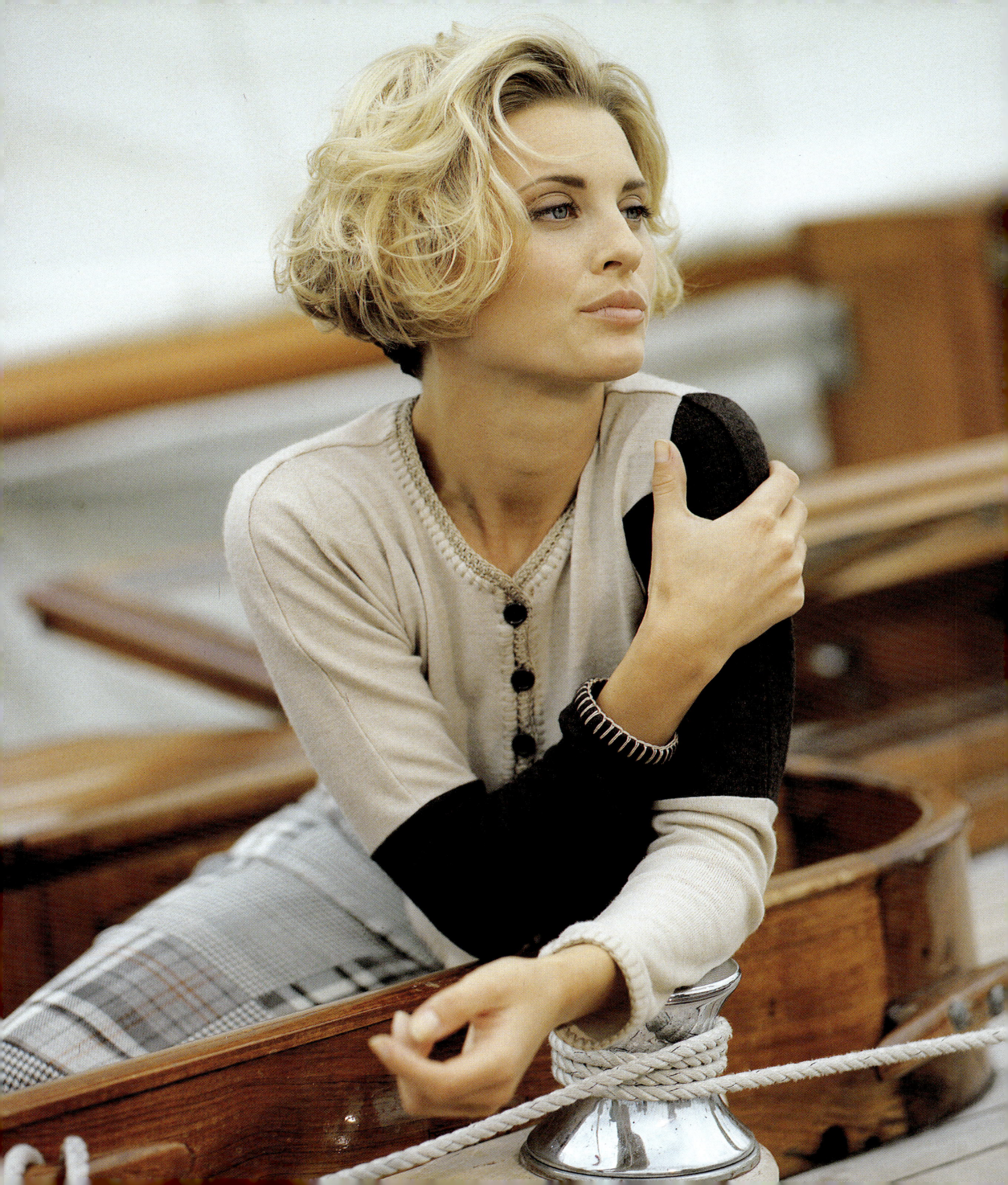

PERMANENT SOLUTIONS

Whether you want cascading curls or just a little extra volume, a perm will inject vitality into your hair-style.

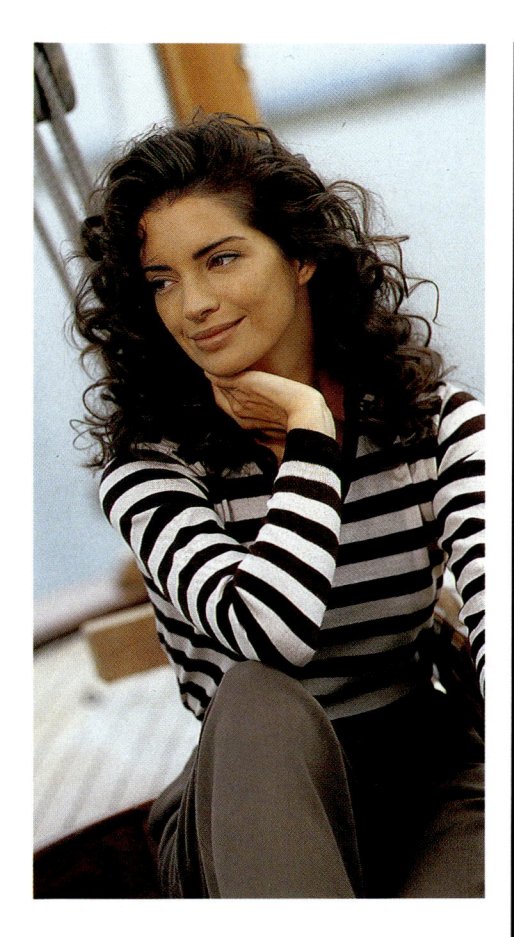

Modern perms are incredibly versatile. You can have your hair permed for volume, to give bounce, curls or ringlets, for root movement (which is good for limp hair) and to give support to a style without any curl at all. They work on almost any length of hair, too.

Perming process

Perming alters the hair's chemical bonds so that new links are forged around the curler. After the perm has taken, the perming solution is rinsed out with water and the curls are then locked into place with a neutralising lotion.

The softness of the perm depends on the size of the perming rod that is used. Large curlers produce softer perms, while small curlers give tight perms. Varying sizes and shapes of perming rods can be used, according to your hair type and the effect required. The hair can also be wound in different directions to achieve different styles.

Pre-perm tips

A skin allergy test and test curl are advisable if you are new to perming or if your hair is in bad condition. As perming is a complicated technical process, it is wise to have it done professionally.

Hairdressers frequently use a deep-cleansing treatment before perming in order to remove residues from conditioners and styling products from the hair.

Perm types

'Acid' and 'alkaline' perms are available. 'Alkaline' perms are more successful, in general, on virgin hair as it is stronger than 'acid' perming lotion. Hair itself is acid-based, so 'acid' perms are considered safer for coloured and highlighted hair. Both types of perm can last the same length of time – there is no set lifespan for a perm, it depends on how quickly your hair grows.

Some perms claim to restructure the hair, restoring up to 90 per cent of its original strength, and to provide on-going conditioning.

Keratin, the protein found in hair itself, and natural moisturizing factors are locked into the hair cortex and so act as a system of 'molecular mending'.

Post-perm tips

- Once a perm has been neutralised properly it is fixed, so there is no need to avoid shampooing it for 24 hours.
- Avoid two-in-one shampoo and conditioner which can be too heavy.
- Have your hair trimmed every 6 weeks, as extra weight will pull the curl down.
- Curl reactivators are effective for restoring bounce.
- Avoid brushing permed hair as this will create static and separate the curls. Use a wide-toothed comb instead.
- Where a perm is too curly you can try setting it on large rollers, or gently blow-dry the curl out using a big round brush.

SHAPE AND STYLE

Get to grips with gels, mousses, lotions and pomades and you'll discover exciting new styling possibilities for your hair.

The new generation of styling aids has revolutionized haircare and styling. Now we can inject life into our hair by building body, boosting shine and fixing styles in just a few minutes.

Mousse
This is a fabulous, instant volume builder. It coats the hair making it easier to control and is especially useful for taming frizzy hair and for shaping the curl in permed hair. It will give energy to fine hair and extra texture to straight hair. Many mousses contain conditioners, which are excellent for dry ends.

Apply mousse by squeezing a golfball-sized knob of foam into the palm of your hand and then applying it with your fingers to the roots. Mousse is best applied to slightly damp hair because it will distribute better. Don't be tempted to use too much or you will overload the hair, and be careful to use very little on fine hair or you could end up with a sticky, heavy result.

Experiment with different strengths of mousse. It is often best to buy a mousse with a high hold factor and use less of it than to apply more of a lighter mousse.

If your hair feels lank later in the day, spraying with a little water will revive it. Shape your hair with your fingers as it dries.

Gels
Gel defines texture on curly hair and will sleek and hold straight hair in place. There are several ways to use it. Gel can be applied to wet hair, combed into shape and then left to set hard. Or you can blow-dry the gelled hair, which gives lots of body and bounce but still leaves it looking silky and natural. Gel spreads more easily when applied to wet or slightly damp hair.

Gels formulated for use on dry hair are good for controlling small areas of hair and for slicking it back at the sides of your face. If the brand you are using becomes flaky, switch to another formulation.

You can combine products such as mousses and gels or mousses and hairspray for extra styling strength.

Styling lotions for blow-drying
These spray-in lotions protect hair from the drying effects of heat when it is blow-dried. They also help to keep the hair cuticle flat, which prevents flyaway ends and increases shine. Many formulations will also help to increase volume.

Sculpting lotions
These ultra-strong hair shapers are designed to be applied either to damp hair, which is then blow-dried into shape, or to dry hair for fullness or uplifting effects.

Hairspray
You can use hairspray for localized styling and to keep your hair sleek. Hairspray holds a polished finish, but allows movement (which sculpting lotions do not). If you simply want to control a few stray ends, spray a little hairspray on to your brush and sweep it through your hair.

Hairspray is indispensable when the atmosphere is humid because it prevents the dampness from making your hair limp. Keep a mini hairspray in your bag – many pump sprays are refillable.

Pomade and wax
These are useful for thick hair, but should not be used on fine hair. Apply a little, using your fingertips to separate and define the hair – for instance, on a spiky fringe. Pomade and wax are terrific for creating shine and for controlling afro hair. Remember that they need to be washed out very thoroughly.

Serums
Fairly new on the market, serums are silicon-based liquids that tame frizzy ends, sleek flyaway hair and enhance shine on all hair types in seconds. You simply need a few drops, smoothed in the palm of your hands, then applied wherever you want. Good ones don't feel sticky.

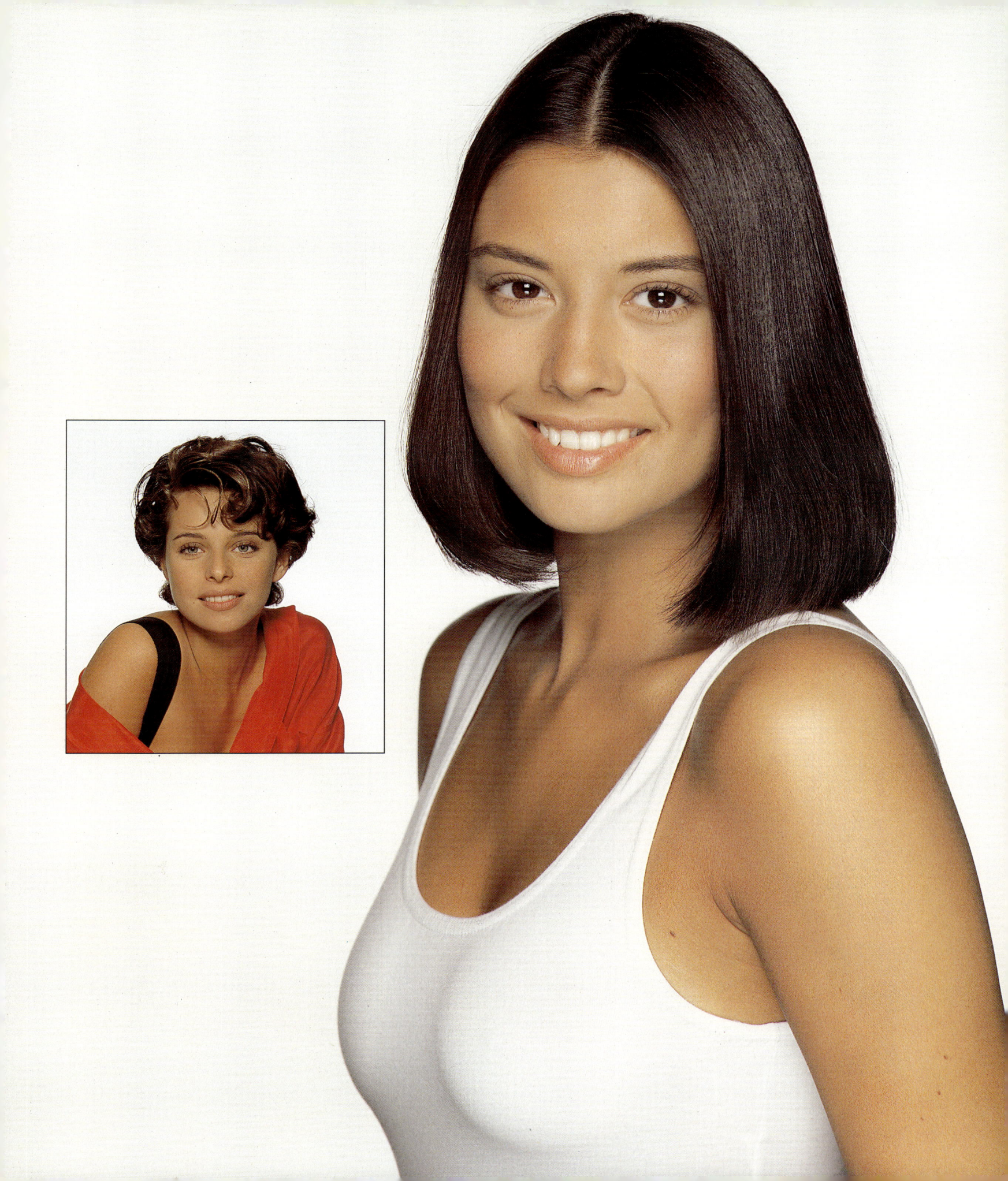

116 SHORT CUTS

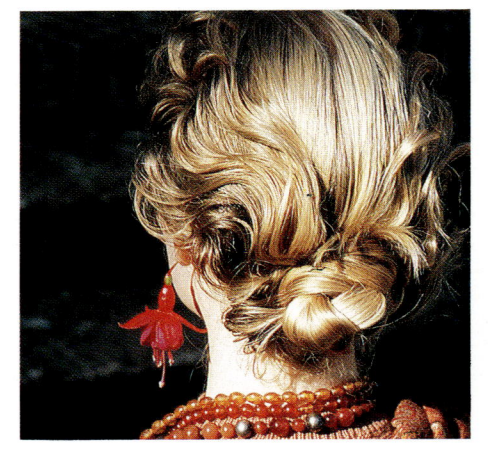

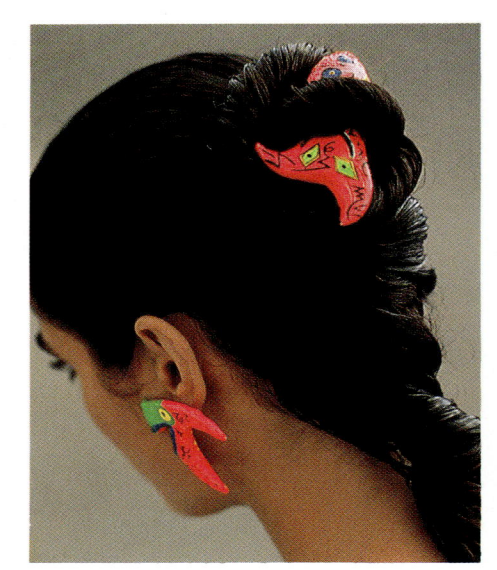

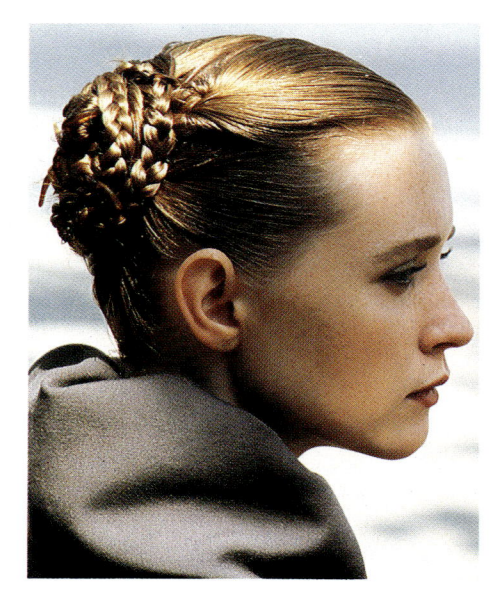

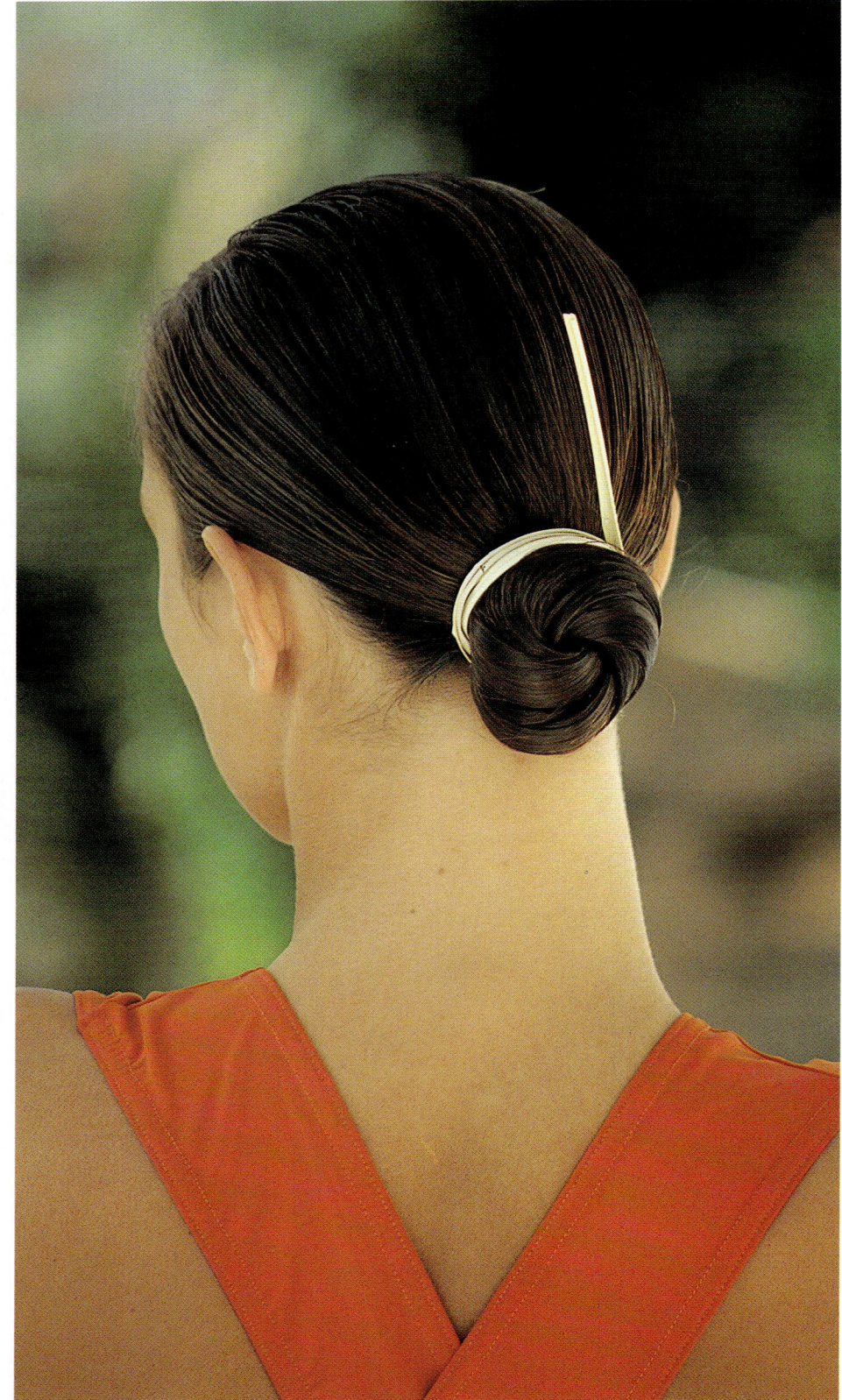

TWISTS, PLAITS AND ROLLS

Modern classicism is today's way with hair looks. There are a multitude of stylish ways to dress mid-length and long hair.

In the same way that we choose accessories to accent a particular outfit, we should consider our hair in terms of an overall look.

The beauty of mid-length and long hair is that it can be styled in an exciting variety of ways. Twists, plaits, braids, rolls and chignons all look super-stylish and can be worn with simple accessories to secure them in place, or decorated ornately to create knock-out looks.

The key to success when styling is to apply a little mousse or gel to control flyaway ends and to sleek your hair before you start. You need to have a selection of long hairpins, Kirby grips and covered elastics.

Twists

Quick to do, twists can be left soft and natural-looking – there is no need to plaster on hairspray!

Simply twist your hair along the side of your head on one side and fasten it at the back with a hair-clip.

Now twist back the other side and clip the two pieces together so that the hair hangs sleek and straight behind, or interweave the two twists at the nape of the neck and fasten with long hairpins.

Twists look pretty when several tortoiseshell chignon pins are placed around the twist.

Combs can be used to help hold twists in place. Look for combs without rough edges. Place them in your hair so that they grip by pushing the teeth up towards the crown of the head, then turn the comb and push it down.

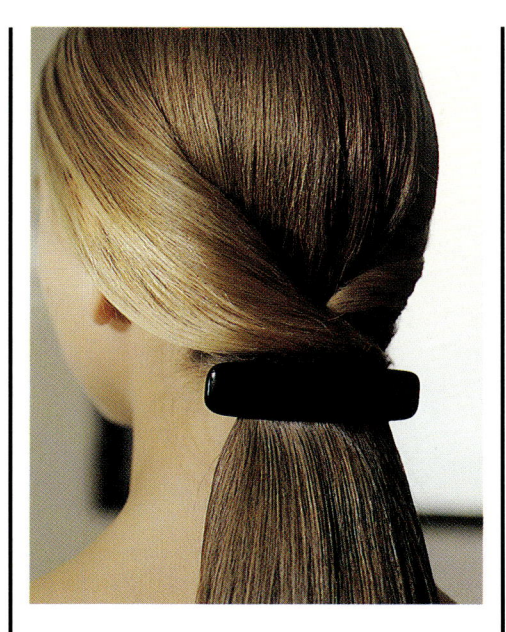

Plaits and braids

Ideally you need to have hair of one length to plait and braid it quickly. Practice makes perfect plaits.

Braids (French plaits) are more tricky to do. Starting just below the crown of your head, divide the centre of your hair into three sections, plait these together and then pick up another section on either side of the centre piece and plait together again. Continue down to the nape of your neck and then plait as usual, fastening with a slide or covered elastic at the end.

Rolls and French pleats

Sharp, stylish and with a touch of formality, rolls are fun to wear with clothes that echo the style of the 1940s and 50s.

For a French pleat, take your hair back into the nape of the neck, twisting along the length of the hair. Roll the twist of hair upwards, turning the ends in, and fasten the pleat in place with pins.

Chignons

These are good on fine to medium-textured hair but take a little more time on heavier hair.

A low chignon placed at the nape of the neck looks modern. You can twist the hair and knot it, pulling the ends through the knot and securing with pins. Alternatively, you can take the hair into a low pony-tail, secure it with a covered elastic and then twist and pin into place.

Look out for hanky knots. These are specially shaped pieces of fabric (raw silk ones look particularly good) which have an elasticated piece at one end. Simply place the fabric over the chignon and twist the elastic around twice to secure it.

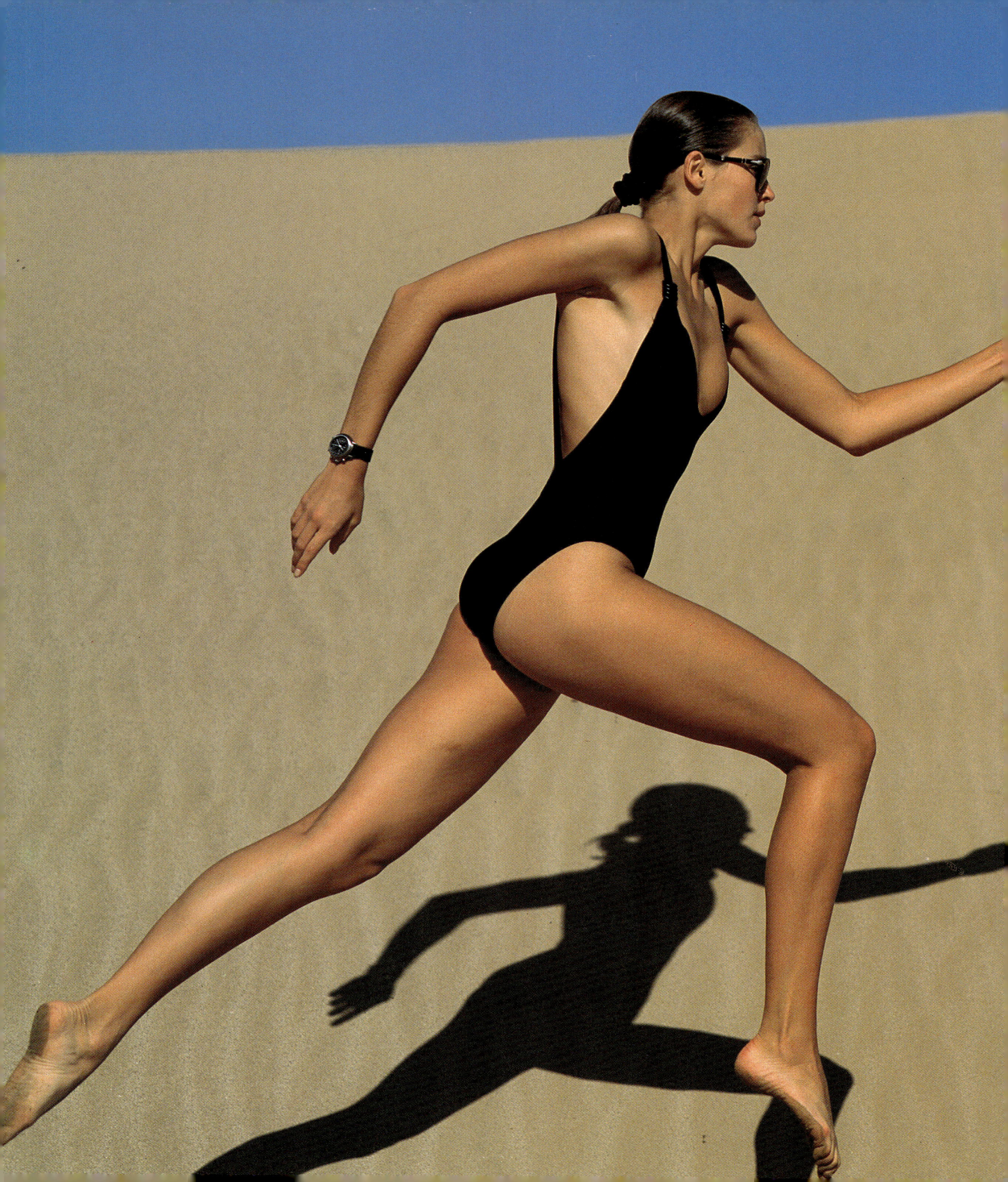

THE BODY BEAUTIFUL

A well-toned body with sleek skin can be achieved through simple exercises and a little regular skincare. By targeting exercise to specific areas you can redefine curves and strengthen muscles – you only need a few spare minutes in your day.

ARM AND SHOULDER SHAPERS   120
BACK STRENGTHENERS   122
BUST BEAUTY   124
STOMACH AND WAIST FLATTENERS   126
HIP, THIGH AND BOTTOM TONERS   130
LEGS WORKOUT   134
HAND AND NAIL SAVERS   136
FEET FIRST   138
SMOOTH HAIR REMOVAL   140

ARM AND SHOULDER SHAPERS

Strong, curvy shoulders and arms will work wonders in balancing your body shape.

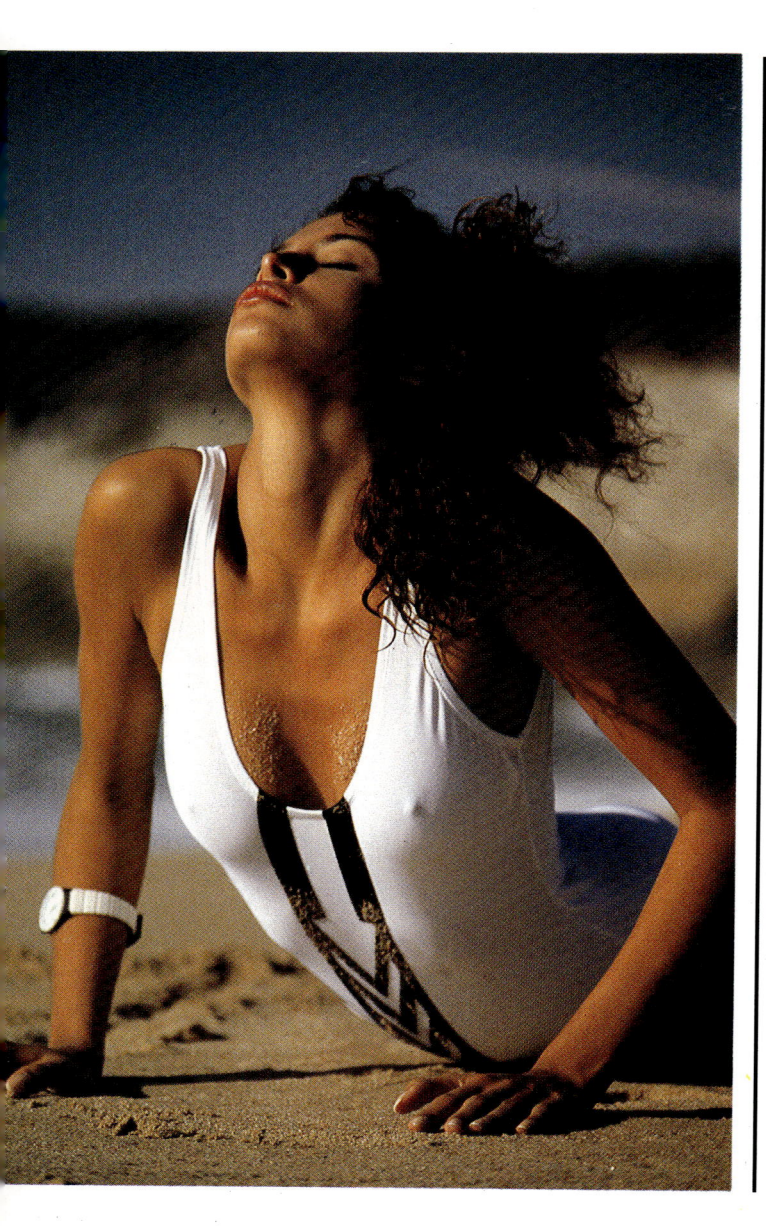

Developing your shoulders makes your waist and hips look at least one size smaller!

You can achieve this by wearing clothes with shoulder details and with exercise. Several popular forms of exercise, such as walking, jogging and cycling, either do not tone the upper body at all or tone it only slightly. (Walking with hand-held weights is popular, but be careful if you suspect you may have any underlying cardio-vascular problems, as you are putting extra strain on your heart.)

The arms, especially the backs of arms, benefit greatly from toning exercises geared to this area. Do them every other day and you'll soon be able to carry your suitcase through the airport without the customary struggle.

Swimming is a fast shoulder shaper. However, you should try to include more than one stroke if you are swimming regularly or you could develop problems later on, as muscles may become overdeveloped or inflamed through overuse.

If you play a lot of tennis, be careful – serving incorrectly can lead to swelling and pain. If this happens to you, ask a tennis professional to check your movements. Otherwise racquet sports are very good for developing and defining your shoulder contours.

Skincare
Care for the skin on your arms by gently exfoliating (removing dead cells from the surface of the skin, see page 54) with a body scrub or hemp mitt, concentrating on the skin on your elbows and any rough skin on the backs of your upper arms.

Short cuts to smooth elbows
Sit with each elbow in half a lemon for a few minutes to whiten the skin. Then rinse and apply moisturizer.

Weights and exercise
Some exercises involve using weights to increase the amount of work done by your muscles. Use dumb-bells (between 1–2kg/2–5lb, depending on what weight feels comfortable) or wrist weights.

Warm up
Always warm up your shoulders before starting any sport that uses your arms, and before doing the exercises here.

Raise and lower your shoulders 4 times. Relax your shoulders down.

Push your shoulders back and forwards 4 times.

Circle your arms back 8 times.

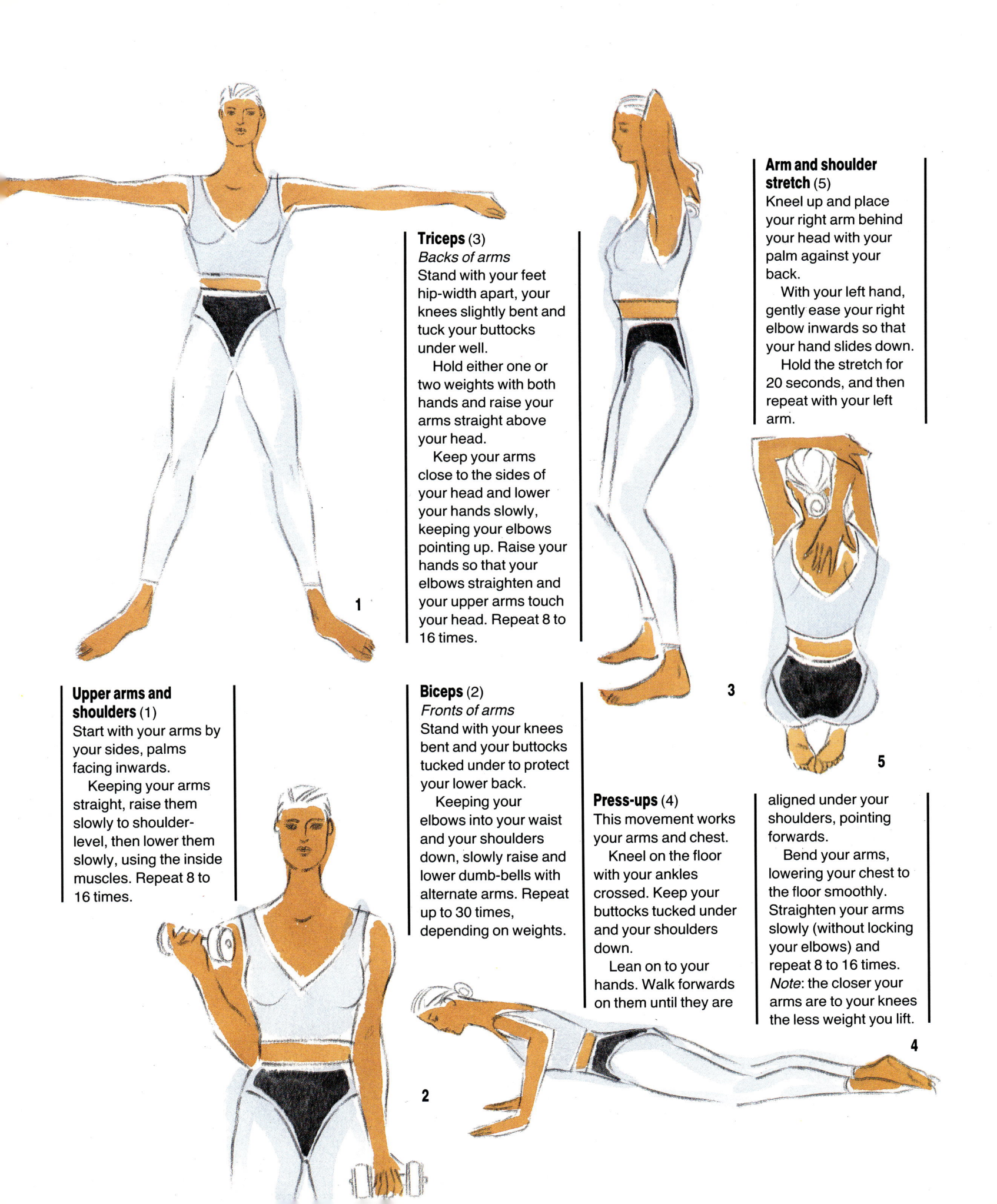

Triceps (3)
Backs of arms
Stand with your feet hip-width apart, your knees slightly bent and tuck your buttocks under well.

Hold either one or two weights with both hands and raise your arms straight above your head.

Keep your arms close to the sides of your head and lower your hands slowly, keeping your elbows pointing up. Raise your hands so that your elbows straighten and your upper arms touch your head. Repeat 8 to 16 times.

Arm and shoulder stretch (5)
Kneel up and place your right arm behind your head with your palm against your back.

With your left hand, gently ease your right elbow inwards so that your hand slides down.

Hold the stretch for 20 seconds, and then repeat with your left arm.

Upper arms and shoulders (1)
Start with your arms by your sides, palms facing inwards.

Keeping your arms straight, raise them slowly to shoulder-level, then lower them slowly, using the inside muscles. Repeat 8 to 16 times.

Biceps (2)
Fronts of arms
Stand with your knees bent and your buttocks tucked under to protect your lower back.

Keeping your elbows into your waist and your shoulders down, slowly raise and lower dumb-bells with alternate arms. Repeat up to 30 times, depending on weights.

Press-ups (4)
This movement works your arms and chest.

Kneel on the floor with your ankles crossed. Keep your buttocks tucked under and your shoulders down.

Lean on to your hands. Walk forwards on them until they are aligned under your shoulders, pointing forwards.

Bend your arms, lowering your chest to the floor smoothly. Straighten your arms slowly (without locking your elbows) and repeat 8 to 16 times.
Note: the closer your arms are to your knees the less weight you lift.

BACK STRENGTHENERS

Gently exercising your upper body and back instantly improves posture and poise – you will look better and feel great.

Our upper bodies are often weaker than we would like. This is because most of our everyday tasks require us to reach forwards (round or over a desk, typewriter or cooker for instance) so that the muscles on the upper back are constantly being stretched while the chest muscles in front often become over-tight. This imbalance not only draws the shoulders forwards, opening out the shoulder blades and rounding the upper back, but also narrows and drops your rib-cage so that you are slumped out of alignment.

The muscles that help you maintain lift in your upper body are in the upper back, working rather like a corset that laces up behind. Tighten the lacing and correct posture is regained – no more rounded shoulders and cramped rib-cage.

Exercise is the key to creating this change. Warm up properly before carrying out any of the exercises here (see page 123).

Skincare
The skin on your back is thicker than that of the face and contains more sebaceous (oil) glands than other areas of the body. Be sure to cleanse the skin here thoroughly, using a back brush, or ask your partner to apply a body scrub once a week.

However, if your skin is *already* spotty, avoid abrading it in these areas or you may spread the infection. Instead, apply topical lotions to dry out the spots and be careful not to pick at them or they may scar.

If your back needs the professional touch, try a 'back facial' in a beauty salon, which will include massage and deep cleansing.

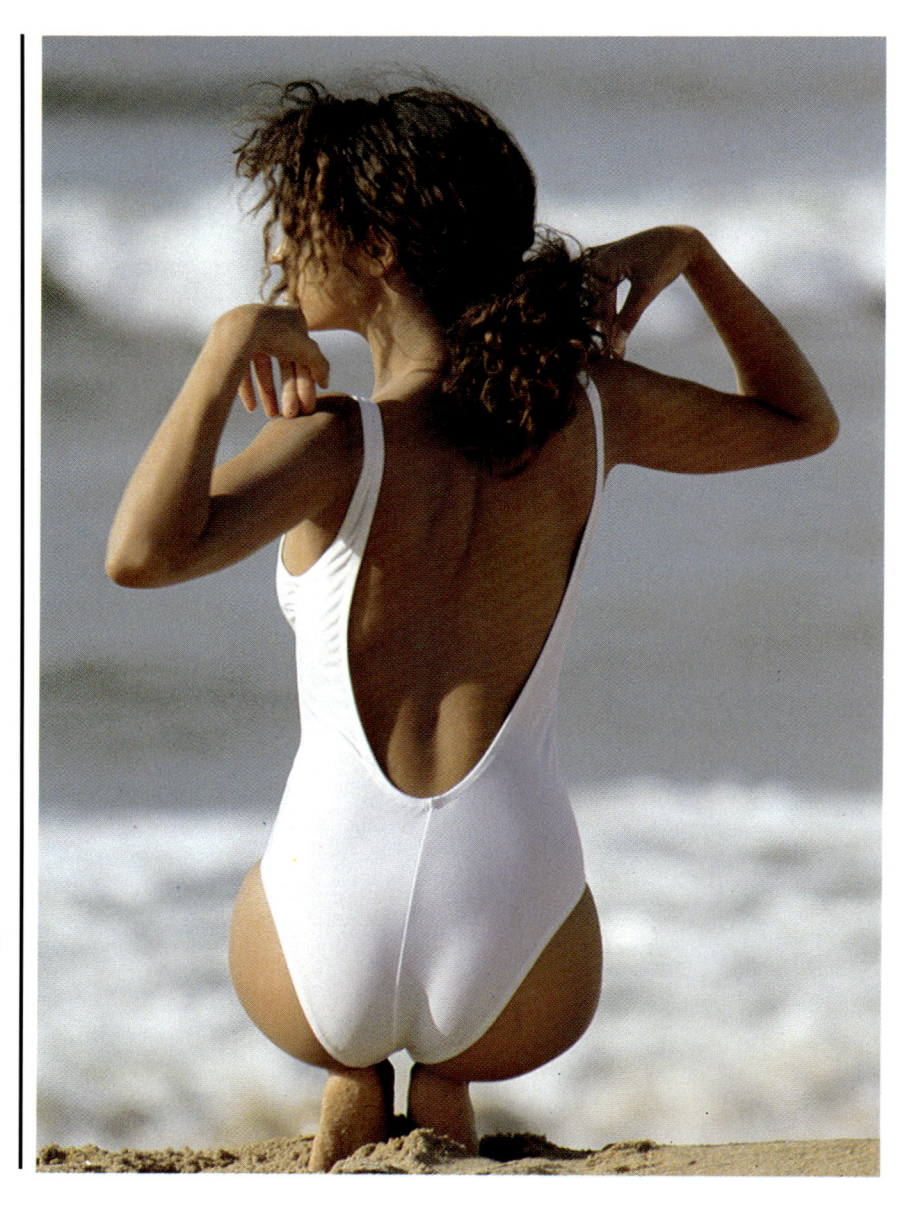

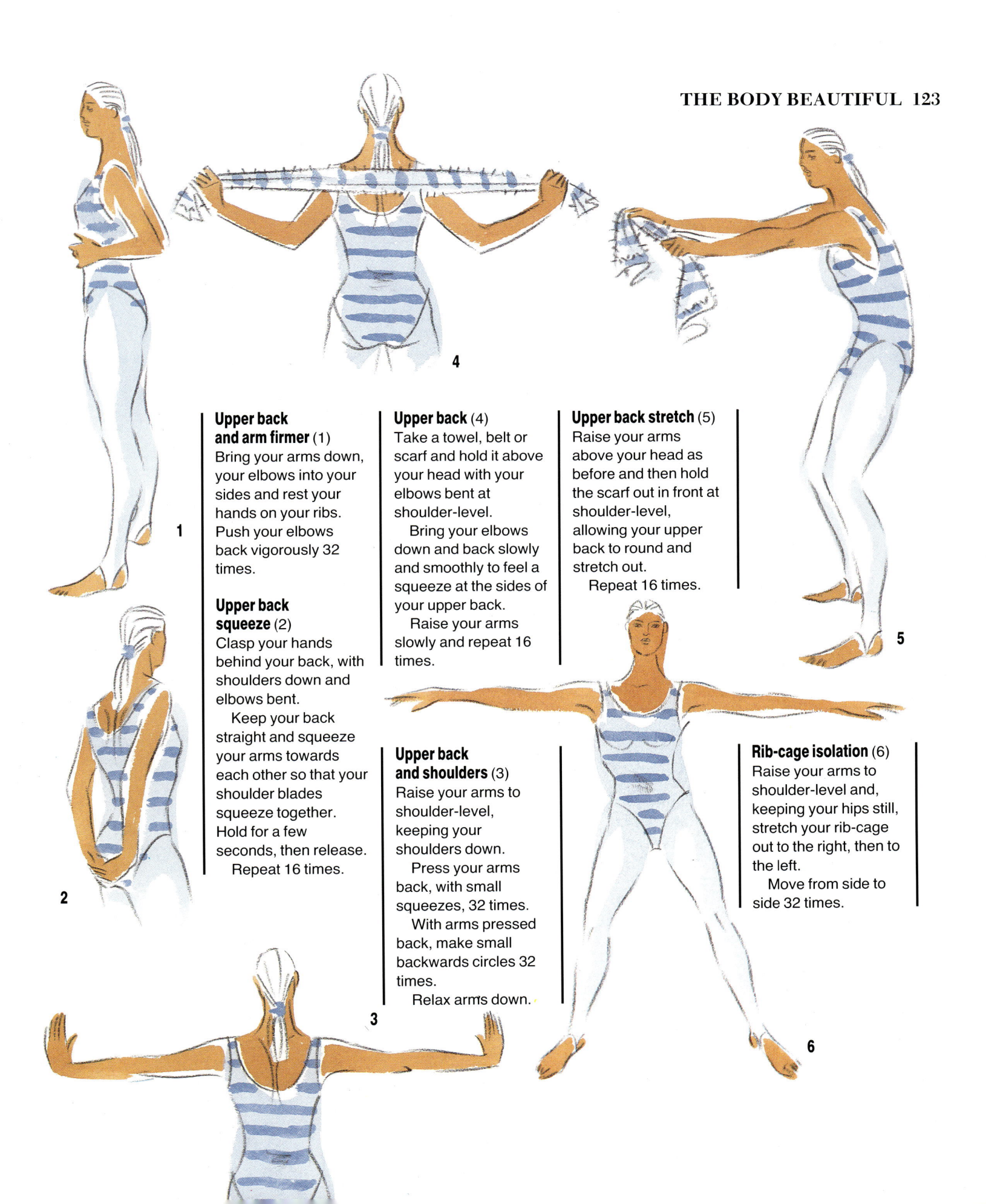

THE BODY BEAUTIFUL 123

Upper back and arm firmer (1)
Bring your arms down, your elbows into your sides and rest your hands on your ribs. Push your elbows back vigorously 32 times.

Upper back squeeze (2)
Clasp your hands behind your back, with shoulders down and elbows bent.
Keep your back straight and squeeze your arms towards each other so that your shoulder blades squeeze together. Hold for a few seconds, then release. Repeat 16 times.

Upper back and shoulders (3)
Raise your arms to shoulder-level, keeping your shoulders down.
Press your arms back, with small squeezes, 32 times.
With arms pressed back, make small backwards circles 32 times.
Relax arms down.

Upper back (4)
Take a towel, belt or scarf and hold it above your head with your elbows bent at shoulder-level.
Bring your elbows down and back slowly and smoothly to feel a squeeze at the sides of your upper back.
Raise your arms slowly and repeat 16 times.

Upper back stretch (5)
Raise your arms above your head as before and then hold the scarf out in front at shoulder-level, allowing your upper back to round and stretch out.
Repeat 16 times.

Rib-cage isolation (6)
Raise your arms to shoulder-level and, keeping your hips still, stretch your rib-cage out to the right, then to the left.
Move from side to side 32 times.

BUST BEAUTY

Make bustcare part of your beauty programme. Good skincare tactics and regular exercise will keep your breasts beautiful.

Care for your bust on a regular basis, with exercise and skincare, and you will be surprised what a difference this makes.

Follow our breast beauty plan and your bustline will always look its natural best.

Tips for beautifying your bust
- The breasts are supported by the fan of skin extending from the tip of the chin to just beneath the bust. It is therefore important to keep this skin firm and toned. Apply body lotion daily after bathing and never take baths that are too hot – very hot water breaks down the skin's connective tissues.
- Don't spray your decolleté with perfume – it will cause this delicate skin to dry.
- When sunbathing, always wear sunscreens on your chest and sunblock on your nipples.
- Correcting poor posture is an instant bustline improver (see page 122). Open out your chest by rolling your shoulders back.
- Exercise the chest muscles three times a week.

Exercising the pectoral muscles – the pectoralis major covers much of the upper part of the front of the chest – gives the bust added lift.

Exercise does not increase the size of the breasts as they do not contain any muscle.
- Crash diets are very bad news for bust-conscious women, leading to stretch marks and sagging.
- Choose a bra made from natural fibres that is not too tight (a very tight bra restricts circulation). Avoid wearing padded bras too often as they cause sweating, which is detrimental to the condition of the skin. Always, always wear a bra when exercising.
- It is essential that you check your breasts for any changes or lumps every month from puberty. Do this on the same day each month, a few days after your period, when changes in the feel and size of your bust due to fluctuating hormone levels will have normalized.

Position for exercises
Lie with two pillows under your head and upper back or on a thick exercise mat. Your elbows should be able to dip below chest-level.

Use dumb-bells (see page 120 for weights).

Start with 10 repeats of each exercise and work up to 20 or 30, leaving a day between each workout. Keep your lower back pressed into the floor.

Chest builder (1)
With your hands lightly grasping the weights, extend your arms straight up, your palms facing each other.

Inhale and slowly pull your arms apart, slightly bending your elbows as you lower your arms smoothly towards the floor.

Exhale and bring your hands back together.

THE BODY BEAUTIFUL 125

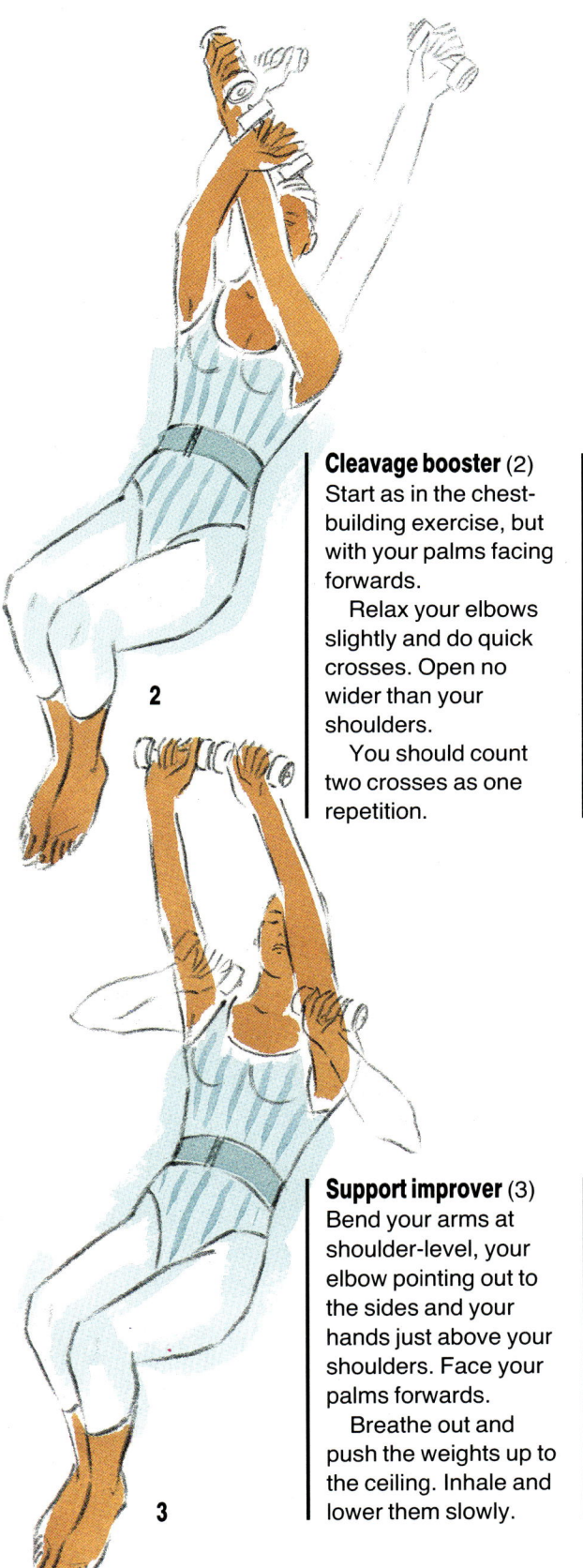

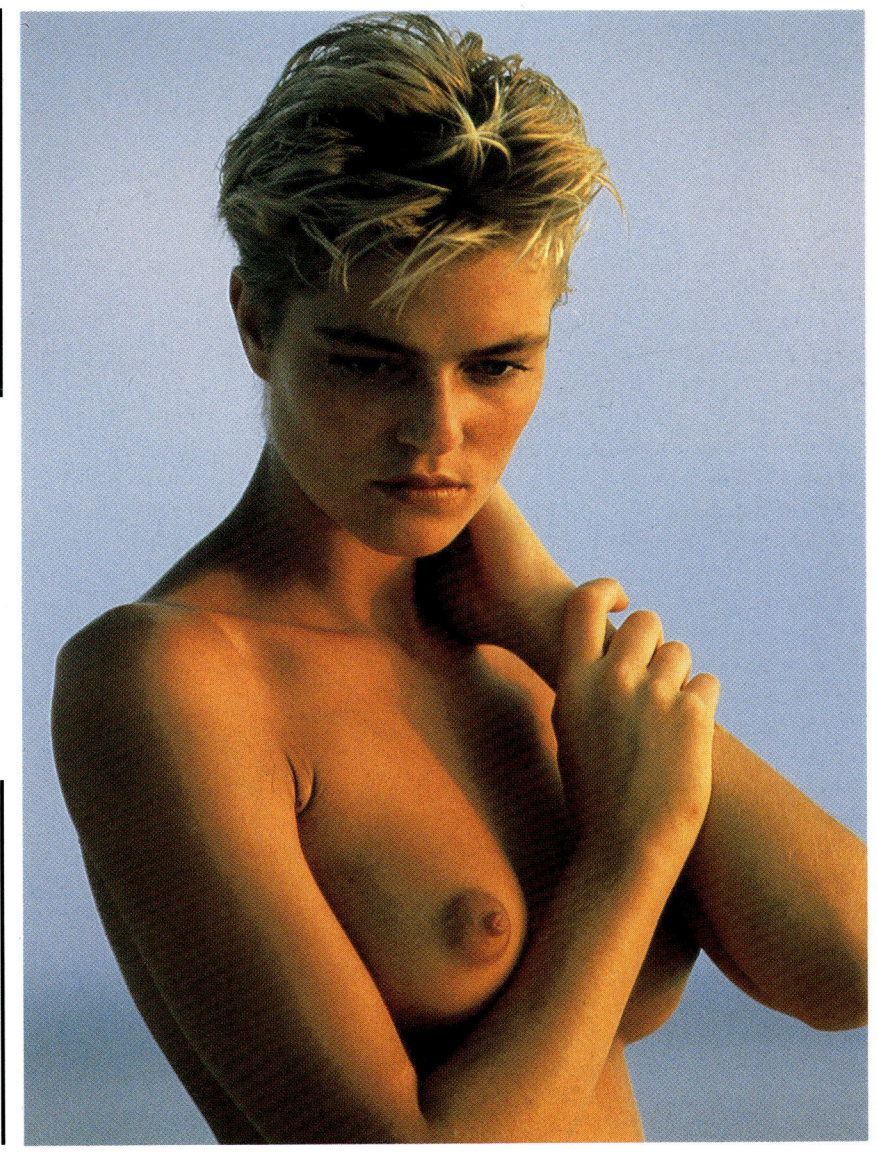

Cleavage booster (2)
Start as in the chest-building exercise, but with your palms facing forwards.
　Relax your elbows slightly and do quick crosses. Open no wider than your shoulders.
　You should count two crosses as one repetition.

Support improver (3)
Bend your arms at shoulder-level, your elbow pointing out to the sides and your hands just above your shoulders. Face your palms forwards.
　Breathe out and push the weights up to the ceiling. Inhale and lower them slowly.

STOMACH AND WAIST FLATTENERS

Developing a stronger, flatter stomach calls for special exercises and a little determination, but we have made it as easy as possible.

Women are designed to have a slightly rounded abdomen, so one has to accept that a totally flat tummy isn't realistic, especially as you get older or have children. Part of the reason why excess fat is so readily deposited in this area is the primitive survival factor – if you were to go short of food, your body would draw on its fat stores for energy. However, all this should not be used as an excuse for having a couple of spare tyres!

To ensure your middle is as trim as it can be, you should follow a healthy, low-fat eating programme. Toning exercises will also help redefine the flab.

● Doing abdominal exercises correctly calls for determination and a fair amount of hard work. The short cut to a flatter stomach is good technique. Done correctly, abdominal exercises are very effective and are definitely worth the effort! Do the exercises regularly and your stomach will be stronger, firmer and flatter.

Straight sit-ups, which are also known as curl-ups, aren't enough. You must also work the upper and lower abdominals and the bands of muscles at the sides. Your stomach muscles should always be pulled in before you add any resistance, and you must hold them in throughout the movement. If you do abdominal exercises with your stomach bulging (for bulging read *straining*), they will develop that way. You will no longer be holding the weight of your body with your abdominal muscles and muscles attached to your lower back will take over. So, if you start to strain you should stop.

● Body-conditioning classes are an excellent place to start if you haven't exercised for a while. The teacher will take you through the movements step-by-step, should check that you are doing them correctly and will motivate you.

● In the gym, most weight-training systems will include some exercises for the stomach area and you may find that simply having a bar to hold on to as you lie on a slanted exercise bench and bend and lower your legs will help you to grit your teeth and carry on!

At-home and salon treatments

You should be very gentle with your stomach: avoid using massage gloves and mitts in this area altogether.

In the salon, the Ionithermie treatment (see also page 131) can be used from

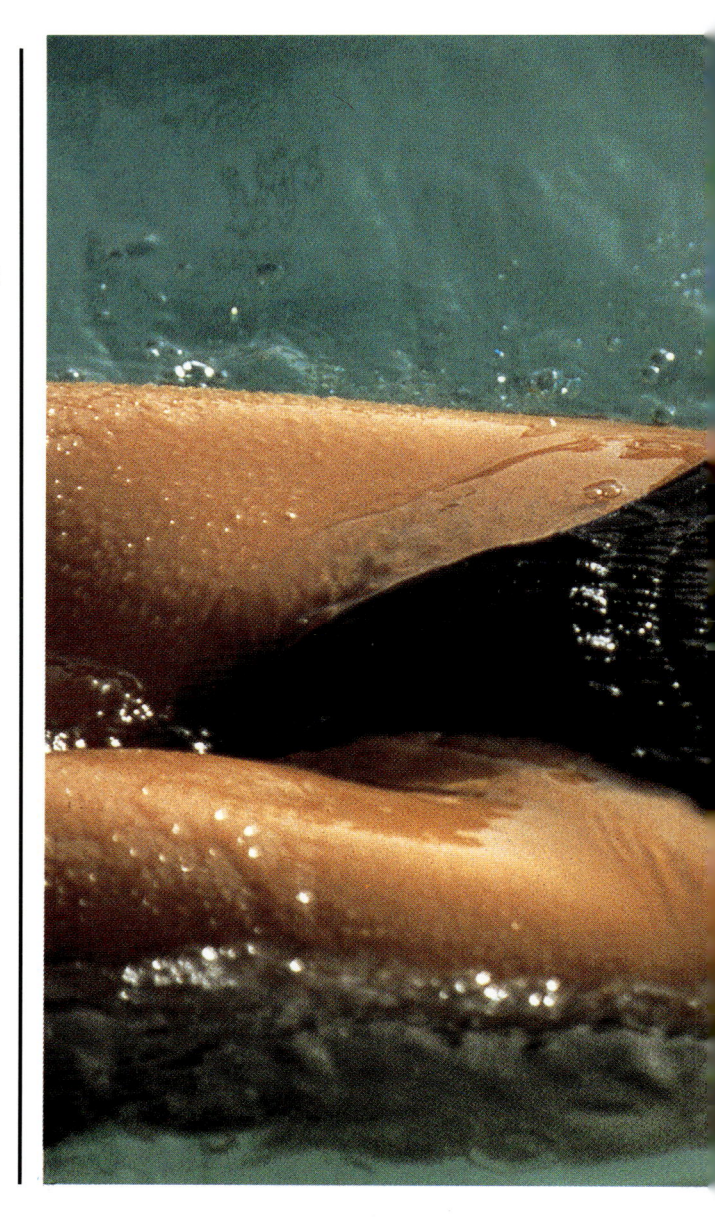

THE BODY BEAUTIFUL 127

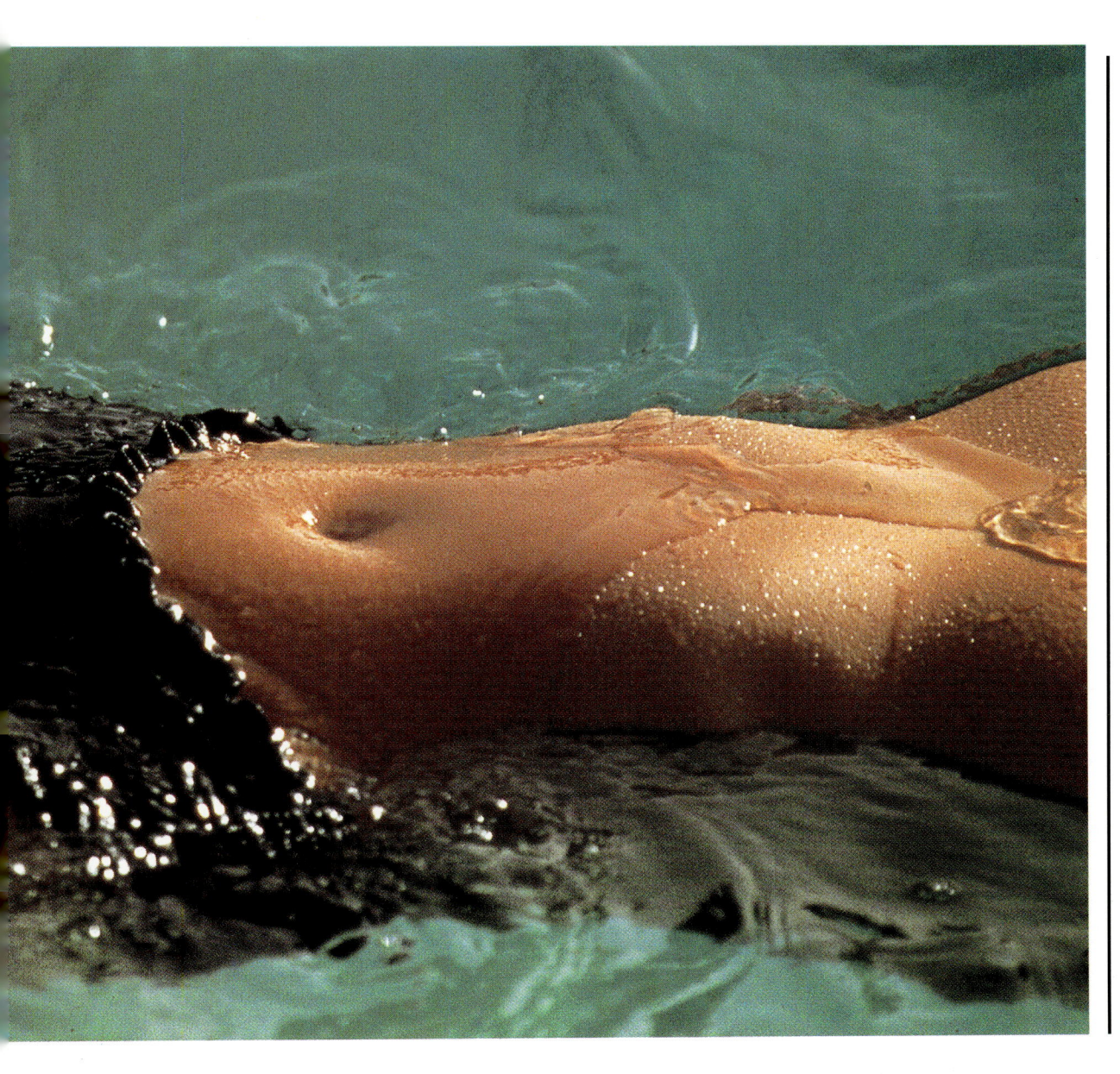

beneath the bust and is useful in reducing the size of the stomach to a small degree.

The exercises described here should, ideally, be done three times a week with a day's rest in between.

Stop exercising if you feel any strain in your lower back or if your stomach bulges and quivers. Don't lock your hands behind your neck as you may strain it as you lift up. If you have a back problem, you should be especially careful when doing stomach exercises. Begin with the first exercise, placing your legs over the seat of a chair, and add the others over a period of time, depending on your level of fitness.

Lie on an exercise mat or on two towels throughout the exercises. You should breathe out as you lift up and in as you go down.

128 SHORT CUTS

Warm up
Walk briskly around the room for a few minutes before you begin.

Pelvic tilt (1)
Lie on your back with your feet flat on the floor, hip-width apart, knees bent.
   Breathe out as you pull your lower stomach in hard and press the small of your back firmly to the floor, lifting your buttocks slightly.
   Repeat this exercise 20 times.

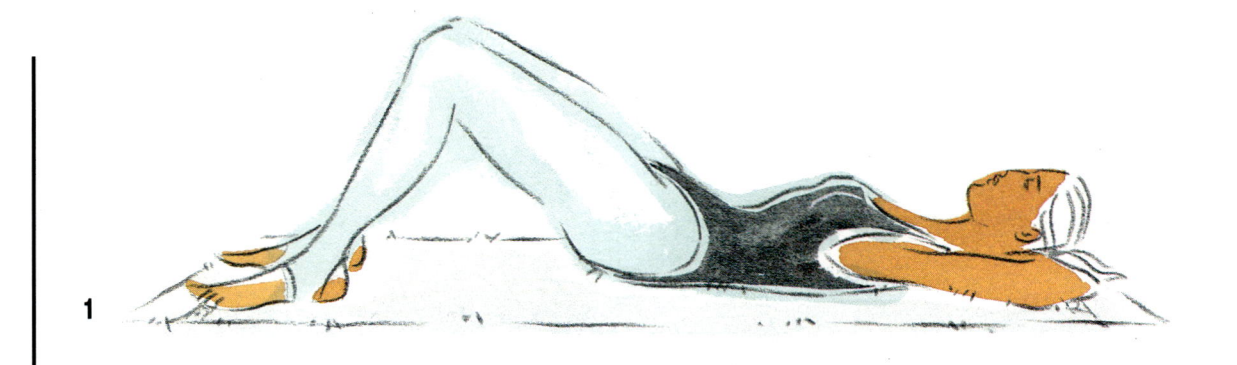

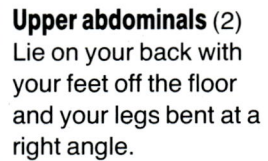

Upper abdominals (2)
Lie on your back with your feet off the floor and your legs bent at a right angle.
   Pull your stomach muscles in so that your pelvis tilts and your lower back presses into the floor.
   Cross your feet.
   Place your hands by the sides of your head, elbows out.
   Gently lift your shoulders from the floor and try to touch your elbows to your knees without moving your thighs.
   Don't allow your legs to drop forwards (if they do, rest your legs over the seat of a chair).
   Return to the start position and repeat 10 to 20 times.

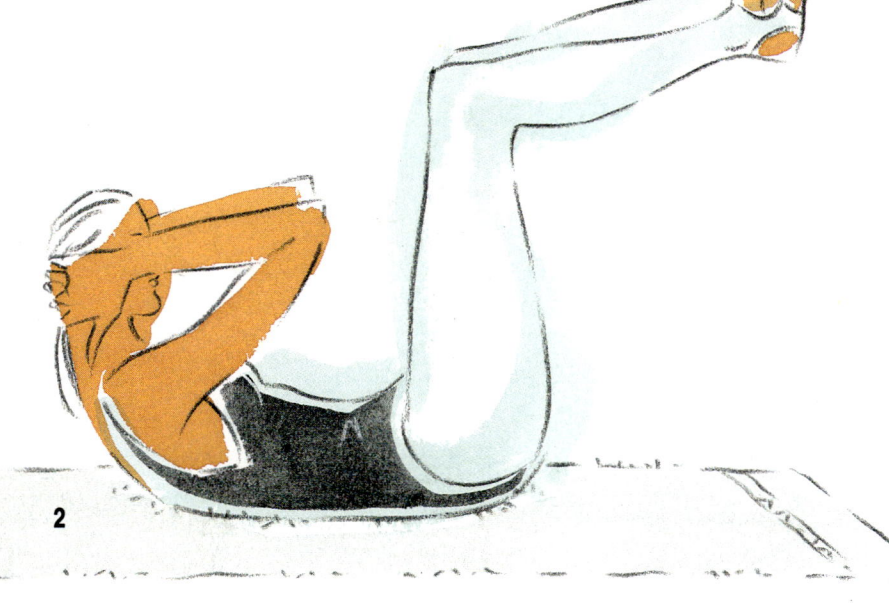

THE BODY BEAUTIFUL 129

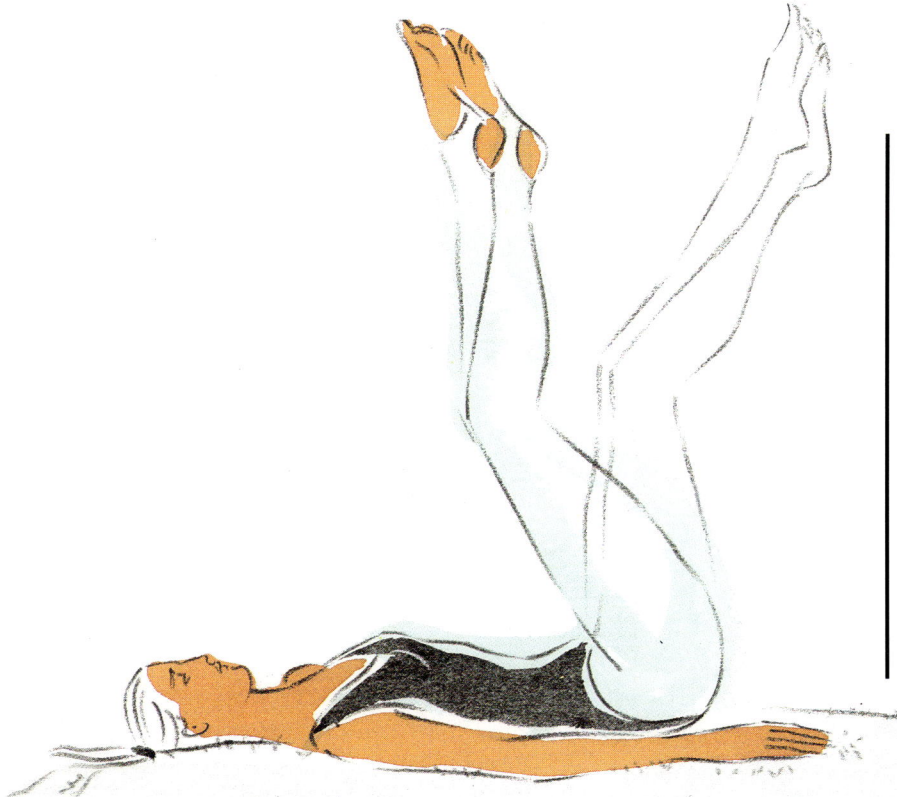

Lower abdominals (3)
Start by lying on your back with your hands by your sides.

Pull in your stomach muscles so that your pelvis tilts and your lower back presses into the floor.

Bend your knees into your chest and lift your legs up until they make a right angle with your upper body.

Cross your ankles.

Without pushing off the floor, lift your hips using your lower abdominals – your knees should come a little way towards your shoulders.

Then, lower your hips back to the floor and repeat 10 to 15 times.

Note: it can take time before you feel any effect in the correct areas, so persevere. You should feel the movement pulling in from the pubic bone and into the lower part of your stomach, but it should not be painful.

Upper abdominals and waist (4)
Start in the same position as for upper abdominals, but only bend one leg, leaving the other extended.

Twist your shoulders so that the opposite elbow points towards the raised knee. Reverse the legs and twist the other way.

Start slowly and gradually increase the speed, getting into a rhythm. Repeat 10 to 20 times.
Note: your straight leg adds the weight for the stomach muscles to resist against. Start with your legs fairly high for less weight. Make sure that you can hold in your stomach against the weight you're adding.

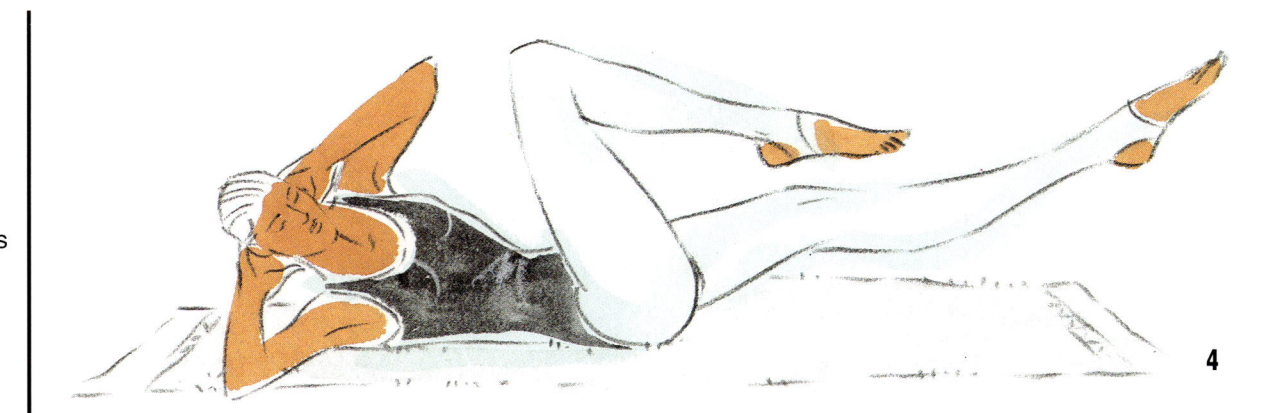

Muscle soother (5)
After performing stomach exercises, relax your muscles by lying on the floor and bringing your knees to your chest, keeping your lower back pressed into the floor. Clasp your hands over your knees.

Breathe in slowly and deeply several times.

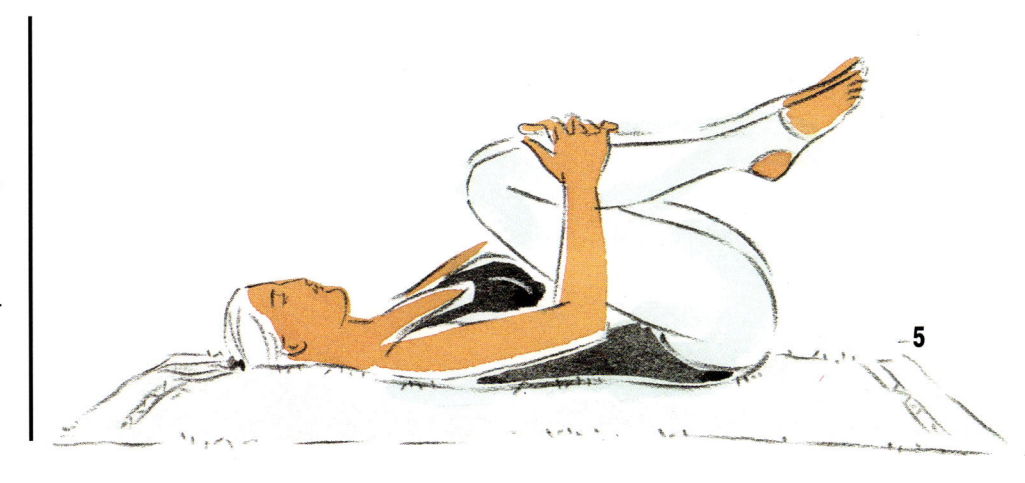

HIP, THIGH AND BOTTOM TONERS

Re-size your thighs, hone your hips and perk up your posterior with these on-the-spot exercises and firming treatments.

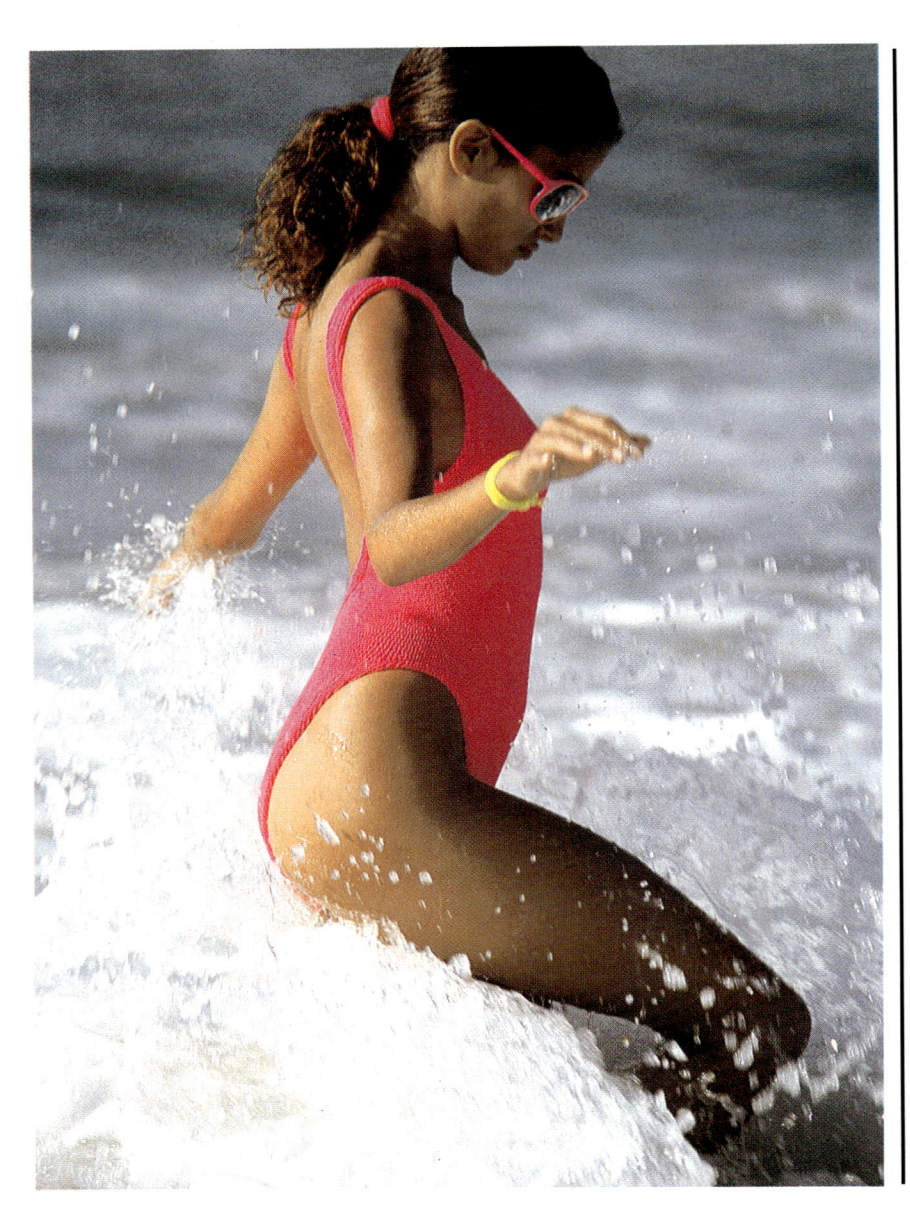

The hips, thighs and bottom are the number one problem area for the majority of women. The simple fact is that we are physiologically built to deposit fat around the hips and buttocks.

You can re-shape this body zone, however, by using the special toning and firming exercises described on the following pages.

WHAT IS CELLULITE?

This is the dimpled, 'orange peel' skin that often forms in puberty, when we increase our weight, and just before the menopause. Toxins, fluid and fat accumulate, weaken the tissues and prematurely age the structure of the skin. While hormonal changes are a prime cause, there are several other contributing factors.

- Toxins are trapped in the area due to poor circulation. When fighting cellulite, you should eat a wholefood diet and drink plenty of water. Give up stimulants such as coffee, nicotine and alcohol that are heavily implicated in the formation of cellulite. Avoid salt, sugar and processed foods and limit the amount of fat, dairy produce and meat you eat.
- A sedentary lifestyle and wearing tight clothes such as jeans leads to poor circulation in the area. Stress can worsen the problem, tense muscles leading to restricted lymph drainage. Walk and swim regularly.

At-home treatments
Regular massage with a mitt and a body-contouring gel will boost the effects of the anti-cellulite tactics above. Don't rub too hard with a massage glove, however, or you may break small

THE BODY BEAUTIFUL 131

capillaries. Simply massaging with your hands helps too. Using your whole hand, gently squeeze the skin, moving it from one hand to the other. Use aromatherapy oils such as cypress and juniper to enhance the action. Remember that whenever you massage you should move towards your heart, in harmony with your circulation.

Dry skin brushing is another cellulite beater. By stimulating lymph drainage this deceptively simple treatment can have tremendous benefits for all-round health. It takes just a few minutes a day.

Before bathing or showering, use a brush made of very stiff, natural bristles to make circular movements all over the hip and thigh area. If you have time, use long, firm movements from your foot up to your knee, and then up to your thigh. Next, focus on your hips and buttocks. Use the brush very gently at first. If it is scratching your skin, soak it in warm water and then leave it to dry before using it again.

Salon treatments
There are a number of salon treatments that speed up the treatment of cellulite.
- Aromatherapists use special blends of essential oils to tackle the area, usually to great effect.
- Health spas and health farms offer a range of solutions from seaweed baths, which have a detoxifying and mild slimming effect, to hydrotherapy, where the aesthetician aims jets of sea-water at the flabby areas.
- G5 massage uses electrically-powered massage heads to improve circulation.
- Treatments such as Ionithermie are very effective at flushing out retained fluid and a reduction of several inches can be achieved over the whole area in one session.

Gels and creams containing active ingredients are applied to the skin, then clay is smoothed on and electrodes inserted in between the layers. Two types of current are then applied: faradic current to exercise the muscles passively – you feel fairly strong tingling and twitching sensations in your muscles – and galvanic current, which increases the absorption of the products. The whole treatment takes about an hour and a half. The inches will stay off if you eat healthily and take regular exercise.
- Lymphatic drainage treatments are becoming increasingly available. The lymph drainage circulation is the body's waste disposal system and it can often become sluggish due to a lack of exercise and other factors. One salon method uses inflatable rubber 'stockings' that are zipped on to the leg from ankle to thigh. As the stockings inflate, the pressure pushes the lymph around the body. Good for total body health.

Warm up (1)
Use the back of a chair for balance.

Start with your outside foot behind you, then swing it forwards and back loosely, allowing your knee to bend.

Do this 16 times.

Then, using small movements, lift a little further up at each end of the swing 16 times.

Change to your left leg and repeat.

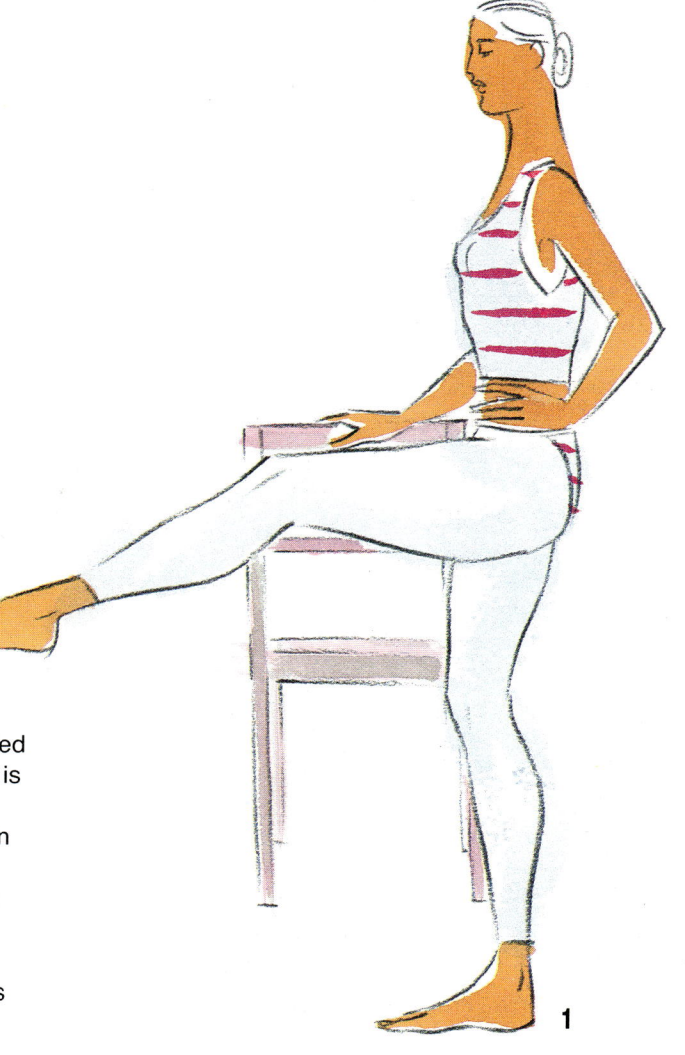

132 SHORT CUTS

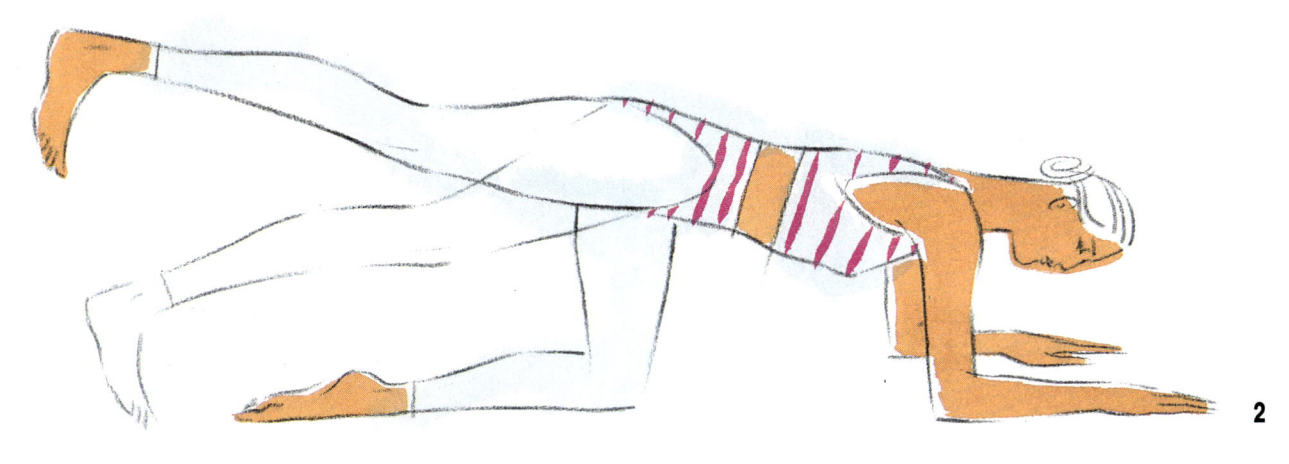

Backs of thighs and bottom

(2) Rest on your knees and forearms.

Hold your stomach in to keep your lower back straight and raise your right leg, keeping your leg straight and your foot flexed at a right-angle to your leg.

Touch the floor with your toe and then raise your leg using the back-of-thigh and buttock muscles.

Do this 16 times.

Then, using small movements, push up a little more at the top of the lift 16 times.

Repeat the exercise using your left leg.

(3) Lying on your front with your head resting on your arms, raise your right leg, keeping your right hip in contact with the floor.

Flex your foot and bend your knee so that your heel comes in towards your bottom.

Straighten your leg a little and repeat the movement 16 times.

Keep your leg bent and raise and lower your thigh 16 times.

Repeat the exercise using your left leg.

Inside thigh (4)

Roll on to your side.

Straighten your underneath leg and turn it out so that your knee faces forwards.

Bend your top leg and place your foot behind your lower leg.

Raise and lower your straight leg, using inside thigh muscles. Repeat 32 times.

Roll over and repeat using your other leg.

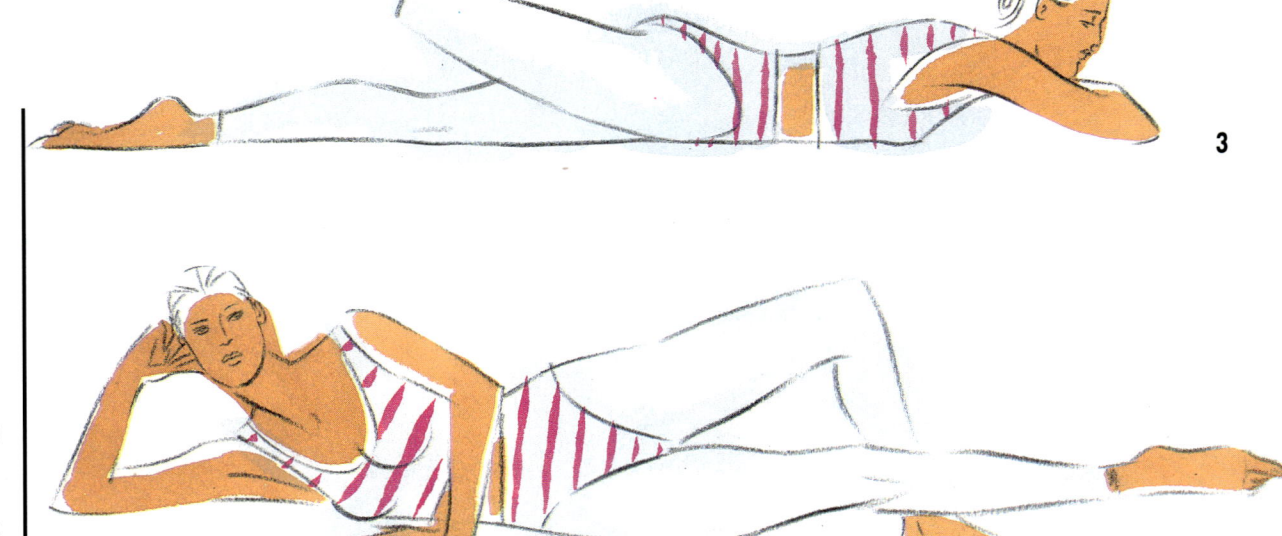

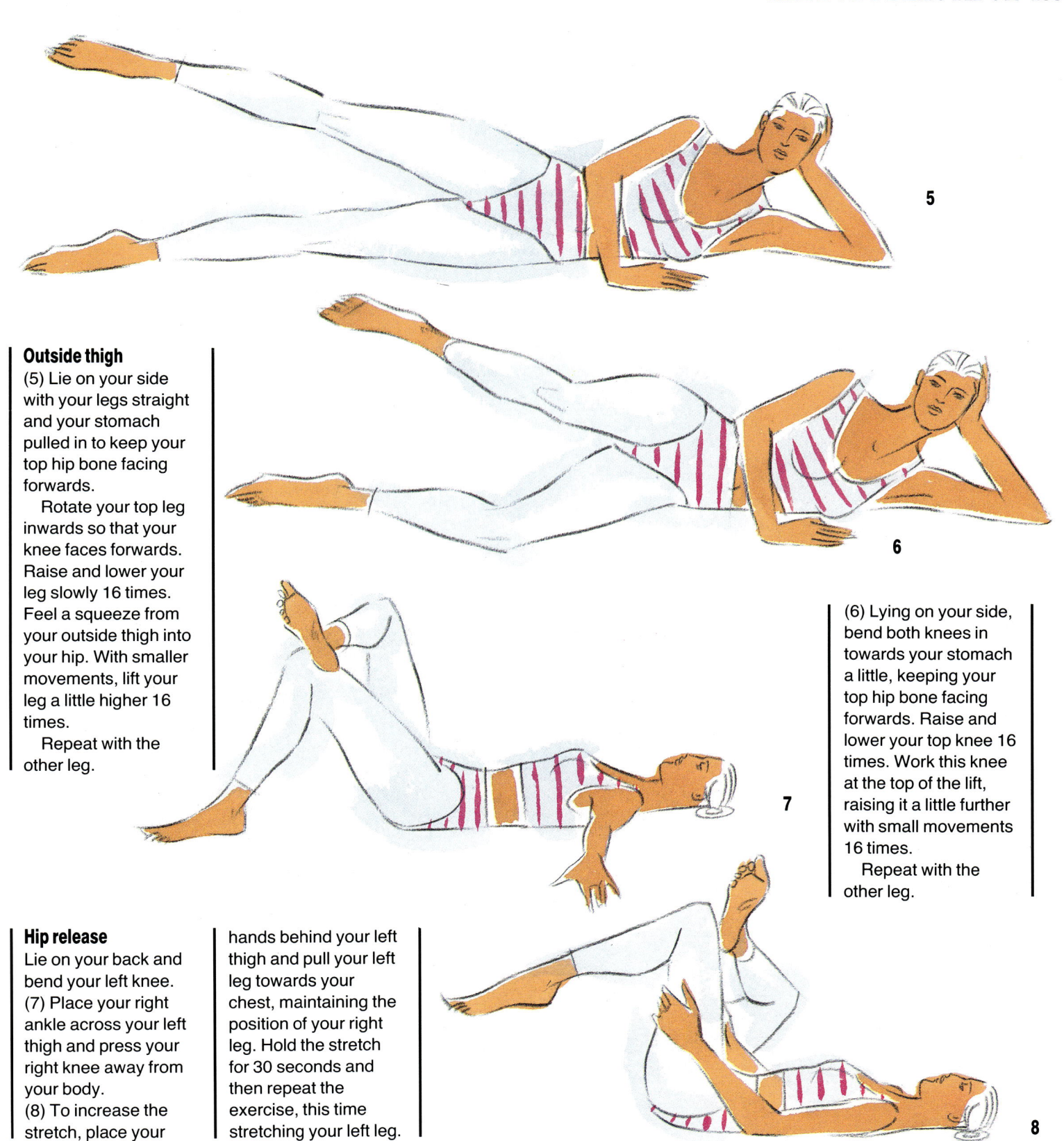

THE BODY BEAUTIFUL 133

Outside thigh
(5) Lie on your side with your legs straight and your stomach pulled in to keep your top hip bone facing forwards.
Rotate your top leg inwards so that your knee faces forwards. Raise and lower your leg slowly 16 times. Feel a squeeze from your outside thigh into your hip. With smaller movements, lift your leg a little higher 16 times.
Repeat with the other leg.

(6) Lying on your side, bend both knees in towards your stomach a little, keeping your top hip bone facing forwards. Raise and lower your top knee 16 times. Work this knee at the top of the lift, raising it a little further with small movements 16 times.
Repeat with the other leg.

Hip release
Lie on your back and bend your left knee.
(7) Place your right ankle across your left thigh and press your right knee away from your body.
(8) To increase the stretch, place your hands behind your left thigh and pull your left leg towards your chest, maintaining the position of your right leg. Hold the stretch for 30 seconds and then repeat the exercise, this time stretching your left leg.

LEGS WORKOUT

Use these exercise and beauty secrets for lovelier legs – they are one of the easiest body areas to firm into shape.

Your basic leg shape is determined by your genes, though you can redefine it to a certain extent. Exercise will strengthen and sculpt, reduce flabbiness and ensure shapely calves and ankles.

As well as the exercises illustrated, make a conscious effort to use your legs more in day-to-day life: walk up and down stairs instead of using escalators and lifts, go on foot or cycle as often as possible. For the sports-minded, swimming, horse-riding, basketball and running are all great leg shapers.

If you are desk-bound all day the chances are that your legs will feel tired and ache and be prone to cramp. This is because sitting slows the circulation. Guard against this by stretching your legs every now and then and don't sit with them tightly crossed.

Try this quick circulation-boosting exercise, which will also firm your thighs and help flabby knees.
- Sit on a chair that supports your back.
- With your left foot flat on the floor, raise your right leg (so that it is parallel to the floor) until your knee locks.
- Bend your right leg a little way then straighten it again.
- Repeat 10 times and then do the same, stretching your left leg.

At-home and salon treatments
Remember that your legs are drier than other areas of your body, so moisturize them after every bath or shower.

Legs like to be exfoliated too, (see page 54), particularly the shin and knee areas. Use a loofah once a week, it will only take a few minutes.

For salon cellulite beaters, see page 131.

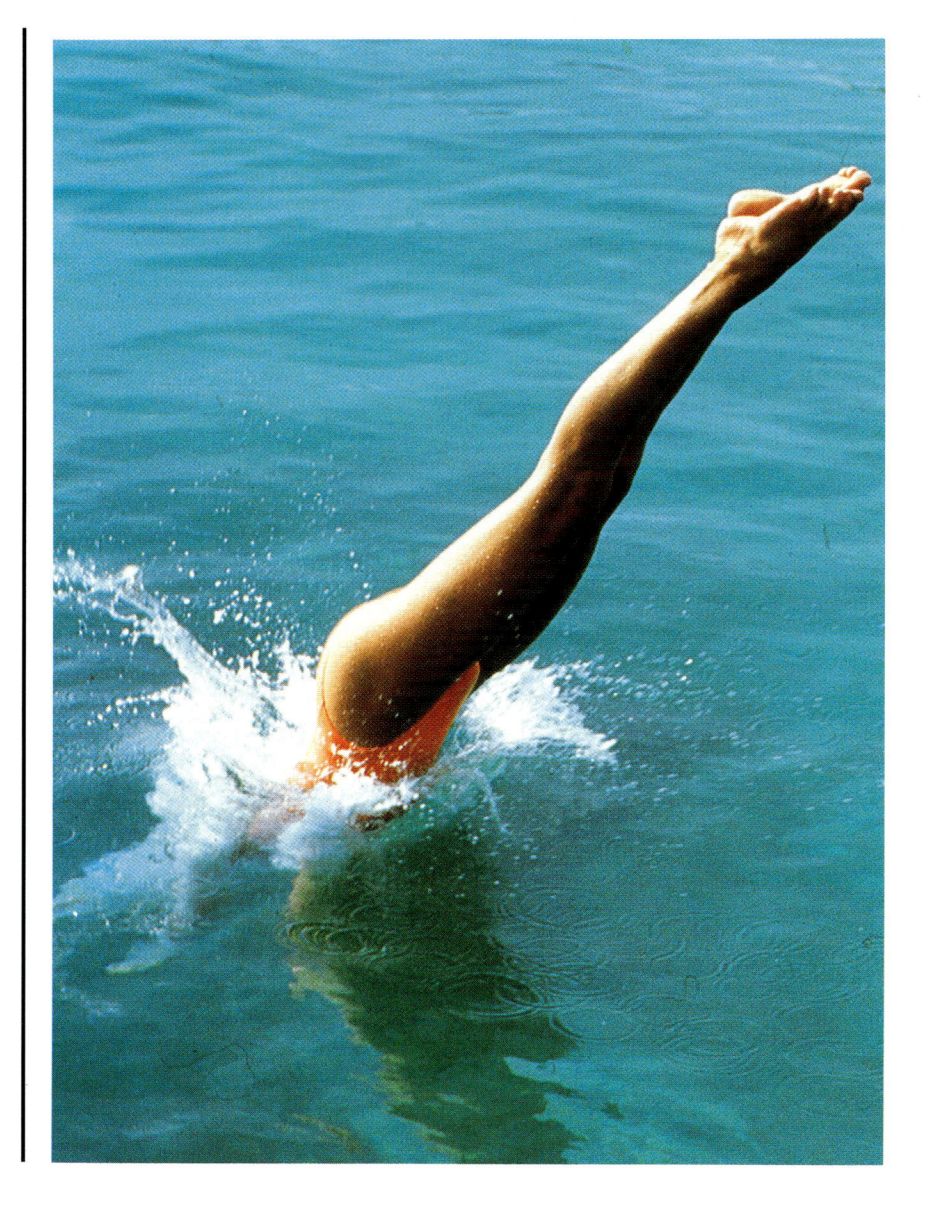

THE BODY BEAUTIFUL 135

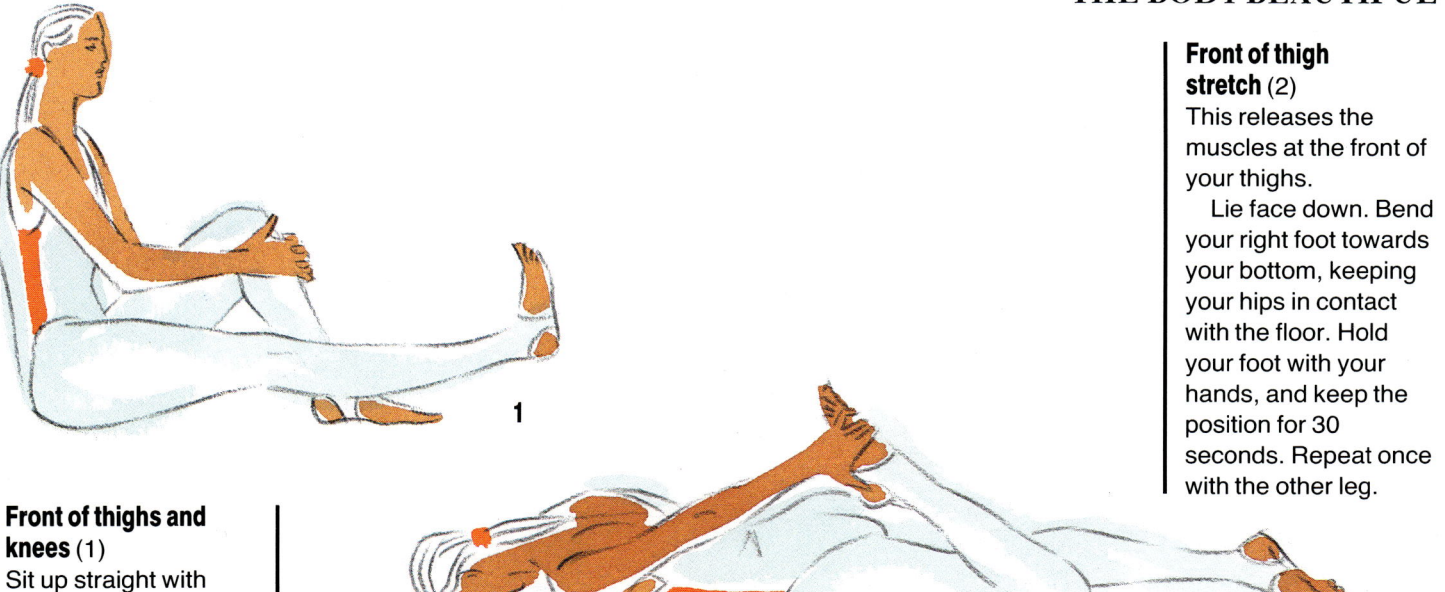

Front of thigh stretch (2)
This releases the muscles at the front of your thighs.
  Lie face down. Bend your right foot towards your bottom, keeping your hips in contact with the floor. Hold your foot with your hands, and keep the position for 30 seconds. Repeat once with the other leg.

Front of thighs and knees (1)
Sit up straight with your left leg bent and your right leg straight out in front of you, with your knee facing up and your foot flexed. Raise and lower your leg smoothly 8 to 16 times. Repeat with your other leg, then do the front of thigh stretch.
Note: the muscles at the front of your thighs – the quadriceps – also support your knees, so by keeping them strong, you keep your knees stable.

Calves (3)
Using the back of a chair for support, place your feet together and tuck in your buttocks.
  Raise and lower your heels smoothly. Repeat 16 to 32 times, then do the calf stretch.

Calf stretch (4)
Standing, slide your right leg back behind you without allowing your hips to twist. Press your heel to the floor and lean your weight forwards, keeping your body straight. Feel the stretch through your calf. Hold this position for 30 seconds. Repeat using your other leg.

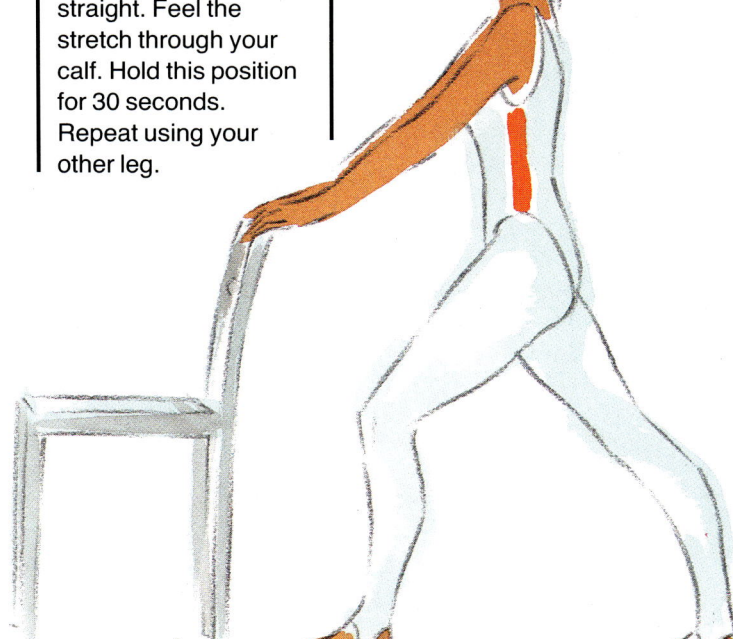

HAND AND NAIL SAVERS

Give your hands and nails the attention they deserve – don't neglect this important part of your total image.

A little regular care will keep your hands and nails looking their polished best. Follow the finger tips below and you'll have no excuse for untidy cuticles, brittle nails or dry hands.

HANDCARE
- Do not plunge unprotected hands and nails into soapy water or household chemicals – wear rubber gloves!
- Apply handcream every time you wash your hands. Keep tubs of handcream beside the sink or basin.
- Remember to exfoliate the skin on the backs of your hands as well when you use a scrub on your body or face.
- Massage your hands with handcream whenever you have a few minutes to spare. Use the first finger and thumb of the opposite hand and work in small circles, moving from tips of fingers to wrist.

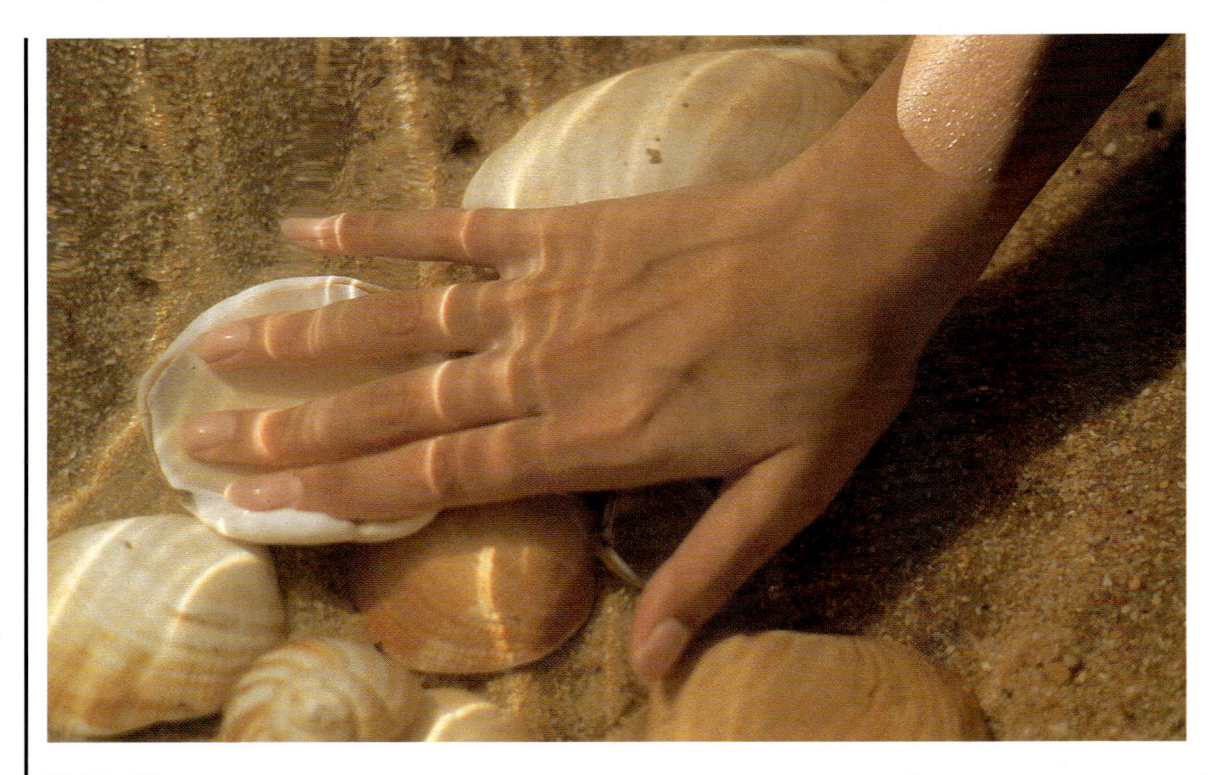

NAILCARE
- When you have a bath, push your cuticles back with your fingertips or a towel (use a light touch) as the warm water will have softened them.
- Nail nourishers are fast to apply and pay big beauty dividends, feeding the nail and surrounding skin with essential vitamins, oils and protein, helping the nails to grow.
- Manicure your nails fully approximately every 10 days, re-applying nail polish as necessary. Treat the cuticles very gently as they protect the growth centre of the nail. Never tear the skin or cut the cuticles.
- After removing nail polish you should wait a few minutes before filing. The nails may split if they aren't completely dry.
- Filing straight up against your nail can peel the tip: you should hold the emery board at a 45 degree angle under the free edge of the nail.
- The fastest way to prevent soft, weak nails from breaking is to apply hardener once or twice a week. It saves vulnerable nails and gives a high-shine finish.
- Brittle, peeling nails are caused by dryness. Massage handcream into nails frequently.

THE BODY BEAUTIFUL 137

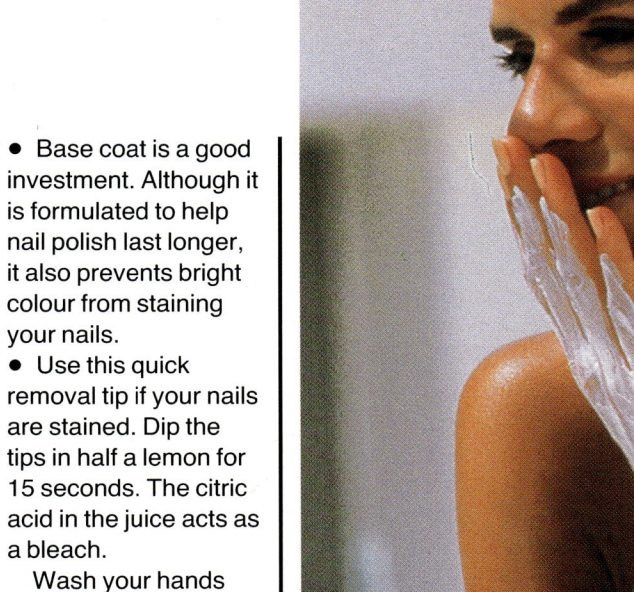

- Base coat is a good investment. Although it is formulated to help nail polish last longer, it also prevents bright colour from staining your nails.
- Use this quick removal tip if your nails are stained. Dip the tips in half a lemon for 15 seconds. The citric acid in the juice acts as a bleach.
  Wash your hands afterwards so that the lemon juice does not dry your nails.
- Nail polish is another good nail protector. When applying polish, especially dark colours, apply two to three thin coats, rather than one thick coat.
- Don't take polish right to the edges of the nails: it's quicker and neater to leave a thin strip down the side. Try this three-stroke method: apply the first stroke along the centre of the nail; then apply polish along both sides.

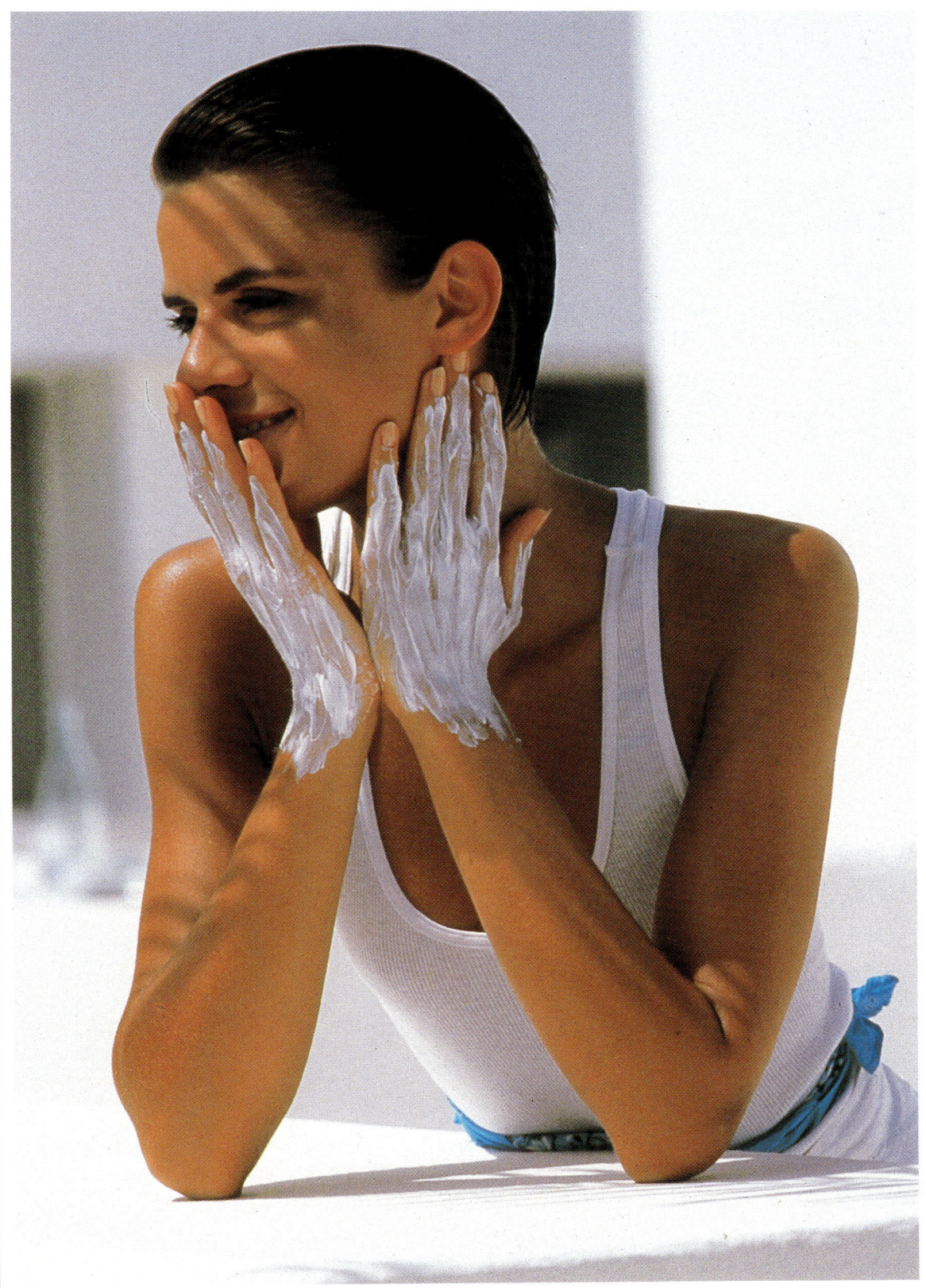

FEET FIRST

Pamper your feet as much as you can – not only will they look better but you'll ward off problems too.

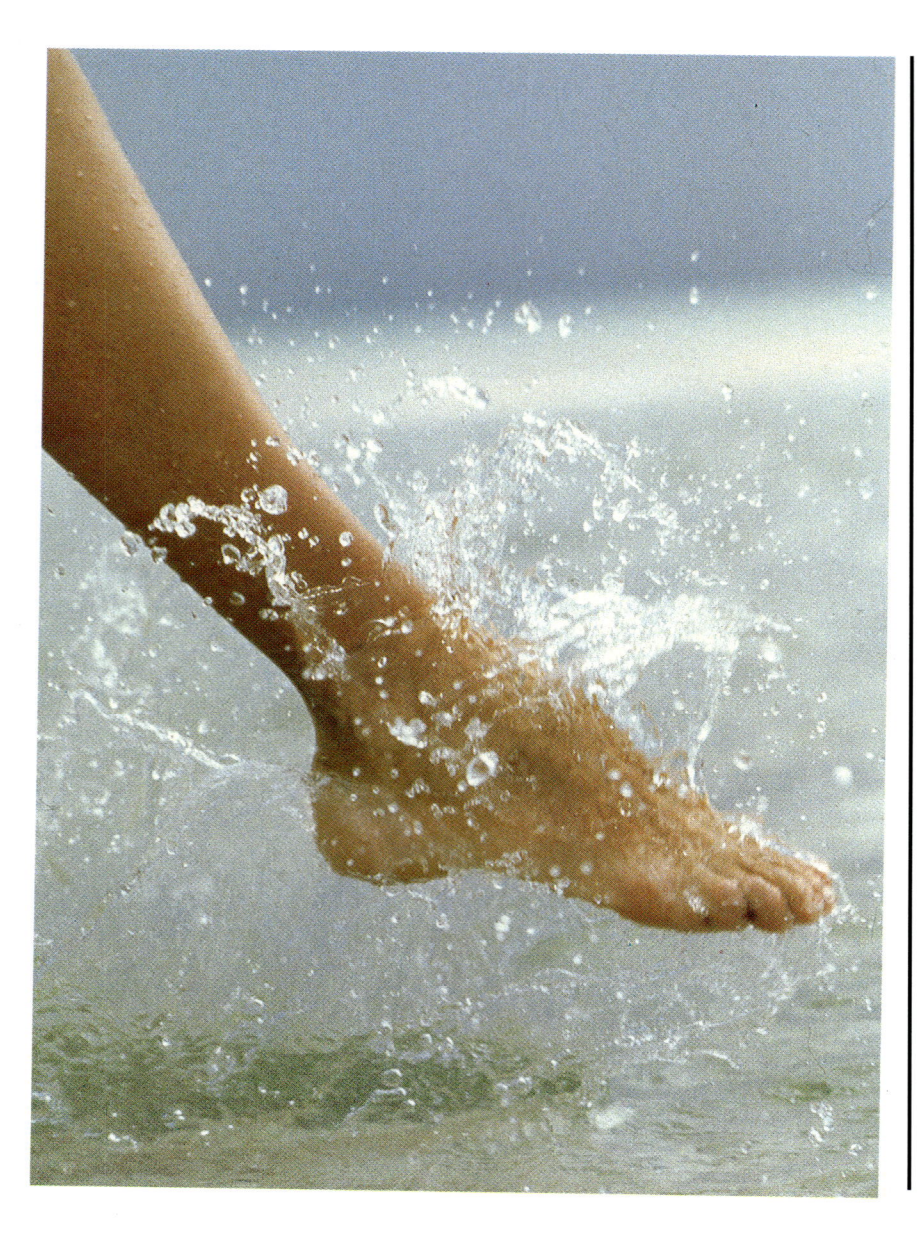

Feet are usually forgotten during a busy day, but often hurt most at the end of it. Looking after them is quick and easy.

FOOT WORKOUT

- Tired feet feel better fast with a massage. Use a refreshing cream or oil (with peppermint for instance) and work your thumbs in a circular motion starting at the ball of the foot, moving backwards towards your heel. Return to the toes, massaging each individually.
- Take the opportunity to walk barefoot whenever you can, allowing your feet free movement. Going barefoot in the sand is particularly good as it shapes the calves and ankles too.
- This exercise will strengthen your arches. Stand up straight with a tennis ball or rolling pin under one foot. Roll it backwards and forwards 10 times and then swap to the other foot and repeat.
- Stretch your feet out frequently, alternately flexing from the ankle and then pointing the toes.
- Circle your foot to the right eight times and then to the left eight times.

SHOE SENSE

The ideal shoe, allowing for toe shape, is 1.5 cm (½ in) longer than your foot. It should fit comfortably round the heel, over the instep and big toe. Leather is the best material, as it is permeable, allowing absorption of perspiration. A low, broad heel stresses the foot least. Sandals are good news for feet, too, as they don't restrict the toes and allow air to circulate.

Changing your shoes once or twice a day ensures that no one part of the foot has too much strain exerted on it.

Choosing shoes
During the day your feet swell. If you are choosing shoes, buy them in the afternoon to allow for this.

PERFECT PEDICURE
Keep your feet looking good with a once weekly treatment. This do-it-yourself pedicure only takes about 10 to 15 minutes.
1 Remove old nail polish, then file or clip your toe-nails straight across.
2 Remove the cuticles with cuticle cream and a wooden manicure stick – these can be found at the chemist.
3 Exfoliate the soles of your feet using water-dampened sea-salt.
4 Soak your feet for a few minutes in a warm foot bath, dry them thoroughly and follow with a massage with oil or moisturizing cream as described in the foot workout above.
5 Before painting your nails, rub off any excess cream or oil, as it may cause the polish to slip.
6 Apply a base coat and two coats of colour for a long-lasting finish. If you haven't the time to allow the polish to dry naturally, use a quick-drying spray or run cold water over your nails.

Quick foot pacifiers for aching feet
- Kick off your shoes and lift your feet on to a desk or table or lie on your bed with your feet raised resting on two pillows.
- Wrap ice cubes in a flannel and rub over your feet up to your ankles. Dry each foot and then dab them with witchhazel.
- Soak your feet in a bowl of lukewarm water containing a foot spa solution.
- Apply a cooling foot lotion over your feet and legs, up to the knees.

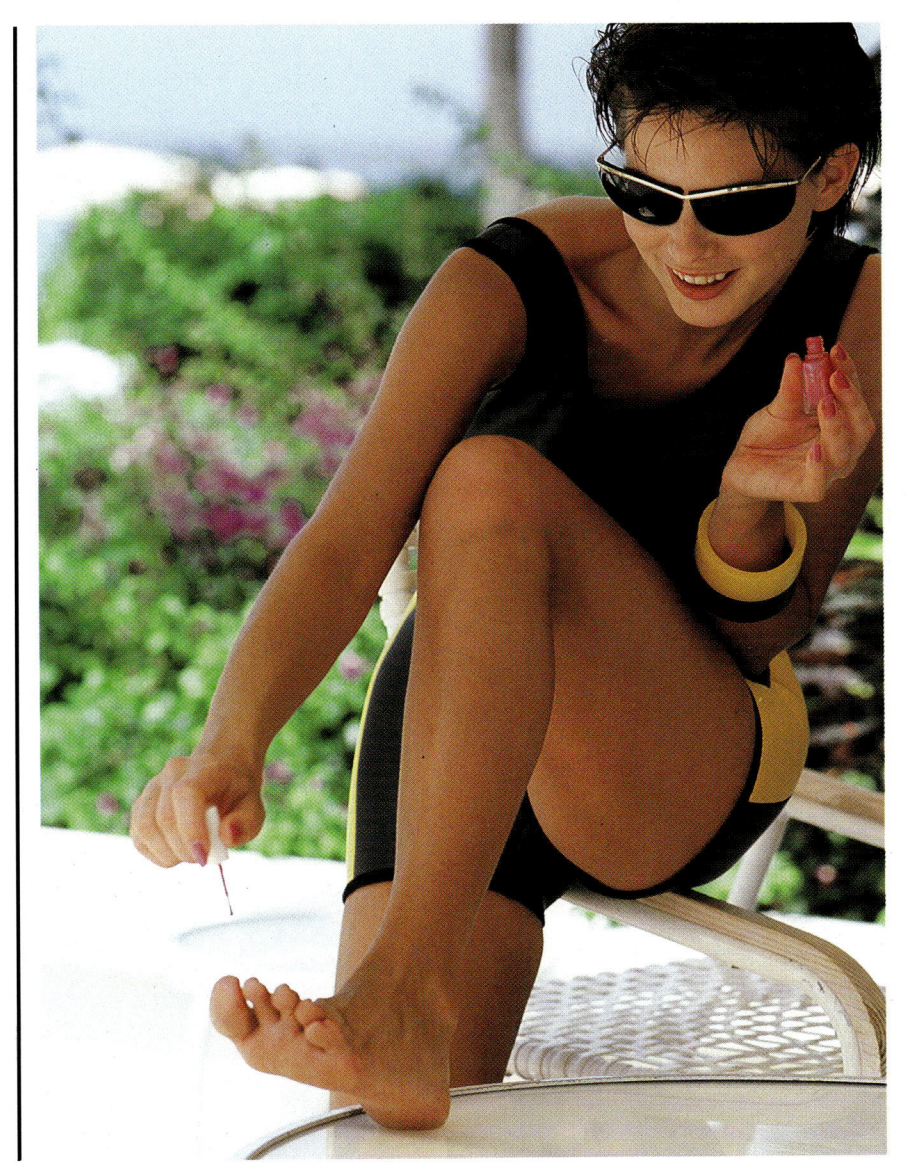

SMOOTH HAIR REMOVAL

Bothered by superfluous hair? Be a smooth operator and choose the best method for trouble-free hair removal.

Electrolysis is the permanent solution to removing unwanted hair, though hormonal changes during the life cycle can cause new hair growth. Other treatments are only temporary.

DEPILATORY CREAMS

These creams dissolve the hair to just below the surface of the skin.

Pain factor
Zero, unless you experience an allergy. It is important, therefore, to do a patch test 24 hours beforehand.
Time factor
5–10 minutes.
Regrowth
Depilation will be necessary again after a week or so.

Depilatory pros and cons
Depilatory creams are quick and effective but fairly messy to use and often smell unpleasant.

SHAVING

Probably the most popular type of at-home hair removal, it cuts the hair down to the surface of the skin, removing some of the skin's outer layer.

Pain factor
Zero, unless you cut yourself.
Time factor
Takes a few minutes.
Regrowth
Starts to look and feel stubbly after a few days. Needs re-doing at least twice a week to keep smooth. Hair grows back coarser.

Shaving tips
- To prevent irritation, use moisturizing shave cream and a razor with a comb guard.
- Use a special electric shaver for the sensitive bikini line.
- If you're off to the beach, shave the day before to allow the skin to recover – soreness can be triggered by chlorine, sunscreens and perspiration.

WAXING

This can be done both at home and in the salon, though salon waxing tends to be more effective.

Wax is usually heated and then pulled off in strips with paper or gauze against the direction of hair growth, pulling hair out from the follicle. Most salons use the 'cold' (in fact, warm) wax system. Hot waxing is less widely available, and is less hygienic as the wax is filtered and re-used.

Pain factor
Ouch! Stings, but it's quick. You get used to it. Your skin will be more sensitive before menstruation.
Time factor
A half-leg wax (both legs, knees to ankles) takes about 10 minutes.
Regrowth
Anything from three to six weeks. Hairs grow back finer after repeated treatments.

Wax fax
- Hair has to be long enough to be covered by the wax. If it's too short, it either won't come out or will be removed patchily to the surface only, with disappointing results.
- Don't wax broken or irritated skin.
- To minimize irritation, the skin should be pulled taut before stripping. Afterwards little pimples may break out, but they generally subside after a few days. To avoid further irritation, for the next 24 hours avoid the sun, very hot showers, products containing alcohol or fragrance, deodorant if the underarms have been waxed and strenuous activity which will cause perspiration.
- If you find you get ingrowing hairs after waxing, use an exfoliator to help them grow correctly.
- Waxing regularly is the best plan.

SUGARING

This is a sugar-and-water putty, applied to a small area at a time and pulled off against the hair growth. It is well known in the Middle East and is becoming increasingly available in salons elsewhere.

Pain factor
Marginally less painful than waxing.
Time factor
Half-leg sugaring takes about 45 minutes.
Regrowth
Anything from four to six weeks depending on the rate of hair growth. Hair grows back slower and finer with successive treatments.

Sugaring savvy
- Sugaring is less expensive than waxing, but it's harder to find a salon that does it.
- Use the same after-care tips as for waxing (see left).

THREADING

An ancient Chinese art that is also very popular in India. The therapist winds a piece of thread around one forefinger, forms a loop with it and whisks the hairs out.

Pain factor
It stings a little.

Time factor
A few seconds or minutes, depending on the size of the area being treated.

Regrowth
Fine hair may not regrow for up to 12 weeks. The regrowth should be much finer than the original hair (if a therapist is unskilled and cuts the hair off at the surface, it looks thicker). Eventually, the hair growth becomes weaker and can stop altogether.

Pros and cons
Threading is best suited to facial hair and much preferred by therapists to wax on this delicate skin.

ELECTROLYSIS

Hair should be treated during its growing cycle. After 2–3 treatments, it is possible to time the sessions to remove new growth.

Electrolysis involves inserting a needle (check your salon uses disposable ones) into the follicle and destroying the hair with heat generated by an electric current. 'The Blend' method combines two currents and is popular as it can produce faster results.

Pain factor
A short, sharp wince. Pain thresholds vary.

Time factor
5 minutes to half an hour depending on the area treated and your pain threshold. As hairs must be caught during an active cycle it can take months to eradicate the hairs completely.

Regrowth
Very slow during treatment. Once treatment is finished, negligible.

Electrolysis pros and cons
● You need to be dedicated to undergo the treatment – it's an effective, but very lengthy process.
● It can become expensive, depending on the area and strength of hair growth being treated. It is not, for example, economically viable to have your legs treated in this manner.
● DON'T use an at-home kit – you could scar yourself permanently. Electrolysis can also produce areas of darker pigment on black skins.
● DON'T schedule your appointment just before a meeting or going out if you are having electrolysis on the face, as there will be a little puffiness and redness afterwards, although this goes after a few hours.

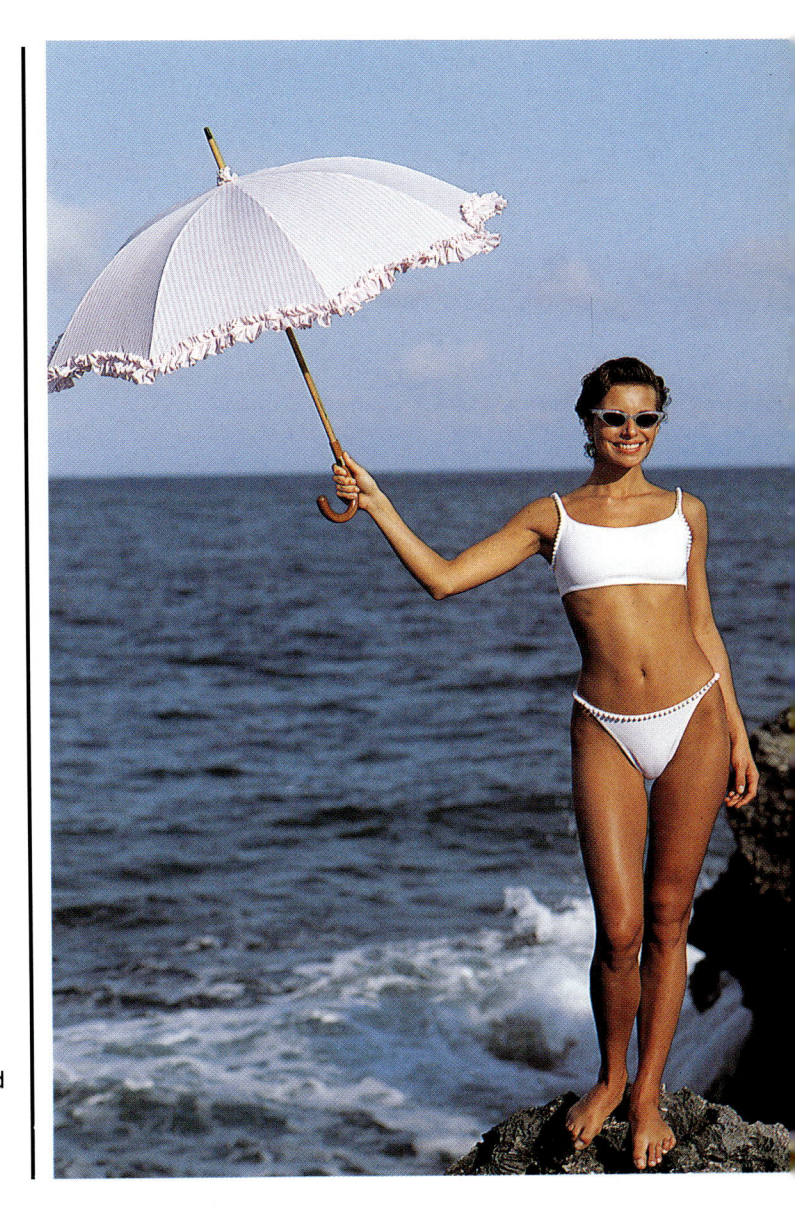

Index

A
abdominal exercises 126–9
acne 45, 59, 70
aerobic exercise 17, 19–20
Afro hair 103
ageing, skincare 58–9
alcohol 37, 130
alpha hydroxy acids 58
alternative therapies:
    aromatherapy 55
    auricular therapy 57
    biofeedback 37
    facials 57
    naturopathy 37
    reflexology 57
    zone therapy 57
arm exercises 120–1
aromatherapy 42–5, 57, 131
    inhalation 45
    in the bath 43
    massage 43
    oil types 44–5
    vaporizers 43

B
back exercises 122–3
biceps exercises 121
biofeedback 37
blackheads 70
black skin 53, 66
bleaching:
    hair 109
    nails 137
blow-drying hair 114
blusher 77
bobs, hairstyles 106
bottom exercises 130–3
boxing circuits 21
braids 117
bras 124
breakfast 13
breathing 35
brushing, dry skin 37, 131, 134
bust-firming exercises 124–5

C
caffeine 37
calcium 15
calf muscles, exercises 135
cancer, skin, 65
cellulite 45, 130
chest muscles 124
chignons 117
cholesterol 16
citric acid 137
cleansing, skincare 50
cleavage, exercises for 125
coffee 130
cold sores 71
cold weather, skincare 60–1
colds 45
collagen treatment 58
colour correction powders 77
combination hair 103
combination skin 45, 52, 60, 75
combs 101, 117
concealers 77
conditioners 100–1
cosmetic dentistry 83
cramp 134
crash diets 124
curl-ups 126
cuticles 136, 139

D
dairy products:
    low-fat yoghurt 17
    skimmed milk 13
damaged hair 102
dance, aerobic 20
dandruff 44, 105
dehydration 69
dental floss 83
dentistry, cosmetic 83
depilatory creams 140
dermatitis 71
diet 12–17
    and fat types 17–17
    and hair 100
    and skincare 58
    and stress 33
    cleansing 37
    weight control 16–17
dry hair 102
dry skin 52, 60, 75
dry skin brushing 37, 131, 134
drying hair 101
dull hair 105
dyeing hair 109–11

E
eczema 45, 71
elbows 120
electrolysis 70, 140–1
environmental problems, skincare 60–3
Epsom salts 35
essential oils 42–5, 55, 131
exercise 17, 19–21
    arms 120–1
    back 122–3
    bikes 20
    bottom toners 130–3
    bust-firming 124–5
    daily routine 25
    feet 138
    15-minute shape-up 26–31
    hips 130–3
    knees 135
    legs 134–5
    shoulders 120–1, 123
    sports 22–3
    stomach and waist flatteners 126–9
    thighs 130–3, 135
    yoga 38–9
exfoliation 54–5
eyeliner 80
eye-pencil 80
eyeshadow 78
eyes:
    dark circles under 71
    make-up 78–81
    moisturizers 50
    sunglasses 63, 67

F
face powder 77
facial massage 40–1
facials 56–7
    ampoule treatment 57
faradic current 131
fasting 37
fat, weight control 16–17
feet, care of 138–9
fibre 13
filing, nails 136
fish 13
floatation 35
foundation 75
free radicals 58
French pleats 117
fringes 106
frown lines 58
fruit 12

G
G5 massage 131
galvanic current 56, 131
gamine hairstyles 106
gels, hair 114
gym circuits 20

H
hair:
    chignons 117
    colour 109–11
    combs 101
    conditioners 100–1
    curls 106
    dandruff 45, 105
    drying 101
    facts 100
    gels 114
    hairspray 114
    long 106
    mid-length 106
    mousse 114
    perms 102, 113
    plaits and braids 117
    pomade and wax 114
    problems 105
    removal of body hair 140–1
    rolls 117

INDEX

sculpting lotions 114
shampoos 100
short cuts 106
styles 106, 117
styling lotions 114
twists 117
types 102–3
hair stylist, choosing 106
handcream 136
hands, care of 136–7
headaches 45
health spas 131
heat exhaustion 69
herpes simplex 71
highlighting hair 110
hip exercises 130–3
humidity, skincare 60, 62
hydrogen peroxide 109
hydrogenated fats 16
hydrotherapy 37, 131

I
iron 15

J
jogging 20

K
knee exercises 135

L
leg exercises 134–5
lemon, bleaching nails 137
lips:
    make-up 83
    sunscreen 67
lonithermie 126, 131
lymph system 37, 56, 131
lymphatic drainage treatments 131

M
magnesium 15
make-up:
    blusher 77
    classic 88
    coloured skin 94–5
    concealers 77
    modern glamour 91
    eyes 78–81
    in 5 minutes 84
    foundation 75
    lips 83
    natural look 87
    party tricks 97
    powder 77
    working girl 92–3
manicures 136
mascara 81
masks, face 55
massage:
    body 130–1
    facial 40–1, 45, 56–7
    feet 138
    hands 136
meat 13
meditation 35
melanin 66
milk 13
minerals 15
moisturizers 50, 58, 62, 75
    tinted 87
mono-unsaturated fats 17
mountain-biking 23
mousse, hair 114

N
nails:
    finger 136–7
    polish 137, 139
    toe 139
naturopathy 37
normal hair 103

O
oils, aromatheraphy 42–5, 57, 131
oily hair 102–3
oily skin 52, 60, 75
olive skin 53, 66
Omega-3 oil 13

P
pectoral muscles, exercises 124
pedicure 139
pelvic tilt 128
pencils:
    eye 80
    lip 83
perms 106, 113
photosensitization 69
plaits 117
polish, nails 137, 139
pollution 62
polymorphic light eruption 69
polyunsaturated fats 16
pomade 114
posture 122, 124
powder 77
    bronzing 87, 95
pre-menstrual tension (PMT) 45
pregnancy, stretch marks 70
press-ups 121
prickly heat 69
psoriasis 71

R
Rags, curling hair 106
rebounding 20
reflexology 57
relaxation 34–7
Retin-A 59
rib-cage exercises 123
riding 22–3
rinses colour 110
rolls, hair 117
rounders 22
rowing 20

S
sailing 23
salads 12
salt deficiency, heat exhaustion 69
saturated fats 16
saunas 63
scalp, itching 105
sclerotherapy 70
sculpting lotions, hair 114
seaweed baths 131
selenium 15
semi-permanent hair colours 110
sensitive skin 45, 52, 60, 69
serums 114
shampoo 100
shaving 140
shoes, fitting 138–9
shoulder exercises 120–1, 123
sit-ups 126
skiing 23
skin cancer 65
skincare:
    anti-ageing 58–9
    arms 120
    back 122
    breasts 124
    cellulite 130
    cleansing 50
    environmental problems 60–3
    exfoliation 54
    facials 56–7
    5-minute skincare programmes 52–3
    hot weather 60, 62
    masks 55
    moisturizers 50, 58
    Retin-A 59
    problems 70–1
    serums 50
skin types 48–9
skin peels 58
sleep 34–5, 58
smoking 58
softball 22
SONA 12
split ends 106
sports 22–3, 63
spots (acne) 70
steaming, skincare 55, 56, 63
step workouts 20, 21
steaming 55, 56, 63
stimulants:
    alcohol 37, 130
    caffeine 37
    nicotine 59, 130
stomach exercises 126–9
streaks, hair 110
stress 32–3, 37, 45, 130
stretch marks 70
stretching exercises 38–9, 123, 124–5, 131, 135
styling lotions 114
sugaring, hair removal 140
sunbathing 65–9, 124
sunbeds 67
sunburn 69
sunglasses 63, 67
sun protection 63, 66–7, 75, 124
sunstroke 69
swimming 20, 120

T
tanning 65–9
    fake 67
teeth, care of 83
tennis 23, 120
thigh exercises 130–3, 135
threading 141
thinning hair 105
thread veins 70
tinting hair 109
toe nails 139
toners 50
toothbrushes 83
toxins 37, 130
travel, skincare 62
tretinoic acid 59
triceps, exercises 121
twists, hair 117

U
ultraviolet filters 58
ultraviolet radiation 65, 69
urchin haircuts 106

V
vegetable colours, hair dyes 111
vegetables 12
veins, thread 70
vitamins 12–15, 33, 58, 100
    anti-oxidant 58
volleyball 23

W
waist exercises 126–9
warming-up exercises 120
wax, hair 114
waxing, hair removal 140
weight control 16–17
weight training 120, 126
windsurfing 23
wrinkles 58, 65

Y
yoga 38–9

Z
zinc 15
zone therapy 57

ACKNOWLEDGMENTS

The publisher thanks the following photographers and organizations for their permission to reproduce the photographs in the book:

12 Transworld Features; 16 Camera Press; 17 Transworld Features; 19 Rapho/Donnezan; 20 left Transworld Features; 20 right Camera Press; 21 left Transworld Features; 22 above Transworld Features; 22 centre Kelly/The Image Bank; 22 below Longfield/The Image Bank; 23 below Rapho/Donnezan; 24 left Marie Claire Idées/Chabaneix/Paillard/Chabaneix; 24 below right Camera press; 34–5 Marie Claire/Chatelain; 36 Marie Claire/Moser; 39 Explorer/Robert Harding Syndication; 42 Cent Idées/Chabaneix/Chabaneix; 43 Marie Claire Idées/Sato Yoichiro/Paillard; 46 Camera Press; 48 Transworld Features; 49 above Transworld Features; 49 below left Transworld Features/Amica; 49 below right Marie Claire/Chatelain; 51 Transworld Features/Grazia; 53 Camera Press; 54 Transworld Features; 55 left Transworld Features; 55 below right Transworld Features/Grazia; 56 Camera Press; 57 above Camera Press; 57 below Transworld Features; 59 Camera Press; 61 Transworld Features; 63 Camera Press; 66 photo courtesy of Uvistat; 67 Camera Press; 68 Marie Claire/Moser; 83 L'Oréal; 88–9 Camera Press; 91 Camera Press; 97 below Camera Press; 98 Transworld Features; 101 Barto/The Image Bank; 102 Camera Press; 104 Syndication International; 105 Camera Press; 107 left Explorer; 107 above and below right L'Oréal Technique Professionnelle; 109 L'Oréal; 110 Camera Press; 111 left Camera Press; 112–113 L'Oréal Technique Professionnelle; 116 above Marie Claire/Moser; 116 centre left Camera Press; 116 below left Marie Claire/Moser; 116 right Camera Press; 117 Camera Press; 118–119 Transworld Features; 125–127 Transworld Features; 134 Transworld Features; 137–138 Camera Press.

The following photographs were specially taken for Cosmopolitan:

1–2 Chris Dawes; 10 Uli Weber; 18 Robert Erdmann; 23 above Steve E. Landis; 24 above right Mauricio Nahas; 33 Constantino Ruspoli; 35 Richard Imrie; 40–1 Jamie Long; 44 Richard Imrie; 55 above right James Brill; 64–5 Tim Bret-Day; 72 Jamie Long; 84–5 Richard Imrie; 86 Barry Hollywood; 87 Richard Imrie; 90 Chris Dawes; 92 Ken Kochey; 93 Anthony Edwin; 94 Peter Wolf; 95 above Paul Alexander; 95 below Tim Bret-Day; 96 David Woolley; 97 above Sara Wilson; 103 Constantino Ruspoli; 108 Chris Dawes; 115 left Paul Alexander; 115 right Jamie Long; 120–122 Constantino Ruspoli; 130 Constantino Ruspoli; 136 Sean Knoz; 139 Robert Erdmann; 141 Richard Imrie.

The following photographs were specially taken for Conran Octopus by Anthony Crickmay and Iain Philpott: 4–5, 6, 8, 21 right, 26, 27, 28, 29, 30, 31, 38, 74, 76–77, 79, 80–81, 82.

Author's Acknowledgments

The authors wish to thank Anne Furniss, Denny Hemming, Karen Bowen, Jessica Walton and Abigail Ahern of Conran Octopus; Marcelle D'Argy Smith of *Cosmopolitan*; Anne Melbourne of the National Magazine Company; Russ Malkin; Stephen Purdew and Peter Bissell of Henlow Grange Health Farm; Peter Cross at L'Oreal Technique Professionnelle; Dance Bizarre; Jesse James; The Conran Shop.